AF443205

The rapid growth of knowledge in molecular biology during the last decade has had far-reaching implications for the understanding, diagnosis and management of haematological malignant disease. The response of many conditions to treatment, and the ease with which patient material can be repeatedly sampled, have made this a fruitful area of study, and in parallel with the expanding contribution of molecular biology there has been growing awareness of the importance of epidemiology, techniques of drug administration, patient support and the evaluation of treatment results.

Haematological Oncology serves as a regular forum for the evaluation and dissemination of this new information, and the topics selected for review range from basic science to clinical applications.

This series provides a comprehensive and up-to-date review of the current state of research and will be an important source of information and knowledge for oncologists, immunologists, postgraduate trainees and other clinical and laboratory workers in the field.

Cambridge Medical Reviews

Haematological Oncology   Volume 3

Cambridge Medical Reviews, a programme of review volumes for the clinical sciences, focuses attention on fields in which rapid and continuing advances in biomedical science have increased significantly our understanding and treatment of disease. Each review series is devoted to a single, clinical discipline. The purpose is to provide a regular evaluation and commentary on the growth of knowledge in that subject. Rigorous standards of selection and editing ensure a reliable and topical series of volumes which will meet the requirements of clinicians and research workers alike.

Haematological Oncology

Series editors

Alan Burnett
Department of Haematology, University of Wales College of Medicine Cardiff, UK

Armand Keating
Autologous Bone Marrow Transplant Program, The Toronto Hospital, Toronto, Ontario, Canada

Adrian Newland
Department of Haematology, The London Hospital, Whitechapel, London, UK

James Armitage
Department of Medicine, University of Nebraska Medical Center, Omaha, Nebraska, USA

Cambridge Medical Reviews

Haematological Oncology
Volume 3

EDITORS

JAMES ARMITAGE
Department of Medicine, University of Nebraska Medical Center
Omaha, Nebraska, USA

ALAN BURNETT
Department of Haematology, University of Wales College of Medicine,
Cardiff, UK

ADRIAN NEWLAND
Department of Haematology, the London Hospital
Whitechapel, London, UK

ARMAND KEATING
Autologous Bone Marrow Transplant Program
The Toronto Hospital, Toronto, Ontario, Canada

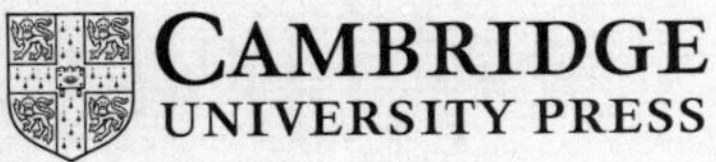

CAMBRIDGE
UNIVERSITY PRESS

Published by the Press Syndicate of the University of Cambridge
The Pitt Building, Trumpington Street, Cambridge CB2 1RP
40 West 20th Street, New York, NY 10011–4211, USA
10 Stamford Road, Oakleigh, Melbourne 3166, Australia

© Cambridge University Press 1994

First published 1994

Printed in Great Britain at the University Press, Cambridge

A catalogue record for this book is available from the British Library

Library of Congress cataloguing in publication data available

ISBN 0 521 44208 7 hardback

WV

Contents

Contributors

BALITRAND, N, Laboratoire de Biol Cell Hémato, Institut d'Hématologie, Lille, France

BARBEY, S, Laboratoire de Biol Cell Hémato, Institut d'Hématologie, Lille, France

ALAN BURNETT, Department of Haematology, University of Wales College of Medicine, Cardiff CF4 4XN, UK

CARTWRIGHT, R A, Leukaemia Research Fund Centre for Clinical Epidemiology, University of Leeds, 17 Springfield Mount, Leeds LS2 9NG, UK

CASTAIGNE, S, Laboratoire de Biol Cell Hémato, Institut d'Hématologie and Service des Maladies du Sang, Lille, France

CHOMIENNE, C, Laboratoire de Biol Cell Hémato, Institut d'Hématologie, Lille, France

CORMIC, M, Laboratoire de Biol Cell Hémato, Institut d'Hématologie, Lille, France

CULLIGAN, D J, Department of Haematology, University Hospital of Wales, Heath Park, Cardiff, UK

DE THE, H, VPR45, Institut d'Hématologie, Hôpital Saint Louis, Lille, France

DUNN, J A, CRC Trials Unit, University of Birmingham Medical School, UK

FENAUX, P, Service d'Hématologie, Lille, France

GORDON, M Y, Leukaemia Research Fund Centre, The Institute of Cancer Research, London, UK

JUTTNER, C A, Hanson Centre for Cancer Research, Institute of Medical and Veterinary Science, Frome Road, Adelaide, South Australia 5000

LEFEBVRE, P, Laboratoire de Biol Cell Hémato, Institut d'Hématologie and Service de Biochimie et Neurobiologie, Lille, France

MACLENNAN, I C M, Department of Immunology, University of Birmingham Medical School, UK

MCNALLY, R J Q, Leukaemia Research Fund Centre for Clinical Epidemiology, University of Leeds, Leeds LS2 9NG, UK

ONIONS, D, Department of Veterinary Pathology, The University of Glasgow, UK

ROGERS, T R, Department of Infectious Diseases and Bacteriology, Royal Postgraduate Medical School, Hammersmith Hospital, Ducane Road, London W12 ONN, UK

SAMSON, D, Department of Haematology, Charing Cross and
Westminster Medical School, London, UK

SECKER-WALKER, L M, Cytogenetics Laboratory, Department of
Haematology, The Royal Free Hospital, Pond Street, London NW3
2QG, UK

TO, L B, Hanson Centre for Cancer Research, Institute of Medical and
Veterinary Science, Frome Road, Adelaide, South Australia 5000

WARBURTON, P, Department of Immunology, University of
Birmingham Medical School, UK

Epidemiology of non-Hodgkin's lymphoma

R A CARTWRIGHT and R J Q MCNALLY

Introduction

Non-Hodgkin's lymphoma has many unsatisfactory features for an epidemiologist: it is not easy to define, its subclassifications are problematical and its natural history is complex. In addition, if the trend of increasing incidence continues, it could in the future be one of the commonest tumours in Europe.

This review deals with the available epidemiological evidence on distribution and causation and briefly points ways towards future research.

Descriptive epidemiology

Age/sex distribution

In the International Classification of Diseases-9 (ICD-9), non-Hodgkin's lymphoma (NHL) is coded 200 (Lymphosarcoma and reticulosarcoma) and 202 (Other lymphoid tissue).

The Leukaemia/Lymphoma Atlas of the United Kingdom, from the Leukaemia Research Fund (LRF) Data Collection Study (DCS),[1] is a major source for population-based incidence figures for NHL. The International Agency for Research on Cancer (IARC) publication *Cancer incidence in five continents, volume V*[2] provides a similar breakdown for all NHL covering all continents, whilst their publication *International incidence of childhood cancer*[3] provides a similar breakdown for all paediatric NHL and Burkitt's Lymphoma, separately, for many countries.

In the UK, following the Kiel classification low-grade NHL shows an absence of cases in children but the age specific incidence rates rise steeply from early adult life (Table 1 (*a*)). There is a suggestion of an adolescent peak in males, and a male excess at all ages. High-grade NHL shows a male predominance at all ages but the age specific incidence shows a substantial incidence in childhood and a much less steep rise with age than the low-grade NHL (Table 1 (*b*)).

All correspondence to: Professor RA Cartwright, Leukaemia Research Fund Centre for Clinical Epidemiology, University of Leeds, 17 Springfield Mount, Leeds LS2 9NG, UK.

Cambridge Medical Reviews: Haematological Oncology Volume 3
© Cambridge University Press 1994

R A Cartwright and R J Q McNally

Table 1 (*a*). *Age specific incidence rates for low-grade NHL*

| | Male | | Female | | Pooled | |
Age	Number	Rate	Number	Rate	Number	Rate
0–4	0	0.00	1	0.04	1	0.02
5–9	0	0.00	0	0.00	0	0.00
10–14	0	0.00	0	0.00	0	0.00
15–19	9	0.30	2	0.07	11	0.18
20–24	16	0.51	3	0.10	19	0.31
25–29	12	0.43	7	0.25	19	0.34
30–34	20	0.78	25	0.99	45	0.89
35–39	59	2.09	41	1.46	100	1.78
40–44	66	2.66	61	2.50	127	2.58
45–49	91	4.19	65	3.01	156	3.60
50–54	111	5.31	78	3.70	189	4.49
55–59	155	7.35	123	5.62	278	6.46
60–64	179	8.67	139	6.21	318	7.37
65–69	205	11.85	199	9.74	404	10.69
70–74	210	14.50	209	10.85	419	12.39
75–79	136	13.56	193	12.05	329	12.61
Total	1269	–	1146	–	2415	–
Standardized Rate	–	4.51	–	3.54	–	4.02

Number of cases/100 000.
From Cartwright RA, Alexander FE, McKinney PA, Ricketts TJ. *Leukaemia and lymphoma. An atlas of distribution within areas of England and Wales 1984–1988.* Leukaemia Research Fund, 1990.

International comparisons show varying rates, with higher rates from those registries that had predominantly fair-skinned populations (Table 2). The age-specific incidence rates again tend to show male excess at all ages.

However, for children (age 0–14) there is a very different pattern (Table 3). No clear geographical associations emerge, except for a tendency towards higher rates around the Mediterranean and in some Latin American registries.[4] The differences cannot be explained by childhood Burkitt's lymphoma (Table 4), which is the most common lymphoma of childhood in Africa and certain other countries.

Burkitt's lymphoma
Burkitt's lymphoma (BL) is the commonest childhood cancer in tropical Africa. In Uganda, the childhood incidence rate is roughly 13/100 000/year,

2

Table 1 (*b*). *Age specific incidence rates for high-grade NHL*

| Age | Male | | Female | | Pooled | |
---	Number	Rate	Number	Rate	Number	Rate
0–4	18	0.73	8	0.34	26	0.54
5–9	23	0.93	9	0.39	32	0.67
10–14	18	0.69	7	0.28	25	0.49
15–19	30	0.98	15	0.51	45	0.75
20–24	38	1.21	14	0.46	52	0.84
25–29	28	0.99	25	0.90	53	0.95
30–34	41	1.60	21	0.83	62	1.22
35–39	67	2.38	26	0.93	93	1.65
40–44	62	2.50	29	1.19	91	1.85
45–49	80	3.69	40	1.86	120	2.77
50–54	121	5.79	66	3.13	187	4.44
55–59	156	7.40	114	5.20	270	6.27
60–64	193	9.34	143	6.39	336	7.87
65–69	212	12.26	187	9.15	399	10.70
70–74	223	15.40	183	9.50	406	11.99
75–79	158	15.76	195	12.17	353	13.97
Total	1468	–	1082	–	2550	–
Standardised Rate	–	5.10	–	3.33	–	4.22

Number of cases/100 000.
From Cartwright RA, Alexander FE, McKinney PA, Ricketts TJ. *Leukaemia and lymphoma. An atlas of distribution within areas of England and Wales 1984–1988.* Leukaemia Research Fund, 1990.

and there is a similar rate in Nigeria.[5] BL is common in children of ages 5–10 years with a peak in incidence at 7–8 years old. There is a tendency for male predominance, but this seems to be diminishing.[6] In tropical Africa it is spread across a belt encompassed by latitudes 10°–15° north and south of the equator and confined to warm, moist areas. Outside Africa, BL is found in areas with similar climatic conditions, such as Papua New Guinea. It is rarely seen in highland areas with altitude greater than 5000 ft, and unknown in arid areas with rainfall less than 20 in or in cold areas where diurnal temperatures fall below 60 °F. African BL has an association with EBV and with endemic malaria. Some doubt has been cast over the role of EBV in the aetiology of BL. Serological surveys were carried out in Uganda and Tanzania[7] to see whether variation in BL incidence from high to low areas is paralleled by a variation in the extent of the infection with EBV. The results showed both the prevalence and strength of the EBV positive titres

Table 2. *Age-specific incidence rates of NHL: international comparisons: Males*

	0–	1–	5–	10–	15–	20–	25–	30–	35–	40–	45–	50–	55–	60–	65–	70–	75–	80–	85+	CR
Brazil (SP)	2.3	2.6	3.7	1.7	1.8	1.8	3.5	5.5	3.3	5.8	7.6	8.6	14.5	23.1	16.3		24.9			5.7
Colombia (CA)		2.6	2.4	0.8	2.7	0.8	1.0	3.6	4.3	2.4	4.2	7.5	12.2	18.9	27.1	18.2	19.5	18.8	22.7	3.7
USA (Conn-W)		1.0	1.2	1.8	2.0	1.7	2.7	3.9	3.4	9.3	11.4	19.2	32.8	36.0	48.5	53.9	80.5	83.8	65.7	13.4
USA (Conn-B)		0.0	0.0	0.0	0.0	0.0	0.0	2.5	0.0	7.4	4.3	23.4	26.7	21.9	30.6	49.1	56.3	0.0	89.3	4.9
Hong Kong		2.0	1.8	1.6	2.1	2.1	2.8	4.7	6.1	7.4	9.3	12.7	12.7	20.4	21.3	30.4	29.4	27.0	6.5	5.9
India (BO)		0.9	1.1	1.4	1.2	1.1	1.0	1.2	2.1	1.7	3.3	5.7	6.8	8.3	11.2	9.0	18.9	86.7		2.0
Israel (All Jews)	0.6	2.0	2.7	2.4	1.9	2.6	3.1	4.3	6.2	10.0	13.3	15.9	21.9	28.1	43.8	54.5	60.8	80.8	71.1	10.6
Israel (Jews-ISR)	0.6	1.9	2.7	2.3	1.5	2.2	2.0	7.8	6.2	12.0	17.8	22.2	34.4	20.3	37.6	52.5		25.7		3.5
Israel (Jews-EU/AM)	0.0	0.0	0.0	4.2	3.5	3.7	3.0	2.2	6.5	10.3	17.6	16.6	21.8	27.2	50.3	60.1		79.2		26.1
Israel (Jews-AF/AS)	0.0	42.1	0.0	0.0	3.2	3.6	6.0	2.8	6.2	8.5	8.0	12.9	19.4	28.6	21.0	34.9		38.4		10.9
Israel (Non-Jews)	0.0	6.6	4.8	1.4	3.8	1.4	2.0	3.9	1.5	7.3	4.6	6.1	24.3	12.1	0.0	40.9	56.4	82.1	46.0	5.0
Japan (Miyagi)	1.6	0.8	0.3	1.0	0.9	1.9	0.9	1.1	1.6	3.3	6.4	4.9	13.0	11.2	15.9	37.4	16.2	19.1	8.7	4.3
Singapore (Ch)	1.4	0.6	1.2	1.4	1.4	1.3	1.2	4.0	2.3	4.0	4.0	5.5	13.9	22.4	20.0	22.1	30.6	50.5	38.4	3.9
Singapore (Ma)	0.0	0.0	0.0	0.0	0.8	0.9	1.3	1.8	0.0	2.7	12.3	8.6	10.3	15.0	43.7	28.3	0.0	0.0	165.3	3.1
Singapore (In)	0.0	0.0	0.0	0.0	0.0	0.0	0.0	0.0	5.1	5.1	3.8	6.6	16.0	35.7	21.8	0.0	205.1	0.0	266.7	5.5
Denmark		1.1	2.0	1.3	1.6	1.4	1.7	3.1	5.4	4.7	8.9	10.4	15.8	24.1	23.9	42.3	44.7	49.7	41.7	9.2
Hungary (Vas)		0.0	0.0	0.0	0.0	0.0	3.2	1.8	6.6	0.0	2.5	0.0	9.3	7.8	3.2	11.7	12.6	12.9	0.0	2.9
Spain (ZA)	0.0	0.0	7.9	1.2	2.3	1.9	0.7	2.1	5.8	5.2	2.8	10.8	7.0	14.5	24.4	10.7	13.0	5.2	15.6	6.1
UK (Birmingham)	0.0	1.4	1.8	0.8	0.9	1.5	1.7	2.0	2.9	5.0	6.2	8.6	15.6	18.7	20.8	25.7	38.0	34.5	20.1	6.9
Australia (NSW)		2.2	1.6	1.9	1.4	1.7	2.7	3.3	5.3	6.8	10.7	16.3	25.1	32.0	42.9	55.8	59.8	74.8	51.6	10.4

Table 2(*a*). *Age-specific incidence rates of NHL: international comparisons: Females*

	0–	1–	5–	10–	15–	20–	25–	30–	35–	40–	45–	50–	55–	60–	65–	70–	75–	80–	85+	CR
Brazil(SP)	0.0	4.1	0.9	1.3	2.2	1.5	1.6	1.1	2.2	4.0	5.3	8.3	11.0	23.2	25.6			25.1		4.7
Colombia (CA)		1.2	0.3	0.8	0.2	0.9	0.4	1.0	0.6	1.4	7.0	4.4	7.5	10.7	25.3	14.4	20.6	22.8	35.8	2.1
USA (Conn-W)		0.7	0.2	0.2	1.1	1.0	0.8	2.1	3.9	6.3	7.5	12.4	21.6	29.5	38.5	37.7	54.4	62.9	56.6	12.2
USA (Conn-B)		0.0	0.0	1.6	1.5	0.0	7.7	4.2	2.5	0.0	7.2	8.0	9.2	11.8	29.5	32.4	46.6	0.0	38.6	4.7
Hong Kong		1.1	0.9	1.2	1.4	2.0	3.7	2.7	6.3	4.6	7.0	10.0	12.1	15.6	13.0	19.5	18.2	20.3	21.5	5.0
India (BO)		0.3	0.3	0.2	0.2	0.4	0.5	0.8	0.8	1.6	2.5	4.4	5.2	5.7	8.7	8.1	6.8	28.4		1.1
Israel (All Jews)	0.0	1.4	1.0	0.5	1.5	1.6	1.7	4.6	3.7	5.0	7.3	9.4	16.0	27.2	34.4	45.4	50.7	67.5	37.0	8.3
Israel (Jews-ISR)	0.0	1.2	1.1	0.7	2.0	2.0	1.4	4.8	5.3	6.0	1.7	15.8	31.2	0.0	72.3	73.4		43.2		2.4
Israel (Jews-Eu/Am)	0.0	7.0	0.0	0.0	0.0	1.2	2.7	6.0	6.0	3.4	8.5	10.0	13.9	29.8	35.7	43.4		57.9		19.4
Israel (Jews-Af/As)	0.0	0.0	0.0	0.0	0.0	0.0	1.2	3.2	1.7	5.2	7.6	5.8	16.6	19.6	20.5	43.4		37.1		8.5
Israel (Non-Jews)	1.8	1.0	1.2	1.0	1.8	0.8	3.9	2.6	4.6	5.4	2.2	11.1	10.8	0.0	26.6	13.6	19.2	18.7	0.0	2.9
Japan (Miyagi)	3.3	0.0	0.6	0.3	0.6	0.0	0.9	0.3	2.7	3.1	2.0	2.2	6.6	6.2	7.1	10.3	17.6	11.3	4.0	2.5
Singapore (Ch)	1.6	1.1	0.4	0.4	0.4	1.0	1.0	1.3	2.7	1.6	4.0	5.2	8.8	10.4	12.6	17.7	4.2	8.6	0.0	2.5
Singapore (Ma)	7.1	0.0	1.2	0.0	0.8	0.0	0.0	0.0	0.0	12.4	0.0	6.7	18.8	6.8	10.5	16.4	0.0	0.0	0.0	2.1
Singapore (IN)	0.0	0.0	0.0	0.0	2.2	0.0	0.0	0.0	5.9	10.8	20.3	0.0	25.6	0.0	0.0	0.0	0.0	0.0	0.0	2.9
Denmark		1.1	0.2	0.4	0.8	0.4	0.9	1.7	4.3	3.4	4.8	7.8	11.5	14.1	20.0	25.9	33.6	36.8	28.1	7.3
Hungary (Vas)		0.0	0.0	0.0	2.4	0.0	1.7	2.0	0.0	0.0	0.0	2.1	2.0	22.7	15.8	8.5	0.0	22.0	0.0	3.3
Spain (Za)	0.0	2.7	1.8	0.0	0.0	0.7	0.0	0.7	0.0	1.8	0.0	2.2	2.1	1.6	7.4	10.1	5.0	3.3	3.3	1.8
UK (Birmingham)	0.8	0.2	0.0	0.4	0.4	0.5	1.2	1.7	1.6	2.2	3.9	6.1	7.7	12.4	15.4	17.3	21.1	22.1	27.8	5.2
Australia (NSW)		1.1	0.3	0.4	0.4	1.0	1.4	2.5	3.3	4.9	8.4	14.0	19.3	22.8	33.3	41.0	51.8	43.8	31.7	8.8

From Muir C, Waterhouse J, Mack T, Powell J, Whelan S. *Cancer incidence in Five Continents, volume V.* IARC, 1987.

R A Cartwright and R J Q McNally

Table 3. *Age standardized (ASR) and cumulative rates (CUM) for childhood NHL* (ages 0–14)

	Registry	Male		Female		Both	
		ASR	CUM	ASR	CUM	ASR	CUM
1	Canada, Atlant Provs	6.6	97.0	2.7	39.0	4.7	69.0
2	Canada, West Provs	9.4	141.0	4.0	61.0	6.8	102.0
3	USA, Delaware W	5.4	85.0	2.9	43.0	4.2	65.0
	NW	3.0	48.0	3.9	58.0	3.5	53.0
4	USA, LA County (B)	4.8	77.0	1.0	18.0	2.9	47.0
5	USA, LA County (HIS)	9.0	138.0	1.9	29.0	5.5	84.0
6	USA, LA County (OW)	7.6	119.0	4.1	64.0	5.9	92.0
7	USA, NY (C & S) (W)	6.8	106.0	2.3	36.0	4.6	72.0
8	USA, NY (C & S) (B)	5.4	85.0	1.6	26.0	3.5	56.0
9	USA, SEER (W)	6.9	107.0	2.8	42.0	4.9	75.0
10	USA, SEER (B)	3.9	61.0	1.5	21.0	2.7	41.0
11	Brazil, Fortaleza	23.9	366.0	11.9	174.0	17.8	268.0
12	Brazil, Recife	9.8	145.0	6.3	95.0	3.1	120.0
13	Brazil, Sao Paulo	22.7	336.0	12.5	183.0	17.6	260.0
14	Colombia, Cali	3.4	54.0	5.5	82.0	4.4	68.0
15	Costa Rica	10.8	150.0	5.9	81.0	8.4	116.0
16	Cuba	19.8	287.0	9.0	27.0	14.5	209.0
17	Jamaica	7.9	128.0	3.9	60.0	5.9	94.0
18	Puerto Rico	6.0	91.0	3.2	48.0	4.6	70.0
19	China, Shanghai	7.1	111.0	2.8	4.6	5.0	79.0
20	China, Taipei	4.4	68.0	3.4	51.0	3.9	60.0
21	Hong Kong	11.0	166.0	7.1	106.0	9.1	137.0
22	India, Bangalore	8.5	130.0	2.8	43.0	5.7	86.0
23	India, Bombay	7.2	110	1.8	27.0	4.6	70.0
24	Israel, (Jews)	16.8	248.0	6.0	85.0	11.5	169.0
25	Israel, (non-Jews)	17.2	252.0	2.5	39.0	10.1	150.0
26	Japan, Kanagawa	1.4	22.0	2.0	31.0	1.7	26.0
27	Japan, Miyagi	1.8	29.0	–	–	0.9	15.0
28	Japan, Osaka	5.6	83.0	3.0	46.0	4.3	65.0
29	Kuwait, Kuwaiti	15.2	236.0	4.9	73.0	10.1	155.0
30	Kuwait, non-Kuwaiti	14.3	213.0	11.9	178.0	13.2	196.0
31	Philippines	3.7	57.0	0.9	14.0	2.3	36.0
32	Singapore – Chinese	7.1	109.0	5.4	79.0	6.2	94.0
	– Malay	7.0	111.0	3.5	51.0	5.3	81.0
33	Czechoslovakia	8.6	131.0	2.5	36.0	5.6	85.0
34	Denmark	4.1	64.0	1.5	22.0	2.8	44.0
35	Finland	7.7	116.0	4.6	66.0	6.2	92.0
36	France, Bas-Rhin	9.2	143.0	8.2	124.0	8.7	134.0
37	France, Paediatric	4.0	64.0	2.4	38.0	3.2	51.0
38	DDR	9.5	148.0	4.5	69.0	7.1	109.0

Table 3 (*cont.*)

Registry	Male		Female		Both	
	ASR	CUM	ASR	CUM	ASR	CUM
39 FDR	7.4	114.0	2.5	37.0	5.0	77.0
40 FDR, Saarland	7.7	116.0	2.1	32.0	5.0	75.0
41 Hungary	0.6	9.0	0.3	4.0	0.4	6.0
42 Italy, Torino	9.7	146.0	3.8	57.0	6.8	103.0
43 Netherlands	12.8	193.0	4.4	62.0	8.7	129.0
44 Norway	5.0	80.0	2.1	30.0	3.6	55.0
45 Poland	3.4	52.0	2.1	30.0	2.8	41.0
46 Spain, Zaragoza	19.2	292.0	6.9	100.0	13.3	199.0
47 Sweden	8.8	133.0	4.0	59.0	6.4	97.0
48 Switzerland	6.8	106.0	2.2	33.0	4.6	70.0
49 UK, E & W	7.9	121.0	3.4	52.0	5.7	88.0
50 UK, Manchester	7.2	107.0	4.1	62.0	5.7	85.0
51 UK, Scotland	6.6	101.0	3.3	51.0	5.0	76.0
52 Yugo., Slovenia	10.8	166.0	3.5	51.0	7.2	110.0
53 Australia, NSW	10.4	159.0	3.3	48.0	6.9	105.0
54 Australia, Queensland	9.5	143.0	2.7	40.0	6.2	93.0
55 New Zealand, Maori	13.6	203.0	5.7	78.0	9.7	142.0
56 New Zealand, non-Maori	10.5	156.0	2.5	39.0	6.6	98.0

From Parkin DM, Stiller CA, Draper GJ, Beiber CA, Terracini B, Young JL. *International incidence of childhood cancer*. IARC, Lyon, 1988.

are nearly similar in the lowlands and on the high plateaux in East Africa. This fails to support a simple causal association between the virus and BL but does not totally exclude the possibility since some other environmental factor essential for BL development may have a geographical distribution that parallels that of BL.

Various studies[8-11] have shown a geographical relationship between high incidence of malaria and BL. A malaria suppression trial was carried out in Tanzania,[12] 1977–1982. An apparent association between malaria engendered suppression of the immune system and decline in BL incidence seemed to occur several years before chloroquine prophylaxis began, thus it appears that malaria could not have been the sole cause of BL decline.

Space–time clustering of BL strengthens the hypothesis of an infective agent being involved in the aetiology.[13-16] The incidence of BL was shown to be several times higher in the low than in the medium and high socioeconomic groups in Ibadan, Nigeria,[17] indicating that the lifestyle of the low socioeconomic group appears to predispose them to the development of BL. Incidence of Burkitt tumours in both white and non-white racial groups in

Table 4(*a*). *Childhood Burkitt's lymphoma as % of all lymphomas (ages 0–14)*

	Registry	Male	Female
1	Madagascar	7.8	11.0
2	Malawi	63.2	60.7
3	Morocco	15.2	39.4
4	Nigeria, Ibadan	78.8	90.0
5	Sudan, Rick, Arab	14.7	5.9
6	Sudan, Rick, Sudanic	36.1	20.0
7	Tanzania	46.2	45.9
8	Tunisia	22.5	34.3
9	Uganda, Kampala	34.3	20.0
10	Uganda, West Nile	90.3	90.3
11	Zimbabwe, Bulawayo	13.0	10.3
12	Canada, Atlant. Provs	0.0	9.1
13	Canada, West Provs	2.7	0.0
14	USA, Delaware (W)	6.5	1.3
15	USA, Delaware (B)	6.9	0.0
16	USA, LA (B)	4.5	0.0
17	USA, LA (His)	6.8	0.0
18	USA, LA (OW)	7.1	3.4
19	USA, NY (C&S) (W)	8.0	8.3
20	USA, NY (C&S) (B)	4.9	0.0
21	USA, SEER, (W)	16.6	3.3
22	USA, SEER, (B)	4.5	0.0
23	Brazil, Fortaleza	3.3	0.0
24	Brazil, Recife	0.0	0.0
25	Brazil, Sao Paulo	2.1	0.5
26	Colombia, Cali	41.4	0.0
27	Costa Rica	1.4	3.3
28	Cuba	1.2	1.1
29	Jamaica	0.0	0.0
30	Puerto Rico	9.3	5.6
31	Bangladesh, CERP	0.0	0.0
32	China, Shanghai	0.0	0.0
33	China, Taipai	0.0	0.0
34	Hong Kong	4.0	9.4
35	India, Bangalore	5.1	0.0
36	India, Bombay	1.0	11.8
37	India, Tata (Bombay)	0.5	2.1
38	Indonesia	0.0	4.2
39	Iraq	29.3	35.4
40	Israel (Jews)	15.5	14.1
41	Israel (non-Jews)	21.1	31.3

Table 4(a) (*cont.*)

	Registry	Male	Female
42	Japan, Kanagawa	6.7	0.0
43	Japan, Miyagi	9.1	0.0
44	Japan, Osaka	2.4	4.5
45	Kuwait, Kuwaiti	2.9	31.6
46	Kuwait, non-Kuwaiti	10.5	0.0
47	Pakistan, JPMC	1.7	0.0
48	Philippines, MM&R	2.9	0.0
49	Singapore, Chinese	5.2	3.3
50	Singapore, Malay	0.0	0.0
51	Thailand	8.0	5.5
52	Vietnam, HCM City	0.0	0.0
53	Czech and Slovak Republics	2.0	0.0
54	Denmark	25.5	8.7
55	FRG, Children's	0.3	0.0
56	FRG, Saarland	9.7	16.7
57	Finland	0.0	0.0
58	France, Bas-Rhin	4.8	0.0
59	France, Paediatric regs	35.5	5.3
60	GDR	6.0	3.7
61	GB, E & W	1.9	2.2
62	GB, Manchester	1.0	1.9
63	GB, Scotland	1.0	2.3
64	Hungary	11.2	6.6
65	Italy, Torino	0.0	0.0
66	Netherlands, Sooz, Eindhoven	0.0	0.0
67	Norway	8.5	4.5
68	Poland, Warsaw city	0.0	8.3
69	Spain, CCR	28.3	18.0
70	Spain, Zaragoza	10.0	18.2
71	Sweden	0.0	0.0
72	Switzerland, 3 Western Cantons	10.5	0.0
73	Yugoslavia, Slovenia	0.0	0.0
74	Australia, NSW	1.9	0.0
75	Australia, Queensland	0.0	3.8
76	Fiji, Fijian	10.0	0.0
77	Fiji, Indian	0.0	0.0
78	New Zealand, Maori	0.0	12.5
79	New Zealand, non-Maori	0.0	7.7
80	Papua New Guinea	55.4	52.4

From Parkin DM, Stiller CA, Draper GJ, Bieber CA, Terracini B, Young JL. *International incidence of childhood cancer*. IARC, Lyon, 1988.

Table 4(*b*). *Age-standardized (ASR) and cumulative rates (CUM) for childhood Burkitt's lymphoma* (ages 0–14)

Registry		Male		Female		Both	
		ASR	CUM	ASR	CUM	ASR	CUM
1	Canada, Atlan. Provs	0.0	0.0	0.7	10.0	0.3	5.0
2	Canada, West Provs	0.6	9.0	0.0	0.0	0.3	4.0
3	USA, Delaware (W)	1.2	18.0	0.1	2.0	0.7	10.0
4	USA, Delaware (N-W)	1.1	16.0	0.0	0.0	0.6	8.0
5	USA, LA, (B)	0.5	9.0	0.0	0.0	0.3	4.0
6	USA, LA, (HIS)	1.9	27.0	0.0	0.0	1.0	14.0
7	USA, LA, (OW)	1.5	24.0	0.5	7.0	1.0	16.0
8	USA, NY (C & S), (W)	1.7	26.0	0.9	14.0	1.3	20.0
9	USA, NY (C & S), (B)	0.8	13.0	0.0	0.0	0.4	6.0
10	USA, SEER, (W)	3.5	54.0	0.4	6.0	2.0	31.0
11	USA, SEER, (B)	0.6	10.0	0.0	0.0	0.3	5.0
12	Brazil, Fortaleza	1.2	19.0	0.0	0.0	0.6	10.0
13	Brazil, Recife	0.0	0.0	0.0	0.0	0.0	0.0
14	Brazil, Sao Paulo	0.8	12.0	0.1	2.0	0.5	7.0
15	Colombia, Cali	11.9	169.0	0.0	0.0	6.0	85.0
16	Costa Rica	0.6	8.0	0.6	9.0	0.6	8.0
17	Cuba	0.3	5.0	0.2	2.0	0.3	4.0
18	Jamaica	0.0	0.0	0.0	0.0	0.0	0.0
19	Puerto Rico	2.0	29.0	0.6	9.0	1.3	19.0
20	China, Shanghai	0.0	0.0	0.0	0.0	0.0	0.0
21	China, Taipei	0.0	0.0	0.0	0.0	0.0	0.0
22	Hong Kong	0.9	14.0	1.3	19.0	1.1	17.0
23	India, Bangalore	1.2	16.0	0.0	0.0	0.6	8.0
24	India, Bombay	0.2	3.0	0.6	8.0	0.4	5.0
25	Israel, Jews	5.6	81.0	2.6	37.0	4.2	60.0
26	Israel, non-Jews	9.0	120.0	4.0	52.0	6.6	87.0
27	Japan, Kanagawa	0.5	9.0	0.0	0.0	0.3	5.0
28	Japan, Miyagi	0.4	7.0	0.0	0.0	0.2	4.0
29	Japan, Osaka	0.3	4.0	0.3	5.0	0.3	5.0
30	Kuwait, Kuwaiti	0.9	12.0	5.7	81.0	3.3	46.0
31	Kuwait, non-Kuwaiti	3.9	55.0	0.0	0.0	2.0	28.0
32	Philippines, MM & R	0.3	4.0	0.0	0.0	0.2	2.0
33	Singapore, Chinese	0.7	11.0	0.2	4.0	0.5	7.0
34	Singapore, Malay	0.0	0.0	0.0	0.0	0.0	0.0
35	Czech and Slovak Republics	0.5	7.0	0.0	0.0	0.2	4.0
36	Denmark	4.8	71.0	0.9	12.0	2.8	42.0
37	FRG, Children's	0.0	1.0	0.0	0.0	0.0	0.0
38	FRG, Saarland	1.7	24.0	1.2	17.0	1.5	21.0
39	Finland	0.0	0.0	0.0	0.0	0.0	0.0
40	France, Bas-Rhin	1.0	15.0	0.0	0.0	0.5	8.0

Table 4(b) *(cont.)*

Registry	Male		Female		Both	
	ASR	CUM	ASR	CUM	ASR	CUM
41 France, Pediatric	6.5	98.0	0.8	10.0	3.7	55.0
42 GDR	1.4	21.0	0.6	8.0	1.0	15.0
43 GB, E & W	0.3	4.0	0.2	2.0	0.2	4.0
44 GB, Manchester	0.2	3.0	0.1	2.0	0.2	2.0
45 GB, Scotland	0.1	2.0	0.1	2.0	0.1	2.0
46 Hungary	2.1	32.0	0.5	7.0	1.3	19.0
47 Italy, Torino	0.0	0.0	0.0	0.0	0.0	0.0
48 Netherlands, Sooz, Eindhoven	0.0	0.0	0.0	0.0	0.0	0.0
49 Norway	0.9	15.0	0.2	3.0	0.6	9.0
50 Poland, Warsaw City	0.0	0.0	0.7	10.0	0.3	5.0
51 Spain, Zaragoza	2.9	46.0	2.3	33.0	2.6	40.0
52 Sweden	0.0	0.0	0.0	0.0	0.0	0.0
53 Switzerland, 3 Western Cantons	2.2	31.0	0.0	0.0	1.1	16.0
54 Yugoslavia, Slovenia	0.0	0.0	0.0	0.0	0.0	0.0
55 Australia, NSW	0.4	6.0	0.0	0.0	0.2	3.0
56 Australia, Queensland	0.0	0.0	0.3	6.0	0.2	3.0
57 New Zealand, Maori	0.0	0.0	1.5	27.0	0.8	13.0
58 New Zealand, non-Maori	0.0	0.0	0.5	8.0	0.2	4.0

Rates/1 000 000. (From Parkin DM, Stiller CA, Draper GJ, Bieber CA, Terracini B, Young JL. *International incidence of childhood cancer*. IARC, Lyon, 1988.)

Cape Province and Namibia suggest that the incidence was not confined to the indigenous African population.[18]

Sporadic BL (non-African type) has been reported in many countries outside Africa and Papua New Guinea. Most cases occur in regions which are not endemic for malaria. The Epstein–Barr Virus (EBV) appears to be present in only 20% of cases of sporadic BL.[19] The absence of EBV and malarial infection in some cases of American BL indicate that they are neither necessary nor sufficient causes of the tumour in all settings.[20] Sporadic BL has been associated with immunosuppressed homosexual men in San Francisco.[21]

In Jordan,[22] where there is no malaria, a space-cluster of sporadic BL was evident, the disease was similar to African BL. The same pattern was also found in other Middle Eastern countries.[23] In contrast to the American form, patients were younger with median age similar to that of African BL.

Similarities between American and African BL included abrupt clinical presentation with involvement of the GI tract, jaw, gonads and central nervous system.[24] Time–space clustering and absence of cases in high-altitude regions are seen in both American and African patients. American patients have bone-marrow and peripheral lymph-node involvement more frequently and are less likely to have EBV genome in their tumours. Most are white. Several other US surveys demonstrated a more marked predominance of BL in young males than had been found in the American Burkitt's lymphoma registry.[25] All data sources indicate a broad age spectrum and a relative paucity of cases in nonwhite US populations. The relative rarity of BL in Singapore is of interest as the climatic conditions conform to observed requirements for endemicity of the disease in Africa.[26]

A reason for the prevalence of BL in males is a possible x-linked susceptibility to EBV or other oncogenes.[27] One suggestion is that BL may be caused by multiple factors, all of which occur in tropical Africa, but only some of which occur elsewhere.[28]

Migration

Migration studies are useful in determining whether a possible aetiology is genetic or environmental. Several studies have been conducted in Japanese migrants in Hawaii, Vietnamese in Los Angeles County, USA, and migrants in Israel.[29–32]

A retrospective morphological survey[30] was carried out, 1973–1983, on Japanese migrants to Hawaii and their offspring. Age-adjusted incidence rates for malignant lymphoma among Hawaii–Japanese (H–J) were similar to rates for US whites. NHL among H–J resembled those of western countries rather than those of Japan. The age-adjusted incidence rates for nodal lymphomas were for Japanese 2.8, H–J 3.6, and US whites 10/100 000 year.

There have been several studies of migrant populations in Israel. In a study carried out 1960–1964[31] there was shown to be an abrupt rise in the incidence of NHL around the age of 50 and a steady increase in older age groups. The incidence was higher among patients of North African origin in younger age groups and among European patients in older age groups, with an intermediate pattern in the Asian group. No differences were observed in the incidence between newly arrived and more veteran immigrants. When the Israeli-born were classified by place of father's origin and added to the immigrant population, each of the ethnic categories followed the parental distribution. Another study,[32] carried out 1967–1968, confirmed these findings, but also noted the unusually high frequency of small intestinal lymphomas in both Jews and non-Jews born in Asia or Africa.

A study comparing Vietnamese and Chinese men and women in Los Angeles County[29] did not indicate any significant excess for NHL.

Clusters

Non-Hodgkin's lymphomas are sometimes termed 'clustered'. Since this is a somewhat vague description the reader should be careful about interpretation. The phenomena can be classified into two broad types: (1) having a possible environmental/genetic cause, and (2) having no obvious or an obscure cause.

Careful consideration of 'reported' case clusters often results in its elimination due to incorrect diagnoses.

Having possible environmental/genetic cause Very few apparent clusters of NHL have an obvious cause. The one exception is the space–time clustering of BL, which has been a distinctive feature of the epidemiology of this disease, though it has not been seen in all areas where BL is endemic.[33] This favours the aetiology for African BL that the disease is a result of the interaction between EBV and malaria. Clustering was first reported in the West Nile district of Uganda for patients with disease onset in the period 1961–65. There was also strong evidence for clustering in the West Nile for the period 1972–73. Seasonal variation in the incidence of BL has been reported and persons who migrate as adults from high altitude areas, where BL and mosquitos are both rare into areas of lower altitude, where BL is endemic and mosquitos are common, develop BL as adults. Some apparent clustering of BL has been reported in temperate areas where the disease is much rarer. If infection with malaria is a cofactor, which determines the time of onset of BL, the clustering of cases of BL probably relates to the patterns of infection with malaria in the community.

Having no obvious or obscure cause A few studies have specifically reported NHL clusters.

In a study carried out in the Yorkshire health region of England, 1978–82, the possibilities of clustering between adjacent electoral wards which display higher than expected incidences of NHL were examined.[34,35] Clusters were defined in two ways. First, they were defined as being those wards with cases in excess (p <10%) which are geographically adjacent to each other, and secondly a separate analysis was done which extended the definition of cluster to include high incidence wards that are adjacent or separated by one other ward. Excessive rates for high grade NHL were found in parts of Leeds and York, and for low grade NHL were found in Scarborough. There was an excess of NHL in rural areas, particularly of follicular subtypes. No aetiological agent could be identified.

A study carried out in three areas of West Virginia,[36] 1964–65, found that several patients with NHL could be interlinked into social clusters. Close personal associations, antedating the onset of disease in one or both individuals of each linkage pair were detected in 61%, 68% and 75% of patients for these three areas during the ten year period. This gives an indication for a possible viral aetiology.

A study in Kingston, Surrey, 1958–64,[37] found that cases of malignant reticuloses were distributed in small residential foci of approximately 2–4 cases in the same and neighbouring streets, which again may indicate a virus. A possible cluster was found in the Liverpool region,[38] where the number of children with NHL was found to be 4–5 times greater than expected, whereas the number of leukaemias was not excessive. Another cluster was identified in India,[39] where four patients with NHL were identified during a period of five months. Three children lived within 60 km in a rural area of Tamilnadu. Two patients were studying in the same school, but there was no other contact, and limited opportunity for environmental exposures.

Anatomical sites

Any associations of NHL site can be extremely dubious as sometimes the site is not the primary one, so conclusions based on site must be treated with caution.

There was a high frequency of primary abdominal lymphoma in Saudi Arabs, which is comparable with that found in Israel among Arabs and Sephardic Jews, and suggests a common environmental or ethnic factor.[40] Histologically the lesions tend to be poorly differentiated lymphocytic or histocytic.[41]

NHL occasionally appears in the oral cavity.[42] The actual frequency occurring primarily in and confined to the head and neck region is difficult to assess due to lack of comprehensive studies in the literature. 17 cases of extranodal head and neck NHL were found in children under 15 years in Finland.[43] An evaluation of 225 untreated patients with lymphoreticular sarcomas with primary involvement of Waldeyer's ring,[44] showed that the primary growth originated from the tonsil (40%), nasopharynx (27.5%), base of tongue (2.7%), soft palate (2.7%), oropharynx (0.9%), and other sites (26.2%).

Cutaneous lymphomas other than mycosis fungoides are a rare and heterogenous group of lymphomas.[45] 27/52 patients presented with skin disease alone, and 25 had concurrent cutaneous and extracutaneous disease. A population-based registry containing 580 patients with NHL[46] had 236 with primary extranodal lymphoma (41%). The initial localization of the primary extranodal sites varied markedly with 36% as primary gastrointestinal lymphomas. 12% of patients with nodal NHL had a localized disease, in contrast to 40% with primary extranodal NHL.

Adult T-cell lymphoma

Adult T-cell lymphoma (ATL) is mainly a disease of the lymph nodes. Some case reports suggest a rare link between ATL and organ transplantation.[47,48] One report has found a link between rheumatoid arthritis and ATL.[49] ATL caused by infection with HTLV-I is relatively common in Japan, Taiwan and the Caribbean.[50–52]

NHL subtype

A European study [53] showed that bcl-2 gene rearrangements were exclusively confined to centroblastic-centrocytic lymphomas. The chromosomal translocation t(14; 18) was reported to occur in up to 85% of follicular lymphomas.

In Iceland there was a high incidence of large cell lymphomas, especially of the immunoblastic type (35%).[54] A study in Norway and other European countries [55] showed that all lymphosarcoma in patients under age 30, was poorly differentiated and diffuse. Stem cell lymphomas occurred only in individuals over 40 years of age.

A study in Uganda showed that tumours of the eye and adnexa had a different incidence compared with the Caucasian community.[56]

Histological examination of patients with NHL of the pleural cavity developing from long-standing pyothorax found that most cases were diffuse large cell type, the immunoblastic type dominating.[57,58] These lymphomas have been reported from Japan.

Trends

Incidence data from the USA, specialist surveys, the World Health Organization and other population based data from the US have been used to assess the rates of NHL.[59] Mortality and incidence rates have been increasing for many years. Larger increases among older persons suggest a role for improving diagnosis, particularly during the 1950s and 1960s. Nevertheless, there is evidence of a constant increase in all ages over 30 years of roughly 2% per year for all NHL grouped together, more rapidly than for all other cancers except melanoma and lung cancer among women. Incidence rates increased over all ages except the very young, among whites and blacks, in geographical areas in the USA and internationally and for both sexes.

During the 1980s, the impact of AIDS is apparent among NHL rates for young and middle-aged men in the USA but not the UK. Increases have been more marked for extranodal disease, particularly those arising in the brain, and for high-grade tumours.

There are also racial/ethnic variations. Whilst white male populations have the highest rates, those for Chinese and Hawaiian were 80% of white males, Fillipinos, blacks and Hispanics were 70%, and Puerto Ricans and American Indians were under 50%. There was a similar pattern for female populations.

The highest rates in the world in recent years were among US whites. Incidence among US blacks is somewhat lower, but increasing as rapidly. In three Canadian provinces, rates have increased, converging over time, and were intermediate between those for US whites and blacks. Rates in the UK and New Zealand are lower, but increasing as rapidly in Oxford as in North America, but less rapidly in Birmingham and New Zealand. Incidence in Denmark, Finland, Norway and Sweden has been similar to the UK, with upward trends. Rates in Hamburg and Warsaw are lower and have not increased greatly. Rates among Jews in Israel were very high in the past, but have increased only modestly. Increases among Jews born in Israel have been more marked. Incidence was consistently lower in Bombay, Japan and Singapore Chinese, but rates of increase were similar to North America and Scandinavia. Rates in South America were intermediate between those in Asia and Israel or North America, with increasing trends.

Overall, incidences are increasing in virtually all registries, although the rates of increase vary. Among women, incidence generally increased across all registries except Hamburg, Warsaw, Jews (Israel) and Cali (Colombia). The international pattern was similar to men, although the incidence was lower.

In the UK[60] problems associated with diagnosis of NHL were reviewed in the context of the apparent rise in incidence. It was concluded that a true rise exists, of about 2% year, for all ages over 30. An age-period-cohort analysis[61] was carried out using NHL incidence data from Connecticut for the period 1935–1989, for both males and females. In addition to age, both period and cohort were significant. A 10.3% increase in risk every 5 years since 1965 was found for females and a 9.2% increase for males.

In order to determine whether the trends are real or not consideration needs to be given to the completeness of registration, the impact of changes in disease classification, the relevance of advances in diagnostic technology and possible changes in aetiologically related conditions such as AIDS. The significance of the cohort effect makes it plausible that there have been changes in exposure to unidentified risk factors in the Connecticut population.

NHLs are a diverse group of malignancies.[62] In the 1970s[63] refinement in the histomorphological criteria for the diagnosis of HD resulted in as many as 10–15% of cases which previously would have been diagnosed as HD being diagnosed instead of NHL. Other considerations appear to have added only marginally to the total of reported cases. These changes are not enough to explain the increase in NHL incidence. Use of the Working Formulation and ICD-O, along with immunohistochemistry, will allow the delineation of NHL subgroups, with possible aetiological significance based on the biology of the disease.[64]

Aetiological aspects
Diet
There is evidence from studies in animals that changes in diet, particularly regarding protein and fats, can effect immune response and the growth and development of lymphomas.[65] Dietary factors may explain geographical differences, but are unlikely to explain changes in NHL incidence over time, unless an overall increased intake of food is the relevant factor.

Very few epidemiological studies address this issue. A case-control study was carried out in the Northeastern part of Italy to investigate the relationship between diet and NHL.[66] Dietary histories concerned the frequency of consumption per week of alcohol, beverages that contain methylxanthine, and 14 select food items. The consumption of milk, liver, butter, oil (mainly polyunsaturated), coffee, tea and cola was positively related with risk for NHL. The consumption of whole-grain bread and pasta showed a protective effect. When a logistic model was fitted that included these food items as well as other nondietary covariates, all of the foods, except liver and beverages that contain methylxanthine, remained significant.

Immunosuppression and viruses

Viruses EBV is related to both BL and nasopharyngeal Carcinoma (NPC) in Africa.[67] The role of EBV in the causation of NPC is not well understood. However, EBV infection takes place much earlier in Uganda, where the vast majority of children are infected before aged 3 and BL is prevalent, than in South East Asia, where NPC is more prevalent.[68]

The excess of NHL associated with HIV is well established.[69] The incidence of HIV associated NHL is increasing. Studies in Los Angeles County USA and Italy show a high incidence of high-grade NHL, including BL, among HIV positive patients. The groups concerned comprised homosexuals and intravenous drug users.[70–72] EBV titres were found to be significantly higher in AIDS patients with lymphoma, than in other AIDS patients,[73] suggesting an aetiological role of EBV infection in the development of NHL. As patients with HIV survive longer with profound immunodeficiency, they have an increased cumulative risk of developing NHL.[74,75]

HTLV-I is the cause of most cases of acute T-cell lymphoma leukaemia (ATL).[76] It is restricted in its geographical distribution to Japan and the Caribbean and is thus unlikely to play a role in the overall increase of NHL.[77] A study of T-cell lymphomas in Taiwan Chinese showed that the HTLV-I positive group had significantly higher incidence of skin and pulmonary lesions, bone marrow and peripheral blood involvement, hypercalcemia and elevated LDH levels compared to the HTLV-I negative group. HTLV-II has not been convincingly linked to any malignancy.[78]

The evidence of an underlying viral aetiology for the lymphomas in several different forms of immune impairment may be relevant to the increases in NHL in the general population.[79] It is possible that changes in hygiene and in population density have altered the average age of exposure to a virus, thereby increasing the likelihood of lymphomagenic effect.

Transplantation The risk of neoplasias occurring after solid organ transplantation is markedly increased by immunosuppressive therapy.[80] Lymphoma has been reported to develop in 13% of heart and in 33% of heart–lung transplant recipients treated with cyclosporine. However, one study[81] reports a reduced risk in heart and heart–lung transplant recipients receiving triple-drug immunosuppression. All neoplasias were observed in patients older than 50 years. In a collaborative UK–Australian study[82] of patients treated with such drugs, there was a 60-fold increase of NHL in renal transplant recipients. The series of patients without transplants but also immunosuppressed also showed tumour excess, though to a lesser extent.

Arthritis Analysis of 643 patients with rheumatoid arthritis (RA) found a 13-fold increase of NHL, whether treated with azothioprine or cyclophosphamide.[83] There is also evidence of an increase of NHL in RA in the absence of immunosuppressive treatment. In another study,[84] cytotoxic drugs could not be implicated in the pathogenesis of the lymphoproliferative malignancies.

Other drugs A population-based case-control study,[85] revealed that long-term regular use of aspirin and other pain relievers and also over 2 months' therapy with antibiotics were associated with significantly increased risk of NHL. Other drugs associated with greater risk of NHL included the use of digitalis and oestrogen replacement therapy by women, use of corticosteroids and a greater than 2 months' use of tranquillizers.

Parental/genetic factors

Up to 25% of patients with certain genetically determined immunodeficiencies will develop tumours, primarily B-cell lymphomas, during their lifetime.[86] These include ataxia telangiectasia, Wiskott–Aldrich syndrome, and common variable hypogammaglobulinaemia.[80,87,88]

Preliminary evidence from a study of NHL in families suggests that multiple-case families may be more susceptible to certain environmental exposures.[89] There is a need to clarify the interrelationship of genetic, familial and environmental factors in the study of NHL.

A case-control study of parental occupation and NHL in children[90] in Turin, Italy (1981–84), revealed that both maternal and paternal cigarette smoking (OR=5) was associated with NHL, but without a correlation with numbers of cigarettes smoked. There was a positive association with maternal employment as a baker, and paternal employment as a lorry driver, and as a worker in the building, wood or furniture industry.

Irradiation

There appears to be an increased prevalence of NHL in highly exposed Hiroshima survivors ($\geqslant 100$ rads).[91] Similar relationships and the subsequent development of NHL was not evident in the population of Nagasaki. Possible explanations for this discrepancy include defined physical differences in the radiation spectra emitted by the two bombs and genetic differences between the two populations at risk. No other study of larger doses of irradiation, however, confirms this partial Japanese finding.

There is no evidence of a link between low dose diagnostic radiation and NHL.[92–94] There is conflicting evidence surrounding NHL and proximity to nuclear installations, partly because acute lymphoblastic leukaemia is often added to NHL in studies on younger people.[95–97]

Secondary cancers

Secondary cancers occur both as NHL following another malignancy, and NHL followed by another malignancy. In a study from the Netherlands,[98] 1966–1983, the relative risk for NHL following Hodgkin's Disease (HD) was 31 (95% CI was 14.2–58.9). For NHL, combined modalities of treatment were shown to be the most important risk factors. The risk of NHL increased with time since diagnosis. Patients with NHL are at almost a threefold risk of subsequently having HD.[99] The incidence of second malignancies in cutaneous T-cell lymphomas (CTCL) was evaluated by comparing series of patients to the general population.[100] The overall cancer incidence rate in the CTCL patients was 2.4 times, and in white male patients 3.3 times greater than expected. A history of prior chemotherapy and a family history of malignancy among first degree relatives was more common among those CTCL patients who developed a second malignancy.

Cigarette smoking

The majority of studies have failed to find an association between cigarette smoking and NHL.[101] A recent study,[102] however, showed a slightly raised odds ratio but no dose response or duration response for NHL as a whole, but a significant result confined to high grade or unclassified diseases.

Chemical exposures – Vietnam

An unusual exposure group comprises veterans of the Vietnam war who were exposed to the various defoliants used during that campaign.

The veterans overall have at least a 20% excess of NHL.[103] However it is not known if this is due to potential confounding factors or specifically to wartime exposure. This excess was confirmed by a large case control study[104] which again failed to link the excess to exposures such as Agent Orange.

Other studies using surrogate measures of exposure to Agent Orange[105,106] again failed to link the excess with herbicide exposure.

Occupations and risk of NHL

There are numerous studies on occupational exposures. These are summarized in the Tables 5 and 6 cohort design and case-control design studies, respectively.[107–121,122–157]

Table 5. *NHL risk for occupational exposure – cohort studies*

(Cohort) Ref no	Time	Place	Occupation/exposure	Risk measure	Risk estimate (95% CI)
107	1961–79	Sweden	Land/animal husbandry	SIR	0.97 (0.89–1.06)
	1961–79	Sweden	Horticulture	SIR	0.71 (0.45–1.08)
	1961–79	Sweden	Other agri. occup.	SIR	1.11 (0.78–1.52)
	1961–79	Sweden	Silviculture	SIR	0.66 (0.32–1.22)
	1961–79	Sweden	Timber cutting	SIR	0.87 (0.72–1.05)
	1961–79	Sweden	Other forestry occup.	SIR	0.81 (0.40–1.46)
108	1965–82	Sweden	Pesticide appliers	SIR	1.01 (0.63–1.54)
109	1940–82	Michigan	Chemical workers (higher chlorinated dioxins)	SMR	1.92 (0.62–4.49)
110	1950–82	Ontario	Forestry workers (Phenoxy acid herbicides)	SMR	– NO DEATHS –
111	1963–85	UK	Phenoxy herbicides	SMR	2.72 (0.33–9.83)
112	1971–85	Saskatchewan	Male farm operators	SMR	0.92 (0.75–1.11)
	1971–85	Saskatchewan	(Farm area <1000 acres (Fuel cost, 1970 $900+	RR (death)	2.29 (1.11–4.73)
	1971–85	Saskatchewan	(Farm area <1000 acres (Acres sprayed, 1970 250+	RR (death)	2.17 (1.02–4.62)
113	1974–83	USA	Navy	SIR	0.7 (0.5–0.9)
114	1946–86	New South Wales	Coal miners	SIR	3.27 (1.31–6.74)
115	1972–80	Finland	2,4-D acid & 2,4,5-T acid herbicide applicators	SMR	– NO DEATHS –
116	1981–89	Australia	Petroleum	SIR	1.7 (0.8–3.1)
117	1970–80	Denmark	Building (F)	SIR	28.57 (3.46–103.14)
	1970–80	Denmark	Fitter/metal industry (M)	SIR	2.53 (1.01–5.21)
	1970–80	Denmark	Gold, silver and electroplate workers (M)	SIR	5.17 (1.07–15.12)
	1970–80	Denmark	Self-employed/medical practice (F)	SIR	8.21 (1.00–29.59)
	1970–80	Denmark	Family worker/other transport (F)	SIR	13.61 (1.65–49.12)
	1970–80	Denmark	Family worker/retail trade (F)	SIR	2.75 (1.01–5.99)
	1970–80	Denmark	Cleaning and kitchen staff/trading	SIR	2.82 (1.41–5.05)

117	1970–80	Denmark	Porter/Real estate Admin.	SIR	10.48 (1.27–37.84)
	1970–80	Denmark	Farming (M)	SIR	1.03 (0.88–1.20)
	1970–80	Denmark	Cowman (F)	SIR	3.02 (1.11–6.56)
	1970–80	Denmark	Farming (F)	SIR	0.80 (0.53–1.16)
	1970–80	Denmark	Wood working	SIR	1.15 (0.87–1.52)
	1970–80	Denmark	Farm worker living on farm	SIR	1.46 (0.63–2.87)
	1970–80	Denmark	Self employed/special farms (M)	SIR	1.91 (0.52–4.90)
	1970–80	Denmark	Self employed/large farms (M)	SIR	2.47 (0.67–6.32)
118	1950–79	USA, Washington	Farmers	PMR	1.01
	1951–61	USA, California	Farmers	PMR	0.81
	1971–78	USA, Iowa	Farmers	PMR	1.14 ($p<0.05$)
	1950–78	British Colombia	Farmers	PMR	0.99
	1950	USA	Farmers	SMR	0.89 ($p<0.05$)
	1970–72	+England & Wales+ (lymphosarcoma only)	Farmers	SMR	1.12+
	1965–69	Canada	Farmers	SMR	0.62
	1961–70	Sweden	Farmers	SMR	1.02
	1961–79	Sweden	Farmers	SIR	1.04
119	Various	Various	Clorophenoxy herbicides and chlorophenols – exposed	SMR	0.97 (0.48–1.73)
	Various	Various	– probably exposed	SMR	0.0 (0–14.76)
	Various	Various	– non-exposed	SMR	1.78 (0.48–4.55)
	Various	Various	– unknown	SMR	0.0 (0–17.57)
120	1945–83	Midland, MI	2, 4 – D Acid	SMR (ICD200)	3.91 (0.44–14.11)
121	1970–79	Denmark	Farmers	SIR	1.01/1.02
	1981–82	Italy	Farmers	MOR	1.27/1.34 (Self-employed/ employee)

Table 6. *NHL risk for occupational exposure – case-control studies*

Ref no	Time	Place	Occupation/exposure	Risk measure	Risk estimate (95% CI)
122	1970–79	USA	Forest and soil conservationists	PMR	2.4 (1.5–3.6)
123	1977–81	New Zealand	Farming	OR	1.0 (0.8–1.4) + (90% CI)
	1977–81	New Zealand	Fencing work	OR	1.4 (1–2) + (90% CI)
	1977–81	New Zealand	Meat works	OR	1.8 (1.2–2.6) + (90% CI)
	1977–81	New Zealand	Orchard	OR	3.7 (1.1–12.1) + (90% CI)
124	1981–84	Western Washington	*Phenoxyherbicide and chlorinated phenol exposure*		
	1981–84	Western Washington	Farmer – medium exposure	OR	1.33 (1.03–1.7)
	1981–84	Western Washington	Herbicides – high exposure	OR	4.8 (1.2–19.4)
	1981–84	Western Washington	DDT	OR	1.82 (1.04–3.2)
	1981–84	Western Washington	Organic solvents	OR	1.35 (1.06–1.7)
	1981–84	Western Washington	Lead-lead arsenate	OR	1.60 (1.1–2.3)
	1981–84	Western Washington	Welding-metal fumes	OR	1.31 (1.03–1.7)
125	1955–85	USA	Flour industry *Nested Case-Control*	OR	4.2 (1.2–14.0)
126	1982–86	Massachusetts	Firefighters	SMOR (police ref)	3.27 (1.19–8.98)
	1982–86	Massachusetts	Firefighters	SMOR (State ref)	1.59 (0.89–2.84)
127	1983–86	E Nebraska	Herbicide 2, 4-D	OR	1.5 (0.9–2.5)
128	1984–88	USA	Dog owners use of 2, 4-D herbicides	OR (canine malig lymphoma)	1.3 (1.04–1.67)
129	1983–86	E Nabraska	Hair colouring products (F)	OR	1.5 (1.1–2.2)
130	1980–83	Iowa & Minnesota	Proximity to industrial plant	RR	1.4 (1.0–1.8)
131	1970–79	USA	Agricultural extension agents	PMR	2.32 (1.72–2.97)
132	1958–83	Ohio	Farmers	OR	1.6 (0.8–3.4)
133	1980–84	New Zealand	Forestry workers	OR	1.84 (0.85–3.97)
134	1984–88	Missouri	Farmers	OR	1.40 (1.04–1.85)
135	1940–78	USA	*Chemical manufacturing*		
	1940–78		Foremen and others	OR	3.2 (1.47–7.2)
	1940–78		Strong acid prod.	OR	8.3 (2.3–30.7)

136	1980–83	Iowa/Minnesota	*Pesticides/agri. risk factors*	OR	1.2 (1.0–1.5)
	1980–83	Iowa/Minnesota	Chlorinated hydrocarbons *Livestock*	OR	1.3 (1.0–1.7)
	1980–83	Iowa/Minnesota	Cyclodienes	OR	1.7 (1.0–2.8)
	1980–83	Iowa/Minnesota	Natural products	OR	1.5 (1.0–2.2)
	1980–83	Iowa/Minnesota	Organophosphates	OR	1.5 (1.0–2.1)
	1980–83	Iowa/Minnesota	Halogenated aromatics	OR	2.0 (1.1, 3.7)
	1980–83	Iowa/Minnesota	Chlorinated hydrocarbons *Crops*	OR	1.4 (1.0, 1.9)
	1980–83	Iowa/Minnesota	Chlorinated hydrocarbons *Crops and/or livestock*	OR	1.3 (1.0, 1.7)
			Organophosphates	OR	1.5 (1.1–2.0)
	1980–83	Iowa/Minnesota	Nonhalogenated aliphatics	OR	1.4 (1.0–2.0)
137	1983–86	E Nebraska	2, 4-D	OR	1.5 (0.9–2.4)
	1983–86	E Nebraska	Organophosphates	OR	1.9 (1.1–3.1)
	1983–86	E Nebraska	Carbamates	OR	1.8 (1.0–3.2)
	1983–86	E Nebraska	Chlorinated hydrocarbons	OR	1.4 (0.8–2.3)
138	1973–77	England & Wales	Forestry workers	RR	1.85 (1.25–2.78)
139	1980–83	Iowa/Minnesota	Hair dyes	RR	2.0 (1.3–3.0)
140	1978–81	Sweden	Organic solvents	OR	3.3 (1.9–5.8)
141	1980–83	Iowa/Minnesota	Embalmers/funeral directors	OR	3.2 (0.8–13.4)
142	1983–88	Milan, Italy	Agriculture/food processing	OR	1.9 (1.2–3.0)
143	1968–76	Wisconsin	Farming	OR	1.22 (0.98, 1.51)
144	1976–82	Kansas	Agricultural herbicide use	OR	1.6 (0.9, 2.6)
			>20 days/year	OR	6.0 (1.9, 19.5)
			Frequent use	OR	8.0 (2.3, 27.9)
145	1973–77	England & Wlaes	Road transport workers	OR (ICD200)	1.16 (0.60–2.26)
			(Bus & coaches)	OR (ICD202)	1.63 (0.62–4.52)
			(Other drivers)	OR (ICD202)	1.67 (0.68–4.32)
146	1974–83	Italy	Agriculture	OR	3.42 (1.10, 10.7)
147	1977–81	New Zealand	Agriculture/forestry	OR (ICD202)	1.76 (1.03, 3.02)

Table 6 (*cont.*)

Ref no	Time	Place	Occupation/exposure	Risk measure	Risk estimate (95% CI)
148	1964–86	Sweden	Solvents	Logistic OR	1.9 (1.1, 3.2) + (90%)
			Carpenters/cabinet makers	Logistic OR	2.8 (1.1, 7.1) + (90%)
			Phenoxy acids	Logistic OR	4.9 (1.3, 18.0) + (90%)
			Creosote	Logistic OR	9.4 (1.2, 69.0) + (90%)
			Pets	Logistic OR	3.4 (1.4, 7.9) + (90%)
149	1968–70)		Professional (whites)	OR	2.7 (1.95, 3.72) + (90%)
	1975–77 }	North Carolina			
	1980–82]		Machine trades (blacks)	OR	3.63 (1.32, 9.97) + (90%)
150	1961–79	Sweden	Cotton	SIR	6.7 (p<0.01)
	1961–79		Trolley/Bus transport (Mycosis Fungoides)	SIR	5.5 (p<0.01)
	1961–79		Streetcar driver (Mycosis Fungoides)	SIR	2.0 (p<0.05)
	1961–79		Circular saw operator, plane operator etc. (Mycosis Fungoides)	SIR	6.1 (p<0.05)
151	1965–76	Connecticut	Manufacturing/construction industries (Mycosis fungoides)	RR	4.3
152	1984–85	Missouri	Farmers	OR	1.11 (0.70–1.77)
153	1967–82	Utah	Farmers	OR	1.3 (0.9–2.3) + (90%)
154	1964–78	Iowa	Farming	OR	1.26 (p<0.05)
155	1977–81	New Zealand	(Fencing	OR	2.0 (1.3–3.0) + (90%)
			(Meat	OR	1.8 (1.1–3.1) + (90%)
			(Fencing and meat	OR	5.7 (2.3–14.3) + (90%)
156	1974–78	Sweden	(Phenoxy acids	RR	4.8
			(Chlorophenols	RR	8.4
			(Organic solvents	RR	2.8
157	1953–86	S Finland	*Chlorophenol exposure*		
			Fish	RR	∞(1.1, ∞)
			Drinking water or fish	RR	6.9 (1.1, 74)

Broadly speaking, the majority of scientific interest over the last 15 years has focussed on exposures to agrichemicals, on the one hand, and petrochemical on the other.

There are at least 9 cohort and 21 case control studies examining different aspects of agricultural activities. Overall, 4 of the cohorts and 15 of the case control studies report statistically significantly raised risk measures. The association between agricultural workers including horticulture and pesticide application seems a reproducible phenomenon. There is no consensus as to what the risk might be, ie which (if any) agrichemical is implicated. To this end studies on phenoxyherbicide manufacture[111,120] were undertaken and all show no risk but with quite wide confidence limits. Further, a large international study of herbicide users and workers[119] showed no excess of NHL.

It may be that only some subtypes of NHL are at risk and that when future studies disentangle the complexity of the multiple exposure with the numerous types of NHL, that a clear link will be found. Possible mechanism for a causal link with agrichemicals have been hypothesized.[158]

However, a good deal of attention has been devoted to the possible harmful effects of the dioxins. These substances are found as contaminants, particularly in the phenoxyherbicides. Several studies are now reported on those who have experienced high levels of dioxin contamination. The main population exposure was consequential on the accident at Seveso in 1976. Here no NHL excess has ever been described.[159]

In addition, workers exposed to dioxins have been reported by Manz,[160] Fingerhut[161] and Zober.[162] The latter study found no excess of NHL, likewise there was no obvious excess of NHL reported by Manz[160] or Fingerhut,[161] although other cancers may be in excess.

It is unlikely therefore that the risks of agrichemical workers are easily explained by dioxin or exposure to related herbicides.

Petrochemical and solvent exposure have been examined in 2 cohort and 4 case-control studies. The 2 cohorts,[109,116] show raised risks which were not statistically significant whilst all 4 case-control studies show statistically significantly raised risks.

A variety of other cohort studies examining other occupations have shown no risk of NHL. An exception was that of coal miners[114] in a single study. Various raised risks from a Danish study are difficult to interpret and may be the result of confounding.[117]

Case control studies have produced risks of firefighters[126], flour industry workers,[125] hair colourants,[129,139] proximity to industrial plant, road transport workers and several other occupations.

These are difficult to interpret unless reproduced and could be due to chance consequential on numerous comparisons. There may also be a publication bias towards positive results.

Conclusion

There is evidence pathologically and epidemiologically that NHL is a heterogeneous group of conditions which are increasing in incidence and which demonstrate unusual geographical distribution. It is thus of prime importance that a clearer understanding is achieved of the causes of NHL and related conditions such as chronic lymphocytic leukaemia.

Presently, much of the aetiology is obscure, although there are numerous clues pointing towards risks associated with various aspects of immune dysfunction. One way forward would be to test for hypotheses linked in with the clues we already possess. Studies linking viruses, inherited susceptibility and responses to specific chemicals, physical agents or gross aspects of diet with the oncogenetically defined groups of NHL, should be more meaningful than past studies based on other disease subclassification. Similarly the molecular expression of environmental influences if available could be more reliable than recalled events. A new era of molecular-based epidemiology could be a way forward to understand this increasingly common group of malignances.

Acknowledgements

The authors are supported by the Leukaemia Research Fund. Agnes McKeating and Ann Pickles are thanked for the typing of this document.

References

(1) Cartwright RA, Alexander FE, McKinney PA, Ricketts TJ. *Leukaemia and lymphoma. An atlas of distribution within areas of England and Wales* 1984–1988. Leukaemia Research Fund, 1990.

(2) Muir C, Waterhouse J, Mack T, Powell J, Whelan S. *Cancer incidence in five continents, volume v.* Lyon: IARC, 1987.

(3) Parkin DM, Stiller CA, Draper GJ, Bieber CA, Terracini B, Young JL. *International incidence of childhood cancer.* IARC, Lyon, 1988.

(4) Stiller CA, Parkin DM. International variations in the incidence of childhood lymphomas. *Paediatr and Perinat Epidemiol* 1990; 4: 303–24.

(5) Olweny, CLM. Lymphomas and leukaemias Part 1: Tropical Africa. *Clin Haematol* 1981; 10: 873–93.

(6) Sinnette CH. Report from a West African teaching hospital with special emphasis on Burkitt's tumour. *Clin Pediatr* 1967; 6: 12, 721–7.

(7) Geser A, Brubaker G, Olwit GW. The frequency of Epstein–Barr virus infection and Burkitt's lymphoma at high and low altitudes in East Africa. *Rev Epidemiol Santé Publ* 1980; 28: 307–21.

(8) Kafuko GW, Baingana N, Knight EM, Tibemanya J. Association of Burkitt's tumour and holoendemic malaria in West Nile District, Uganda: Malaria as a possible aetiologic factor. *E Afr Med J* 1969; 46: 414–36.

(9) Eddington GM. The Burkitt lymphoma in the Northern Savannah of Nigeria. *Prog Clin Biol Res* 1981; 53: 133–49.

(10) Sudarsanam T, Habte D, Asfaw T. Burkitt's lymphoma in Ethiopia. *E Afr Med J* 1972; 49: 502–8.

(11) Edington GM. The pattern of cancer in the Northern Savannah of Nigeria with special reference to primary liver cell carcinoma and the Burkitt lymphoma. *Nig Med J* 1978; 8: 281–9.

(12) Geser A, Brubaker G, Draper CC. Effect of a malaria suppression program on the incidence of African Burkitt's lymphoma. *Am J Epidemiol* 1989; 129: 740–52.

(13) Williams EH, Spit P, Pike MC. Further evidence of space-time clustering of Burkitt's lymphoma patients in the West Nile District of Uganda. *Br J Cancer* 1969; 23: 235–46.

(14) Williams EH, Smith PG, Day NE, Geser A, Ellice J, Tukei P. Space–time clustering of Burkitt's lymphoma in the West Nile District of Uganda: 1961–1975. *Br J Cancer* 1978; 37: 109–22.

(15) Siemiatycki J, Brubaker G, Geser A. Space-time clustering of Burkitt's lymphoma in East Africa: analysis of recent data and a new look at old data. *Int J Cancer* 1980; 25: 197–203.

(16) Pike MC, Williams EH, Wright B. Burkitt's tumour in the West Nile District of Uganda 1961–5. *Br Med J* 1967; 2: 395–9.

(17) Williams CKO. Clustering of Burkitt's lymphoma and other high-grade malignant lymphoproliferative diseases, but not acute lymphoblastic leukaemia among socio-economically deprived Nigerians. *E Afr Med J* 1988; 65: 253–63.

(18) Wood RE, Nortje CJ, Hesseling P, Mouton S. Involvement of the maxillofacial region in African Burkitt's lymphoma in the Cape Province and Namibia. *Dentomaxillofac Radiol* 1988; 17: 57–60.

(19) Ablashi DV, Salahuddin SZ. Viruses associated with non-Hodgkin's lymphomas. In: Magrath IT, ed. *The non-Hodgkin's lymphomas*. London: Edward Arnold, 1990: 160–79.

(20) Evans AS. *Epidemiology of Burkitt's lymphoma: other risk factors*. IARC Sci Publ 1985; 60: 197–204.

(21) Ziegler JL, Miner RC, Rosenbaum E et al. Outbreak of Burkitt's-like lymphoma in homosexual men. *Lancet* 1982; Sept 18: 631–3.

(22) Madanat FF, Amr SS, Tarawneh MS, El-Khateeb MS, Marar B. Burkitt's lymphoma in Jordanian children: Epidemiological and clinical study. *J Trop Med Hygiene* 1986; 89: 189–91.

(23) Anaissie E, Geha S, Allam O, Jabbour J, Khalyl M, Salem P. Burkitt's lymphoma in the Middle East. A study of 34 cases. *Cancer* 1985; 56: 2539–43.

(24) Levine PH, Connelly RR, Berard CW et al. The American Burkitt lymphoma registry: a progress report. *Ann Int Med* 1975; 83: 31–6.

(25) Levine PH, Connelly RR, McKay FW. *Burkitt's lymphoma in the USA: Cases reported to the American Burkitt lymphoma registry compared with population-based incidence and mortality data*. IARC Sci Publ 1985; 60: 217–24.

(26) Shanmugaratnam K, Tan KK, Lee KW. Lymphoma of the Burkitt type in Singapore. *Int J Cancer* 1967; 2: 576–80.

(27) Purtilo DT. Prevalence of Burkitt's lymphoma in males. *N Eng J Med* 1976; 295: 1484.

(28) Wright DH. Burkitt's tumour in England: A comparison with childhood lymphosarcoma. *Int J Cancer* 1966; 1: 503–14.

(29) Ross RD, Bernstein L, Hartnett NM, Boone JR. Cancer patterns among Vietnamese immigrants in Los Angeles County. *Br J Cancer* 1991; 64: 185–6.

(30) Yanagihara ET, Blaisdell RK, Hayashi T, Lukes RJ. Malignant lymphoma in Hawaii–Japanese: a retrospective morphologic survey. *Haematol Oncol* 1989; 7: 219–32.

(31) Modan B, Goldman B, Shani M, Meytes D, Mitchell BS. Epidemiological aspects of neoplastic disorders in Israeli migrant populations. V. The lymphomas. *J Natl Cancer Inst* 1969; 42: 375–81.

(32) Sacks MI, Hulu N, Selzer G, Steinitz R. Malignant lymphoreticular tumours in Israel. *J Natl Cancer Inst* 1973; 50: 1669–79.

(33) Smith PG. Current assessment of 'case clustering' of lymphomas and leukaemias. *Cancer* 1978; 42: 1026–34.

(34) Barnes N, Cartwright RA, O'Brien C et al. Variation in lymphoma incidence within Yorkshire health region. *Br J Cancer* 1987; 55: 81–4.

(35) Barnes N, Cartwright RA, O'Brien C, Roberts B, Richards IDG, Bird CC. Spatial patterns in electoral wards with high lymphoma incidence in Yorkshire health region. *Br J Cancer* 1987; 56: 169–72.

(36) Schimpff SC, Schimpff CR, Brager DM, Wiernik PH. Leukaemia and lymphoma patients interlinked by prior social contact. *Lancet* 1975; Jan 18: 124–9.

(37) Dowsett EG. Leukaemia in Kingston, Surrey, 1958–64: An epidemiological study. *Br J Cancer* 1966; 20: 16–31.

(38) Mainwaring D, Martin J. Leukaemia and Reticuloses. *Br Med J* 1968; Dec 14: 702.

(39) Kolandaivelu G. A cluster of non-Hodgkin's lymphoma. *Indian Paediatr* 1988; 25: 583.

(40) Gelphi AP. Malignant lymphoma in the Saudi Arab. *Cancer* 1970; 25: 892–5.

(41) Al-Saleem T, Al-Bahrani Z. Malignant lymphoma of the small intestine in Iraq (Middle East lymphoma). *Cancer* 1973; 31: 291–4.

(42) Haidar, Z. A review of non-Hodgkin's lymphoma of the oral cavity 1950–1980. *J Oral Med* 1986; 41: 197–200.

(43) Usenius T, Vornanen M, Karaja J, Collan Y. Extranodal head and neck NHLs in children in Finland. *Acta Oncol* 1990; 29: 529–31.

(44) Banfi A, Bonadonna G, Carnevali G, Molinari R, Monfardini S, Salvini E. Lymphoreticular sarcomas with primary involvement of Waldeyer's Ring: clinical evaluation of 225 cases. *Cancer* 1970; 26: 341–51.

(45) Joly P, Charlotte F, Leibowitch M et al. Cutaneous lymphomas other than Mycosis Fungoides: Follow-up study of 52 patients. *J Clin Oncol* 1991; 9: 1994–2001.

(46) Otter R, Gerrits WBJ, Sandt MMVD, Hermans J, Willemze R. Primary extranodal and nodal non-Hodgkin's lymphoma: A survey of a population-based registry. *Eur J Cancer Clin Oncol* 1989; 25: 1203–10.

(47) Kemnitz J, Cremer J, Gebel M, Uysal A, Haverich A, Georgii A. T-cell lymphoma after heart transplantation. *Am J Clin Pathol* 1990; 94: 95–101.

(48) Lippman SM, Grogan TM, Carry P, Ogden DA, Miller TP. Post-transplantation T-cell lymphoblastic lymphoma. *Am J Med* 1987; 82: 814–6.

(49) Weir AB, Herrod HG, Lester EP, Holbert J. Diffuse large-cell lymphoma of B-cell origin and deficient t-cell function in a patient with rheumatoid arthritis. *Arch Intern Med* 1989; 149: 1688–90.

(50) Bunker JD, Freeman JH, Jester JD, Golitz LE. Cutaneous T-cell lymphoma in Colorado 1974–1991. *J Dermatol* 1991; 18: 369–76.

(51) Neugut AI. Epidemiology of T-cell leukaemia/lymphoma. *Lancet* 1982; Sept 4: 557–8.

(52) Gibbs WN, Lofters WS, Campbell M et al. Non-Hodgkin's lymphoma in Jamaica and its relation to adult T-cell leukaemia-lymphoma. *Ann Intern Med* 1987; 106: 361–8.

(53) Ott MM, Muller-Hermelink HK, Schmitt B, Feller AC. Chromosomal translocation detected by bcl–1 and bcl–2 rearrangement in low-grade B-cell lymphomas in a European population. *Histopathology* 1991; 19: 163–7.

(54) Agnarsson BA, Olafsdottir K, Benediktsson H. Tumours in Iceland. *Acta Pathol Microbiol Immunol Scand Sect A* 1987; 95: 23–8.

(55) Stalsberg H. Lymphoreticular tumours in Norway and in other European countries. *J Natl Cancer Inst* 1973; 50: 1685–702.

(56) Templeton AC. Tumours of the eye and adnexa in Africans of Uganda. *Cancer* 1967; 20: 1689–98.

(57) Iuchi K, Ichimiya A, Akashi A et al. Non-Hodgkin's lymphoma of the pleural cavity developing from long-standing pyothorax. *Cancer* 1987; 60: 1771–5.

(58) Iuchi K, Aozasa K, Yamamoto S, et al. Non-Hodgkin's lymphoma of the pleural cavity developing from long-standing pyothorax. Summary of clinical and pathological findings in thirty-seven cases. *Jpn J Clin Oncol* 1989; 19: 249–57.

(59) Devesa SS, Fears T. Non-Hodgkin's lymphoma time trends: United States and international data. *Cancer Research* 1992; 52 (Suppl): 5432–40.

(60) Cartwright RA. Changes in the descriptive epidemiology of non-Hodgkin's lymphoma in Great Britain. *Cancer Res* 1992; 52 (Suppl): 5441–2.

(61) Holford TR, Zheng T, Mayne ST, McKay LA. Time trends of non-Hodgkin's lymphoma: are they real? What do they mean? *Cancer Res* 1992; 52 (Suppl): 5443–6.

(62) Jaffe ES, Raffeld M, Medeiros LJ, Stetler-Stevenson M. An overview of the classification of non-Hodgkin's lymphomas. An integration of morphological and phenotypical concepts. *Cancer Res* 1992; 52 (Suppl): 5447–52.

(63) Banks PM. Changes in diagnosis of non-Hodgkin's lymphomas over time. *Cancer Res* 1992; 52 (Suppl): 5453–5.

(64) Weisenburger DD. Pathological classification of non-Hodgkin's lymphoma for epidemiological studies. *Cancer Res* 1992; 52 (Suppl): 5456–64.

(65) Davis S. Nutritional factors and the development of non-Hodgkin's lymphoma: a review of the evidence. *Cancer Res* 1992; 52 (Suppl): 5492–5.

(66) Franceschi S, Serraino D, Carbone A, Talamini R, La Vecchia C. Dietary factors and non-Hodgkin's lymphoma: A case-control study in the Northeastern part of Italy. *Nutr Cancer* 1989; 12: 333–41.

(67) de-The G. *Virus-associated lymphomas, leukaemias and immunodeficiencies in Africa.* IARC Sci Publ, Lyon 1984; 63: 727–44.

(68) de-The G. Epstein–Barr virus behaviour in different populations and implications for control of Epstein–Barr virus-associated tumours. *Cancer Res* 1976; 36: 692–5.

(69) Obrams GI, Grufferman S. Epidemiology of HIV associated non-Hodgkin's lymphoma. *Cancer Surveys* 1991; 10 (Cancer and AIDS): 91–102.

(70) Bernstein L, Levin D, Menck H, Ross RK. AIDS related secular trends in cancer in Los Angeles County men: A comparison by marital status. *Cancer Res* 1989; 49: 466–70.

(71) Tirelli U, Vaccher E, Ambrosini A et al. HIV-related malignant lymphoma: A report of 46 cases observed in Italy. *Acta Haematol* 1988; 80: 49–51.

(72) Harnly ME, Swan SH, Holly EA, Kelter A, Padian N. Temporal trends in the incidence of non-Hodgkin's lymphoma and selected malignancies in a population with a high incidence of acquired immunodeficiency syndrome (AIDS). *Am J Epidemiol* 1988; 128: 261–7.

(73) Beckhardt RN, Farady N, May M, Torres RA, Strauchen JA. Increased incidence of malignant lymphoma in AIDS: A comparison of risk groups and possible etiologic factors. *Mt Sinai J Med* 1988; 55: 383–9.

(74) Pluda JM, Yarchoan R, Broder S. The occurrence of opportunistic non-Hodgkin's lymphoma in the setting of infection with the human immunodeficiency virus. *Ann Oncol* 1991; 2 (Suppl 2): 191–200.

(75) Rabkin CS, Hilgartner MW, Hedberg KW et al. Incidence of lymphomas and other cancers in HIV-infected and HIV-uninfected patients with hemophilia. *JAMA* 1992; 267: 1090–4.

(76) Levine PH, Blattner WA. The epidemiology of human virus-associated hematologic malignancies. *Leukemia* 1992; 6 (Suppl 3): 54–9.

(77) Mueller NE, Mohar A, Evans A. Viruses other than HIV and non-Hodgkin's lymphoma. *Cancer Res* 1992; 52 (suppl): 5479–81.

(78) Hjelle B, Mills R, Swenson S, Mertz G, Key C, Allen S. Incidence of Hairy Cell leukaemia, mycosis fungoides and chronic lymphocytic leukaemia in first known HTLV-II endemic population. *J Infect Dis* 1991; 163: 435–40.

(79) Kinlen L. Immunosuppressive therapy and acquired immunological disorders. *Cancer Res* 1992; 52 (suppl): 5474–6.

(80) Ioachim HL. Neoplasms associated with immune deficiencies. *Pathol Ann* 1987; 22 (pt 2): 177–222.

(81) Olivari M-T, Diermann RA, Kubo SH, Braunlin E, Jamieson SW, Ring WS. Low incidence of neoplasia in heart and heart-lung transplant recipients receiving triple-drug immunosuppression. *J Heart Transpl* 1990; 9: 618–21.

(82) Kinlen LJ, Shell AGR, Peto J, Doll R. Collaborative United Kingdom-Australasian study of cancer in patients treated with immunosuppressive drugs. *Br Med J* 1979; 2: 1461–6.

(83) Kinlen LF. Incidence of cancer in rheumatoid arthritis and other disorders after immunosuppressive treatment. *Am J Med* 1985; 78 (suppl 1A): 44–9.

(84) Symmons DPM. Neoplasms of the immune system in rheumatoid arthritis. *Am J Med* 1985; 78 (suppl 1A): 22–7.

(85) Bernstein L, Ross RK. Prior medication use and health history as risk factors for non-Hodgkin's lymphoma: Preliminary results from a case-control study in Los Angeles County. *Cancer Res* 1992; 52 (suppl): 5510–5.

(86) Filipovitch AH, Mathur A, Kamat D, Shapiro RS. Primary immunodeficiencies: Genetic risk factors for lymphoma. *Cancer Res* 1992; 52 (Suppl): 5465–7.

(87) Kersey JH, Shapiro RS, Filipovitch AH. Relationship of immunodeficiency to lymphoid malignancy. *Paed Infect Dis J* 1988; 7: 510–2.

(88) Kinlen LJ, Webster ADB, Bird AG et al. Prospective study of cancer in patients with hypogammaglobulinaemia. *Lancet* 1985; Feb 2: 263–5.

(89) Linet MS, Pattern LM. Familial aggregation of hematopoietic malignancies and risk of non-Hodgkin's lymphoma. *Cancer Res* 1992; 52 (Suppl): 5468–73.

(90) Magnani C, Pastore G, Lazzatto L, Terracini B. Parental occupation and other environmental factors in the etiology of leukaemias and NHL's in childhood: A case-control study. *Tumori* 1990; 76: 413–9.

(91) Anderson RE. Malignant lymphoma. *Human Pathol* 1971; 2: 515–9.

(92) Pifer JW, Hempelmann LH, Dodge HJ, Hodges FJ. Neoplasms in the Ann Arbor Series of Thymus-irradiated children: A second survey. *Am J Roentgenol, Radium Therapy Nucl Med* 1968; 103: 13–8.

(93) Li FP, Cassady JR, Barnett E. Cancer mortality following irradiation in infancy for hemangioma. *Radiology* 1974; 113: 177–8.

(94) Boice JD, Morin MM, Glass AG et al. Diagnostic X-ray procedures and risk of leukemia, lymphoma and multiple myeloma. *JAMA* 1991; 254: 1290–4.

(95) Urquhart JD, Black RJ, Muirhead MJ et al. Case-control study of leukaemia and non-Hodgkin's lymphoma in children in Caithness near the Dounreay nuclear installation. Br Med J 1991; 302: 687–92.

(96) Beral V. Leukaemia and nuclear installations: Occupational exposure of fathers to radiation may be the explanation. Br Med J 1990; 300: 411–2.

(97) Gardner MJ, Snee MP, Hall AJ, Powell CA, Downes S, Terrell JD. Results of case-control study of leukaemia and lymphoma among young people near Sellafield nuclear plant in West Cumbria. Br Med J 1990; 300: 423–34.

(98) Van Leeuwen FE, Somers R, Taal BG et al. Increased risk of lung cancer, non-Hodgkin's lymphoma, and leukemia following Hodgkin's disease. *J Clin Oncol* 1989; 7: 1046–58.

(99) Trams LB, Gonzalez CL, Hankey BF, Jaffe ES. Hodgkin's disease following non-Hodgkin's lymphoma. *Cancer* 1992; 69: 2337–42.

(100) Olsen EA, Delzell E, Jegasothy BV. Second malignancies in cutaneous T-cell lymphoma. *J Am Acad Dermatol* 1984; 10: 197–204.

(101) Cartwright RA, McKinney PA, O'Brien C et al. Non-Hodgkin's lymphoma: case control epidemiologic study in Yorkshire. *Leukemia Res* 1988; 12: 81–8.

(102) Brown LM, Everett GD, Gibson R, Burmeister LF, Leonard MS, Blair A. Smoking and risk of non-Hodgkin's lymphoma and multiple myeloma. *Cancer Causes Control* 1991; 3: 49–55.

(103) Namboodiri KK, Harris RE. Hematopoietic and lymphoproliferative cancer among male veterans using the veterans administration medical system. *Cancer* 1991; 68: 1123–30.

(104) Selected Cancers Cooperative Study Group. The association of selected cancers with service in the US military in Vietnam. *Arch Intern Med* 1990; 150: 2473–83.

(105) Dalager NA, Kang HK, Burt VL, Weatherbee L. Non-Hodgkin's lymphoma among Vietnam veterans. *J Occup Med* 1991; 33: 774–9.

(106) O'Brien RT, Decoufle P, Boyle CA. Non-Hodgkin's lymphoma in a cohort of Vietnam veterans. *Am J Public Health* 1991; 81: 758–61.

(107) Wiklund K, Lindefors BM, Holm LE. Risk of malignant lymphoma in Swedish agricultural and forestry workers. *Br J Ind Med* 1988; 45: 19–24.

(108) Wiklund K, Dich J, Holm LE. Risk of malignant lymphoma in Swedish pesticide appliers. *Br J Cancer* 1987; 56: 505–8.

(109) Ott MG, Olson RA, Cook RR, Bond GG. Cohort mortality study of chemical workers with potential exposure to the higher chlorinated dioxins. *J Occup Med* 1987; 29: 422–9.

(110) Green, LM. A cohort mortality study of forestry workers exposed to phenoxy acid herbicides. *Br J Ind Med* 1991; 48: 234–8.

(111) Coggon D, Pannett B, Winter P. Mortality and incidence of cancer at four factories making phenoxy herbicides. *Br J Ind Med* 1991; 48: 173–8.

(112) Wiggle DT, Semencin RM, Wilkins K et al. Mortality study of Canadian male farm operators: non-Hodgkin's lymphoma mortality and agricultural practices in Saskatchewan. *J Natl Cancer Inst* 1990; 82: 575–82.

(113) Garland FC, Gorham ED, Garland CF, Ferns JA. Non-Hodgkin's lymphomas in US navy personnel. *Arch Environ Health* 1988; 43: 425–9.

(114) Corbett S, O'Neill BJ. A cluster of cases of lymphoma in an underground colliery. *Med J Aust* 1988; 149: 178–85.

(115) Riihimaki V, Asp S, Hernberg S. Mortality of 2,4-dichlorophenoxyacetic acid and 2,4,5-trichlorophenoxyacetic acid herbicide applicators in Finland. *Scand J Work Environ Health* 1982; 8: 37–42.

(116) Christie D, Robinson K, Gordon I, Bisby J. A prospective study in the Australian petroleum industry. II. Incidence of cancer. *Br J Ind Med* 1991; 48: 511–4.

(117) Skov T, Lynge E. Non-Hodgkin's lymphoma and occupation in Denmark. *Scand J Soc Med* 1991; 19: 162–9.

(118) Blair A, Malker H, Cantor KP, Burmeister L, Wiklund K. Cancer among farmers. *Scand J Work Environ Health* 1985; 11: 397–407.

(119) Saracci R, Kogevinas M, Bertazzi P-A, et al. Cancer mortality in workers exposed to chlorphenoxy herbicides and chlorophenols. *Lancet* 1991; 338 (Oct 26): 1027–32.

(120) Bond GG, Wetterstroem NH, Roush GJ, McLaren EA, Lipps TE, Cook RR. Cause specific mortality among employees engaged in the manufacture, formulation, or packaging of 2,4-dichlorophenoxyacetic acid and related salts. *Br J Ind Med* 1988; 45: 98–105.

(121) Ronco G, Costa G, Lynge E. Cancer risk among Danish and Italian farmers. *Br J Ind Med* 1992; 49: 220–5.

(122) Alavanja MCR, Blair A, Merkle S, Teske J, Eaton B, Reed B. Mortality among forest and soil conservationists. *Arch Environ Health* 1989; 44: 94–101.

(123) Pearce NE, Sheppard RA, Smith AH, Teague CA. Non-Hodgkin's lymphoma and farming: an expanded case-control study. *Int J Cancer* 1987; 39: 155–61.

(124) Woods JS, Polissar L, Severson RK, Heuser LS, Kulander BG. Soft tissue sarcoma and non-Hodgkin's lymphoma in relation to phenoxyherbicide and chlorinated phenol exposure in western Washington. *J Natl Cancer Inst* 1987; 78: 899–910.

(125) Alavanja MCR, Blair A, Masters MN. Cancer mortality in the US flour industry. *J Natl Cancer Inst* 1990; 82: 840–8.

(126) Sama SR, Martin TR, Davis LK, Kriebel D. Cancer incidence among Massachusetts firefighters, 1982–1986. *Am J Ind Med* 1990; 18: 47–54.

(127) Zahm SH, Weisenburger DD, Babbitt PA et al. A case-control study of

non-Hodgkin's lymphoma and the herbicide 2,4-Dichlorophenoxyacetic acid (2,4-D) in eastern Nebraska. *Epidemiol* 1990; 1: 349–56.

(128) Hayes HM, Tarone RE, Cantor KP, Jensen CR, McCurnin DM, Richardson RC. Case-control study of canine malignant lymphoma: positive association with dog owner's use of 2,4-Dichlorophenoxyacetic acid herbicides. *JNCI* 1991; 83: 1226–31.

(129) Zahm SH, Weisenburger DD, Babbitt PA, Saal RC, Vaught JB, Blair A. Use of hair coloring products and the risk of lymphoma, multiple myeloma and chronic lymphocytic leukemia. *Am J Public Health* 1992; 82: 990–7.

(130) Linos A, Blair A, Gibson RW et al. Leukemia and non-Hodgkin's lymphoma and residential proximity to industrial plants. *Arch Environ Health* 1991; 46: 70–4.

(131) Alavanja MCR, Blair A, Merkle S, Teske J, Eaton B. Mortality among agricultural extension agents. *Am J Ind Med* 1988; 14: 167–76.

(132) Dubrow R, Paulson JO, Windian R. Farming and malignant lymphoma in Hancock County, Ohio. *Br J Ind Med* 1988; 45: 25–8.

(133) Reif J, Pearce N, Kawachi I, Fraser J. Soft-tissue sarcoma, non-Hodgkin's lymphoma and other cancers in New Zealand forestry workers. *Int J Cancer* 1989; 43: 49–54.

(134) Brownson RC, Reif JS, Chang JC, Davis JR. Cancer risks among Missouri farmers. *Cancer* 1989; 64: 2381–6.

(135) Ott MG, Teta MJ, Greenberg HL. Lymphatic and hematopoietic tissue cancer in a chemical manufacturing environment. *Am J Ind Med* 1989; 16: 631–43.

(136) Cantor KP, Blair A, Everett G et al. Pesticides and other agricultural risk factors for non-Hodgkin's lymphoma among men in Iowa and Minnesota. *Cancer Res* 1992; 52: 2447–55.

(137) Weisenburger DD. Environmental epidemiology of non-Hodgkin's lymphoma in Eastern Nebraska. *Am J Ind Med* 1990; 18: 303–5.

(138) Balarajan R. Malignant lymphomas in agricultural and forestry workers in England and Wales. *Public Health* 1988; 102: 585–92.

(139) Cantor KP, Blair A, Everett G et al. Hair dye use and risk of leukaemia and lymphoma. *Am J Pub Health* 1988; 78: 570–1.

(140) Olsson H, Brandt L. Risk of non-Hodgkin's lymphoma among men occupationally exposed to organic solvents. *Scand J Work Environ Health* 1988; 14: 246–51.

(141) Linos A, Blair A, Cantor KP et al. Leukemia and non-Hodgkin's lymphoma among embalmers and funeral directors. *J Natl Cancer Inst* 1990; 82: 66.

(142) La Vecchia C, Negri E, Avanjo BD, Franceschi S. Occupation and lympoid neoplasms. *Br J Cancer* 1989; 60: 385–8.

(143) Cantor KP. Farming and mortality from non-Hodgkin's lymphoma: a case-control study. *Int J Cancer* 1982; 29: 239–47.

(144) Hoar SK, Blair A, Holmes FF et al. Agricultural herbicide use and risk of lymphoma and soft tisssue sarcoma. *JAMA* 1986; 256: 1141–8.

(145) Balarajan R. Malignant lymphomas in road transport workers. *J Epidemiol Community Health* 1983; 37: 279–80.

(146) Binaschi S, Santoro G, Introini U, Fraumeni JF. Sull'ipotesi occupazionale dei linfomi Hodgkin e non-Hodgkin; uno studio caso-controllo. *Ital Med Lav* 1985; 7: 181–6.

(147) Pearce NE, Smith AH, Fisher DO. Malignant lymphoma and multiple myeloma linked with agricultural occupations in a New Zealand cancer registry-based study. *Am J Epidemiol* 1985; 121: 225–37.

(148) Persson B, Dahlander A-M, Fredriksson M, Brage HN, Ohlson CG, Axelson O. Malignant lymphomas and occupational exposures. *Br J Ind Med* 1989; 46: 516–20.

(149) Schumacher MC. A death-certificate case-control study of non-Hodgkin's lymphoma and occupation in men in North Carolina. *Am J Ind Med* 1988; 13: 317–30.

(150) Linet M. Mycosis Fungoides and occupation in Sweden. *J Natl Cancer Inst* 1989; 81: 1842–3.

(151) Cohen SR, Stenn KS, Brauerman IM, Beck GJ. Mycosis fungoides: Clinicopathologic relationships, survival, and therapy in 59 patients with observations on occupation as a new prognostic factor. *Cancer* 1980; 46: 2654–66.

(152) Brownson RC, Reif JS. A cancer registry-based study of occupational risk for lymphoma, multiple myeloma and leukaemia. *Int J Epidemiol* 1988; 17: 27–32.

(153) Schumacher CM. Farming occupations and mortality from non-Hodgkin's lymphoma in Utah. *J Occup Med* 1985; 27: 580–4.

(154) Burmeister LF, Everett GD, van Lier SF, Isacson P. Selected cancer mortality and farm practices in Iowa. *Am J Epidemiol* 1983; 118: 72–7.

(155) Pearce NE, Smith AH, Howard JK, Shepperd RA, Giles HJ, Teague CA. Non-Hodgkin's lymphoma and exposure to phenoxyherbicides, chlorophenols, fencing work, and meat works employment: a case-control study. *Br J Ind Med* 1986; 43: 75–83.

(156) Hardell L, Eriksson M, Lenner P, Lundgren E. Malignant lymphoma and exposure to chemicals, especially organic solvents, chlorophenols and phenoxy acids: a case-control study. *Br J Cancer* 1981; 43: 169–76.

(157) Lampi P, Hakulinen T, Luostarinen T, Pukkala E, Teppo L. Cancer incidence following chlorophenol exposure in a community in Southern Finland. *Arch Environ Health* 1992; 47: 167–75.

(158) Newcombe DS. Immune surveillance, organophosphorus exposure and lymphomagenesis. *Lancet* 1992; 339: 539–41.

(159) Bertazzi PA, Zocchetti C, Pesatori AC, Guercilena S, Sanarico M, Radice L. Ten-year mortality study of the population involved in the Seveso incident in 1976. *Am J Epidemiol* 1989; 129: 1187–200.

(160) Manz A, Berger J, Dwyer JH, Flesch-Janys D, Nagel S, Waltsgott H. Cancer mortality among workers in chemical plant contaminated with dioxin. *Lancet* 1991; 338: 959–64.

(161) Fingerhut MA, Halperin WE, Marlow DA et al. Cancer mortality in workers exposed to 2,3,7,8-tetrachlorodibenzo-*p*-dioxin. *New Eng J Med* 1991; 324: 212–8.

(162) Zober A, Messerer P, Huber P. Thirty-four year mortality follow-up of BASF employees exposed to 2,3,7,8-TCDD after the 1953 accident. *Int Arch Occup Environ Health* 1990; 62: 139–57.

Viruses as the aetiological agents of leukaemia and lymphoma

D ONIONS

Introduction

Leukaemogenesis, like other neoplastic processes, is a multistage event requiring several genetic or epigenetic events before clonal disease becomes clinically apparent. The discovery of leukaemogenic viruses has had a profound impact on unravelling these events in transformation. It was research on the animal retroviruses that led to the discovery of cellular proto-oncogenes and initiated the modern era of molecular investigations of the pathogenesis of neoplasia.

Two main groups of viruses have been associated with leukaemias and lymphomas, the oncogenic retroviruses (oncoviruses) and the herpesviruses. While these viruses are very different in their structure and replication patterns there are features in the biology of leukaemia viruses that are common. Usually these viruses establish persistent infections and neoplastic disease may result only after many years of infection during which the individual may be clinically normal. In most cases leukaemogenic viruses require intimate contact for their transmission, virus being transmitted from a healthy carrier to a susceptible individual usually through contaminated, blood and saliva or perinatally by transplacental or milk transmission.

In naturally occurring virus infections it is usually only a minority of individuals that develop neoplasia following infection, although the proportion varies widely from one virus to another. This feature can make simple epidemiological associations between infection and disease difficult to establish unless a serological marker is available. In cases where the incidence of neoplasia is low, prospective studies may be necessary to establish an epidemiological connection. It is possible that a wider range of viruses than currently envisaged may be involved as uncommon aetiological agents of

All correspondence to: Professor David Onions, Department of Veterinary Pathology, The University of Glasgow, UK.

Cambridge Medical Reviews: Haematological Oncology Volume 3

leukaemia. Such associations are not likely to be revealed by conventional seroepidemiological studies and may only be revealed by detection of viral genomes within the leukaemic cell population.

In those conditions that have a viral aetiology, prophylactic vaccination or therapeutic intervention become realistic prospects. Vaccines are now widely used to control infection by feline leukaemia virus and Marek's disease virus, a commercially important leukaemogenic herpesvirus of chickens. In the near future we may expect to see clinical trials of prophylactic vaccines against the human T-cell leukaemia virus (HTLV-1) and Epstein–Barr Virus (EBV).

Retroviruses

Retroviruses are characterized by their ability to transcribe their RNA genomes into a DNA copy or provirus which can integrate into cellular DNA. Several distinct subgroups exist, the oncoviruses which contain the leukaemogenic viruses, the lentiviruses which are associated with immunosuppressive and degenerative diseases and the spumaviruses which have not been associated definitively with the aetiology of any disease. Traditionally, the oncoviruses have been subdivided into types A through to D on the basis of their morphology and pattern of release from cells. However, as more has become known about the molecular biology of these viruses it is clear that two distinct groups of leukaemogenic viruses can be discerned. One group exemplified by the feline, murine and avian leukaemia viruses replicate efficiently in their hosts establishing high titre viraemias and causing neoplasia through their interaction with cellular proto-oncogenes. HTLV-1 is the paradigm virus for a small subgroup of viruses which includes the bovine leukaemia virus and the simian T-cell leukaemia virus. In contrast to feline leukaemia virus they establish a latent pattern of infection and transformation of cells appears to be dependent on viral encoded genes.[1]

The FeLV/MuLV/ALV subgroup

Structure and replication of the FeLV/MuLV oncoviruses Viruses are essentially replicating agents and it is hardly surprising that the replication strategy of a virus profoundly influences its biology. Amongst the retroviruses there are important differences in replication systems but there are also common themes that are exemplified in the simple oncoviruses like feline leukaemia virus (FeLV).[2]

A unique feature of retroviruses is that their genomes are diploid consisting of two copies of single-stranded RNA. This property may account for the very high frequency of recombination observed for these viruses. The genome is enclosed within an icosahedral core that in turn is surrounded by an envelope derived from a modified cell membrane into which viral glycoproteins become substituted. Between the core and the envelope is a matrix protein that bridges these two structures. The major envelope glycoprotein, termed SU binds, to cognate receptors on the cell surface and entry is mediated by fusion of the viral envelope and cell membrane; the latter process being dependent on the activity of a minor transmembrane (TM) envelope protein. In some retrovirus infections this fusion may occur after endocytosis of the virus and activation in the low pH of the endosome. Once the virus core is released into the cytoplasm, the genomic RNA is transcribed into double stranded DNA by a virion encoded enzyme, reverse transcriptase which is present in the core of the virus. The DNA copy, termed a provirus, migrates to the nucleus as a nucleoprotein complex and becomes covalently integrated into chromosomal DNA through the action of the integrase function of the reverse transcriptase complex (Fig. 1).

The sites of integration of a provirus can essentially be considered to be random although fine structural features of the DNA may influence the precise integration point. Only mitotically active cells can be successfully infected by FeLV or MuLV and between 1 and 30 proviruses may become integrated. Under certain circumstances these proviruses may be transcriptionally silent establishing a latent infection within the cell but usually, transcription proceeds resulting in the production of new virus particles. Viral glycoproteins become incorporated in regions of the cell membrane and nascent virus particles form by budding from these regions. In the case of most oncovirus infections this process is non-cytopathic so the cell continues to function and divide normally, the progeny cells each receiving copies of the provirus in the same chromosomal location. The establishment of persistent infections is favoured by these properties of proviral integration and non-cytopathic release; and also influences oncogenesis which is dependent on integration of the virus at critical sites.

Endogenous proviruses An event unique to this class of viruses is their ability to infect the germ line stem cells and become transmitted as genetic elements called endogenous proviruses. In some strains of laboratory mice these genetically inherited viruses become expressed and eventually lead to the development of leukaemia. In most species, however, endogenous proviruses are under tight transcriptional control in the whole animal and are not usually expressed as infectious virus. Probably all vertebrate species contain endogenous proviruses and transposable elements from which they may have evolved extend far back in evolutionary history.

A positive selection pressure for the retention of endogenous proviruses may be the property of viral interference, in which viral glycoproteins expressed within a cell block the cellular receptors and prevent superinfection. Consequently selective expression of an envelope glycoprotein gene can an act as a viral resistance gene. Indeed, in wild mouse populations this process has been observed[3] and in veterinary medicine

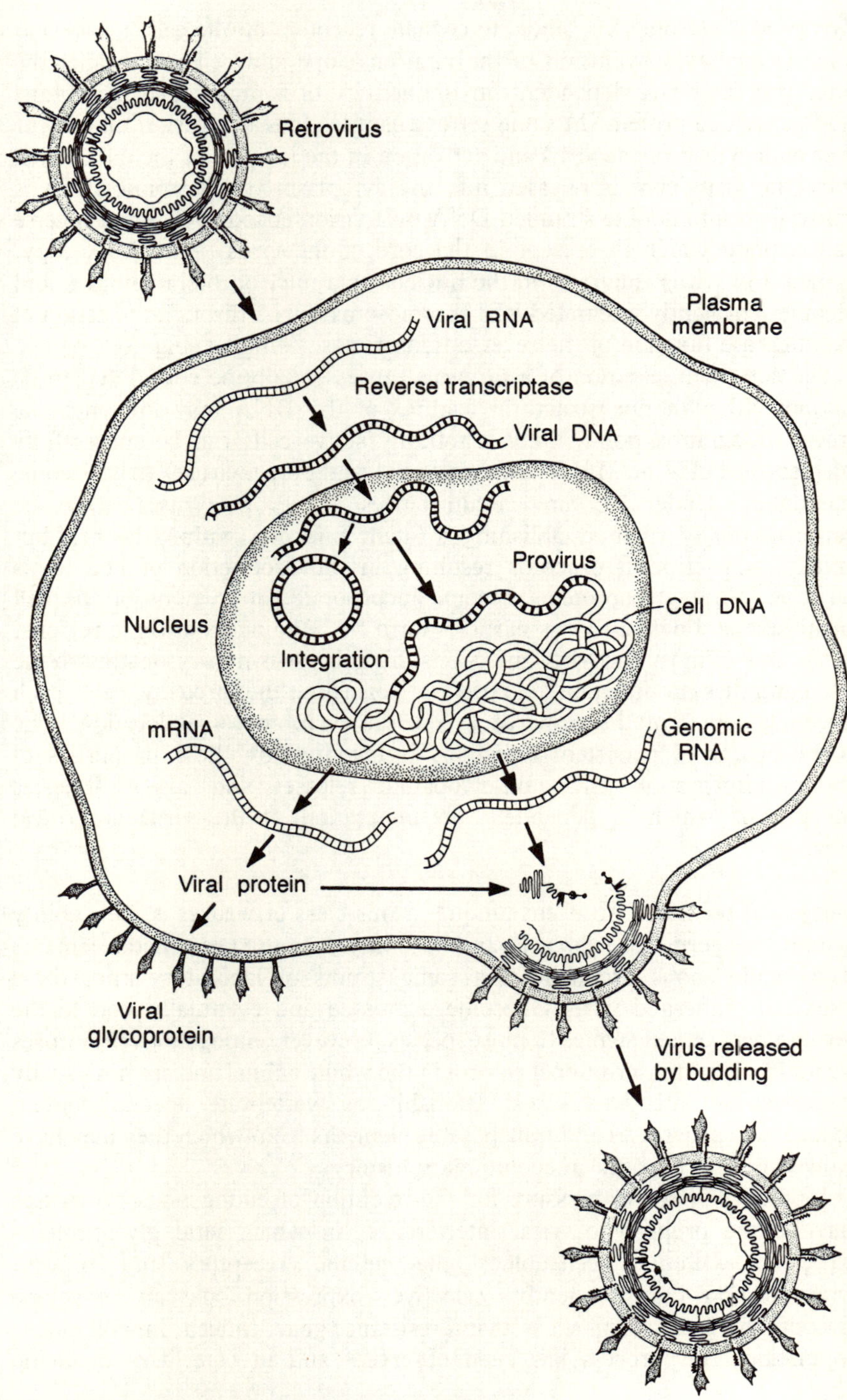

Fig. 1. Replication cycle of a Type-C retrovirus.

transgenic chickens expressing a retroviral envelope gene are being produced to confer resistance to the economically important avian leukosis virus (ALV).

The relationship between endogenous viruses and their horizontally transmitted exogenous counterparts can be complex. The domestic cat contains two principal sets of endogenous viruses. One group is closely related to an endogenous virus of baboons and is found in the germ line of all old world cats but not in the DNA of new world cats like jaguars and snow leopards. It has been suggested that this virus was transmitted to ancestral cat species after the division of the old and new world species several million years ago. The second main proviral family is related to FeLV, the leukaemogenic virus of cats. Endogenous FeLV is not expressed as complete virus particles but envelope message can be detected in certain cells.[4]

In natural cat populations 3 distinct subgroups of FeLV are found. These subgroups are defined by viral interference in that they use different receptors to enter cells and these differences are reflected in the polymorphism of their envelope glycoproteins. In FeLV infections a subgroup A virus is always present but in addition subgroups B and C may also be isolated. It has been demonstrated that the subgroup B viruses arise by recombination between the infecting virus and the endogenous FeLV virus.[5] On the other hand, sequence analysis of the subgroup C viruses indicates that they arise by mutation from the prototype A virus.

It is becoming apparent that the envelope glycoproteins may have a wider series of effects on cells than simply being passive receptors. The Friend murine leukaemia virus contains a defective envelope gene product which is able to bind to and activate the erythropoietin receptor by binding to an internal site.[6] In contrast, FeLV-C is always associated with onset of a fatal pure red cell hypoplasia in which there is a rapid fall in the number of erythroid precursor cells (BFU-E).[7]

In man there are a large number of defective endogenous proviruses which may be divided into broad classes. Class I viruses are related to type C retroviruses like FeLV and MuLV while class II viruses have greater sequence similarity to the mammary tumour virus of mice. Although none of these proviruses can produce virus particles, transcripts of class I proviruses have been observed in normal spleens, placentas and colon carcinomas. Similarly, class I and II transcripts have been detected in breast carcinomas.[8]

In addition to these genetic remnants of once infectious retroviruses, vertebrate cells contain mobile genetic elements; called retroposons, that encode reverse transcriptase and can be mobile within a cell through expression of an RNA copy followed by its reverse transcription and re-insertion into another chromosomal site. In mice, intracisternal type A particles (IAPs) that resemble the cores of retroviruses are frequently expressed in haemopoietic cell lines. Mice contain about 1000 copies of IAP proviral sequences per haploid genome and they have been associated with activation of the *mos* and *myc* proto-oncogenes in myelomas and the IL-3 gene in a myeloid leukaemia line. Mobile genetic elements like IAPs have been classified as type I retroposons which are distinguished from class II retroposons that lack LTRs but which contain reverse transcriptase. The LINE-1 elements are an example of this second group and they constitute up to 3% of the coding capacity of the human genome. LINE insertions have been found in at the c-*myc* locus in canine transmissible venereal tumour and a human breast carcinoma.[9]

Epidemiology of FeLV The epidemiology of FeLV highlights the problems of associating viruses with neoplastic disease even when, as in the case of feline leukaemia virus, the incidence of neoplastic disease can be high. In suburban areas containing cats kept in small household groups, most cats will eventually encounter a carrier cat shedding virus in their saliva. Virus can be transmitted during the relatively brief social contacts between animals. Although most serological surveys suggest that between 50 to 80% of cats become infected by the virus only 1 to 5% become persistently infected and develop disease. The remainder become transiently infected but eventually eliminate the infection and are solidly immune to reinfection.[10]

A quite distinct pattern of infection is observed in closed communities containing breeding cats. Young animals are more susceptible to infection and litters born to infected mothers are immunotolerant to the virus with all the kittens becoming persistently infected.[11] Consequently the incidence of persistent infection can reach 40% or higher and the majority of these cats will die from anaemia, immunosuppression or an FeLV related leukaemia within 3 years of exposure. It was the presence of such cluster households that first indicated that feline leukaemia might have an infectious aetiology. However, it would be extremely hard to determine a viral aetiology from the pattern of disease in the suburban group cats without knowledge of their status of infection.[12]

Neoplastic transformation by the ALV/MuLV/FeLV group The first demonstration that a virus, now known as a retrovirus, could cause leukaemia dates to the formative studies conducted by Ellerman and Bang in 1908 who transmitted leukaemia with cell free filtrates and Peyton Rous who transmitted fibrosarcomas of chickens with a virus that now bears his name. Despite these early origins, it was not until the 1970s that molecular analysis revealed the nature of the interaction of these viruses with cellular genes that leads to their transforming ability.

The structure of a typical murine or feline leukaemia provirus is shown in Fig. 2. It contains three major gene groupings. The *gag* gene encodes internal proteins of the virus; the end of this region contains a contiguous gene *pro*

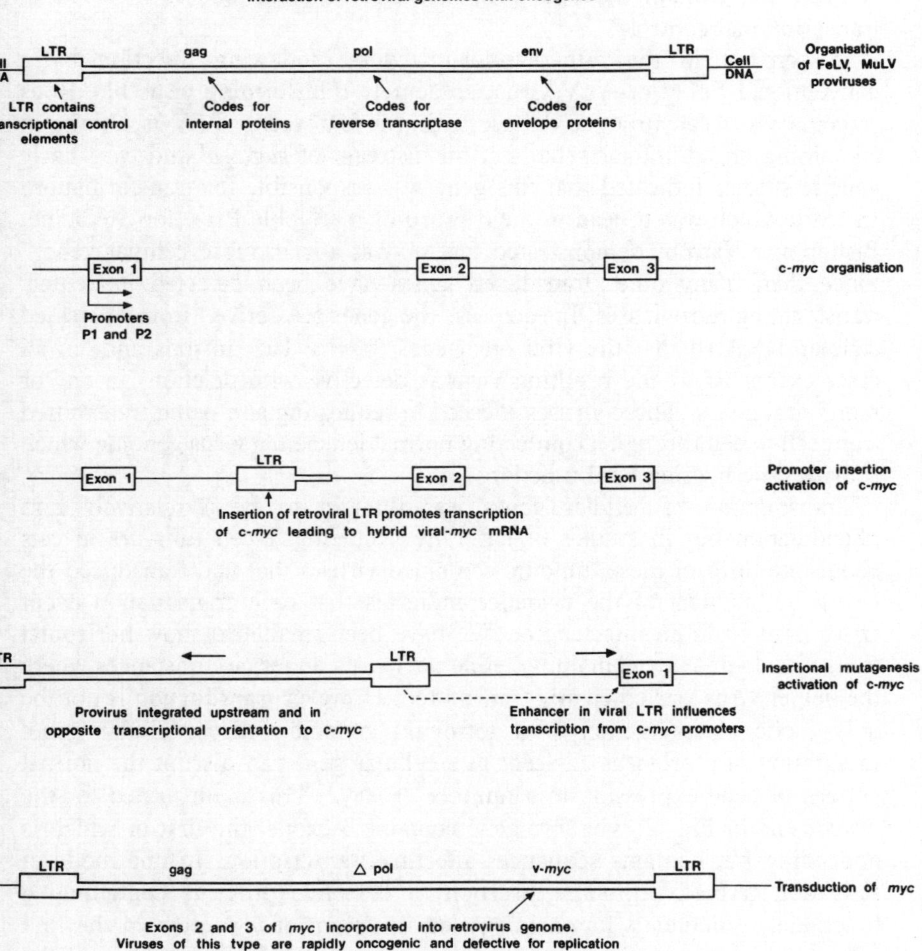

Fig. 2. Structure of an FeLV/MuLV provirus and patterns of insertional mutagenesis and transduction of the *myc* gene.

which encodes a protease responsible for cleaving the *gag* polyprotein into its constituent elements. Downstream from *gag* is the *pol* gene which encodes the reverse transcriptase and the integrase protein, the latter being clipped from the *pol* protein by the viral protease. The *env* gene is in a different reading frame from *pol* and partially overlaps the end of that gene but in a different reading frame. The *env* gene is transcribed from a spliced message, the donor site being in the untranslated region upstream from *gag*. At each end of the virus are two repeated sequences called long terminal repeats

(LTRs) that contain the viral promoter and other sequences involved in transcriptional control.

In contrast to the rather indolent course following infection by a conventional FeLV or ALV virus, an acutely transforming virus like Rous sarcoma virus can produce disease within a few weeks. RSV is unique in containing an additional gene, *src*, downstream of *gag*, *pol* and *env*. Early genetic studies indicated that this gene was responsible for transformation. In work which was to lead to their award of the Noble Prize for Medicine, Bishop and Varmus demonstrated that *src* was a transduced cellular gene.[13] Since then many other transduced genes have been detected in acutely transforming retroviruses. In each case the genes are derived from processed cellular RNA so that the viral oncogenes (*v-oncs*) lack introns and, in all cases except RSV, the resulting virus is defective with deletions in one or more viral genes. These viruses succeed in replicating and being transmitted from cell to cell through a coinfecting normal leukaemia virus genome which provides the missing viral functions.

Transduction of cellular genes was thought to be a relatively rare phenomenon but in studies of naturally occurring T-cell tumours in cats about one-third of these tumours contained viruses that had transduced the *myc* gene.[4,14] Most of the evidence indicates that each transduction event arises *de novo* in an infected cat. We have been unable to show horizontal transmission of a *myc* containing feline retrovirus under circumstances where the helper virus was efficiently transmitted. However transduction is not the only mode of interaction of a retroviral genome with a cellular gene. Integration of a provirus adjacent to a cellular gene can disrupt the normal pattern of gene expression in a number of ways. This is illustrated for the c-*myc* gene in Fig. 2. The *myc* gene contains 3 exons, the first of which is noncoding but contains sequences affecting transcription. In one mode of activation termed promoter insertion, a defective provirus containing a functional promoter is found integrated upstream of *myc* often in the first intron. The transcription of the *myc* gene is now under the control of the viral LTR so that a hybrid viral-*myc* message is produced at a steady state level that may be 50-fold above the normal maximum. Spliced hybrid messages of this form may be packaged into virions and after another round of recombination with the retroviral genome can form the transducing class of viruses.

Proviral insertion can also occur within an exon or in an intron between two coding exons. This results in truncation of either the NH_2-terminal or COOH-terminal regions of the protein, which in turn can affect the stability and function of the protein. For instance truncation of the COOH-terminus of c-*myb* has been observed in MuLV induced myeloid leukaemias.[15] Insertion of a provirus in the 3′ untranslated region of a gene can also affect the stability of the mRNA. This has been observed for the *pim*-1 gene in rodent T-cell tumours induced by MuLV. In this case the insertion results in a message lacking an AUUUA motif, the net effect being to enhance the stability of the *pim*-1 mRNA.[16]

Proviral insertions of the form described above are essentially short range events. However, in some instances, the provirus may be integrated many kilobases away either upstream in the opposite transcriptional orientation or downstream in the same transcriptional orientation as the gene. In these cases transcription proceeds from a normal promoter but the viral enhancer overrides the transcriptional control.

Viral oncogenes fall into broad classes filling niches in the signalling pathway from the cell surface to DNA transcription. They include growth factors, for instance, IL-3, growth factor receptors like EGF, membrane or cytoplasmic proteins involved in signal transduction and nuclear proteins that includes transcription factors like c-*myc*. In the case of growth factors an unequivocal assignment of function has proved possible as the cells expressing these cytokines also possessed functional receptors and an autocrine pathway of stimulation was evident. Growth factor receptors have also been revealed as viral oncogenes but they are usually modified. For instance the v-*erb* B product is the homologue of epidermal growth factor receptor but most of the extracellular domain including the EGF binding site is missing and a small deletion of the intracellular C-terminal region removes a site for autophosphorylation by this protein kinase. The overall effect is to produce a receptor that is constitutively active in the absence of its ligand.[9]

The oncogenes identified by insertional mutagenesis or transduction usually have strong dominant effects and over 50 such genes have now been identified. In general these genes have been found to be involved in other cancers whether viral or not. For instance c-*myc* gene is activated by feline leukaemia virus in T-cell tumours, by ALV in B-cell tumours, whereas it is involved in Burkitt's lymphoma through translocation into the IgH locus.

With the resolution that p53 and Rb proteins are tumour suppressor genes attention has turned to this class of gene as potential targets for retroviral insertion. In this instance one might expect that both alleles would have to be inactivated before a phenotypic effect is observed. Although this might be considered a rare event, inactivation of both p53 alleles has been observed in an erythroleukaemia induced by friend leukaemia virus.

Gene collaboration in leukaemogenesis Retroviral insertion has proved to be a powerful method for identifying new oncogenes and over 50 have been discovered through this route. Moreover, it is becoming clear that retroviruses can contribute more than one genetic event, adding another dimension to the information that can be gleaned from these tumours. For instance when FeLV-*myc* viruses are used to experimentally infect cats, T-cell tumours are produced rapidly but as these tumours are clonal in origin another event other than FeLV-*myc* infection is required.[17] We have analysed the insertion sites of the helper leukaemia viruses in these tumours and by identifying integration sites shared in different tumours we have found a novel site termed *fit*-1 involved in four of nine tumours.[18] In addition another site previously identified as *bim*-1 has been identified as a proviral integration site in combination with *myc* and *fit*-1. In naturally occurring tumours we have also found an instance of two separate FeLV proviruses each containing a transduced gene, one being *myc* and the other turning out to be a completely processed β chain of the T-cell antigen receptor.[19] This is the first instance of an antigen receptor gene being associated with retrovirus activation. Possibly reactivity to a self or viral antigen, conferred by this antigen receptor, was involved in stimulating the leukaemic cells.

The resolving power of this approach has been increased by the ability to target oncogene expression to particular tissue compartments of transgenic mice coupled with identification of collaborating genes through superinfection with MuLV. This approach was used in the formative studies of Cory, Adams and Berns and revealed novel genes collaborating with *myc* in producing B-cell tumours in Eμ-myc mice.[20,21] In similar studies we have targeted the human *myc* expression to the T-cell compartment using the CD2 locus defining sequence.[22] Superinfection of these mice results in a rapid acceleration of tumour development above that observed with virus or transgene alone (Fig. 3) Since the tumours are clonal, they afford an opportunity to identify new genes at proviral integration sites.

Human T-cell leukaemia virus

The discovery of transmissible oncogenic retroviruses in natural occurring outbred species led to an intensive search for related viruses in man. Despite several false starts and a period of disillusionment with this type of work, the persistence and insight of Bob Gallo and his colleagues was rewarded with the discovery of HTLV-1.[23] The original isolate was described as being from a case of mycosis fungoides but later analysis showed that the features of this, and other HTLV-1 related lymphomas, fitted the criteria of adult T-cell leukaemia/lymphoma (ATLL) first defined by Takatsuki.[24] Takatsuki had observed an unusually high incidence of a mature T-cell leukaemia and lymphoma that clustered in the Southern Japanese Islands and later, it became clear that these were associated with infection by HTLV-1. A second HTLV family member, HTLV-II, was originally isolated from a patient with T-cell hairy cell leukaemia. However, the disease associations of this virus are far from clear and it may be less pathogenic than type I virus.

HTLV associated diseases ATLL is an aggressive lymphoproliferative disorder that usually affects patients in the middle and later decades of life. Several

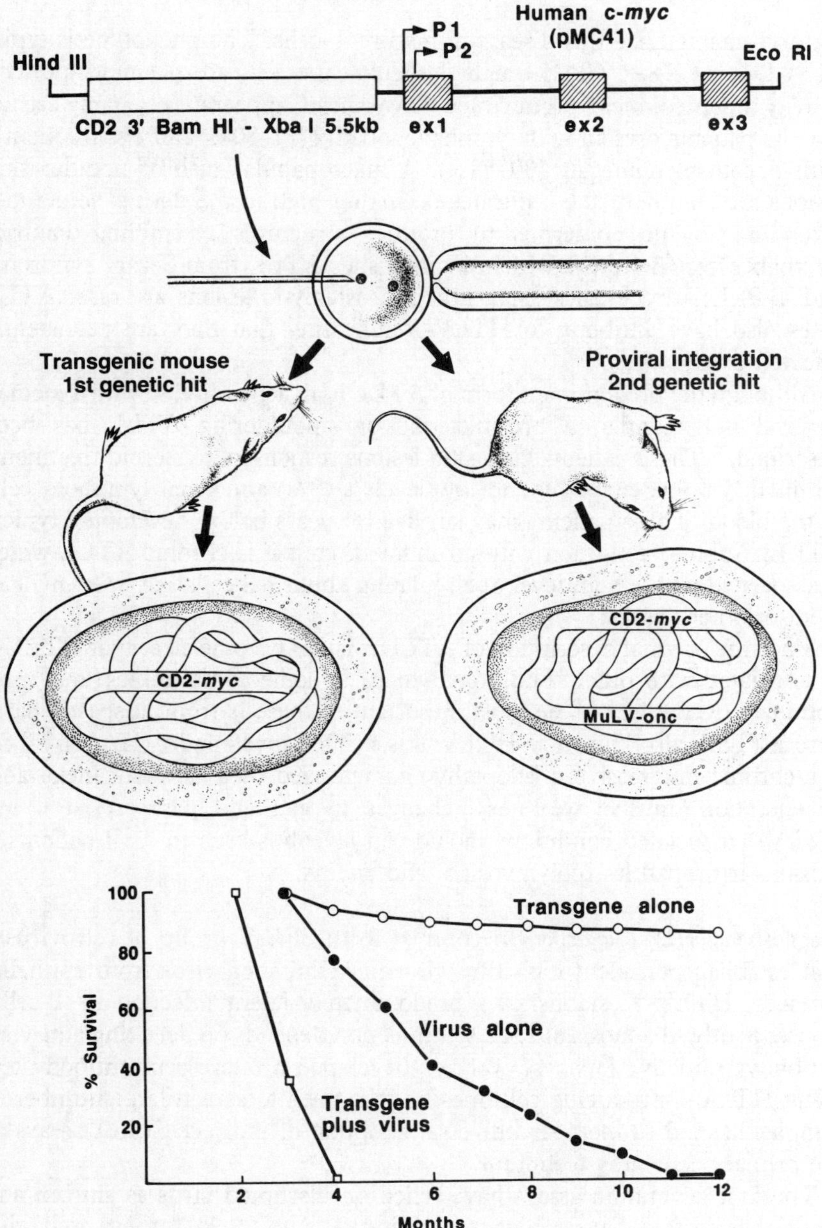

Fig. 3. Production of transgenic mice containing the human c-*myc* gene under the control of the CD2 locus defining sequence. Acceleration of clonal tumour development is shown after superinfection with MuLV indicating that *myc* collaborating oncogenes are activated.

features characterize this disease of mature T-cells. The phenotype is typically CD4+, CD8−, CD25+ and the leukaemic cells are pleomorphic with heavily indented nuclei producing a 'flower head' appearance. Characteristically the patients present with lymphadenopathy (71–80%) and less frequently with hepatosplenomegaly (39–58%). A macropapular rash or nodular skin lesions are common, the infiltrates occurring high in the dermis sometimes extending to the epidermis to produce structures resembling Pautrier microabcesses. A feature which distinguishes ATLL from Sézary syndrome and T-PLL is hypercalcaemia, although osteolytic lesions are rare. ATLL cases also have antibody to HTLV-1 indicating that they are persistently infected by the virus.[25,26]

Although the predominant form of ATLL is an acute disease with a median survival 4.4 months, a preleukaemic or smouldering ATLL has been described.[27] These patients have skin lesions responsive to steroid treatment, minimal lymphadenopathy and low levels (<3%) abnormal lymphoid cells in the blood. These patients may survive for years before developing typical ATLL. Another condition with an indolent course is chronic ATLL which is associated with a high level of circulating abnormal cells but little involvement of other tissues.

Since the original description of ATLL it is has become clear that HTLV-1 is associated with other conditions which, in some communities, may predominate over ATLL. The most important of these is tropical spastic paraparesis (TSP) also known as HTLV-1 associated myelopathy (HAM).[28] TSP is a chronic progressive myelopathy characterized by a slow but inexorable degeneration, muscle weakness, changes in gait and paraparesis. Other HTLV-1 associated conditions include an alveolitis seen in TSP patients,[29] chronic arthropathies, polymyositis, and uveitis.

Diagnosis of HTLV-1 infection In contrast to the FeLV group of retroviruses that establish persistent high titre viraemias and shed virus from epithelial surfaces, HTLV-1 establishes a predominately latent infection in T-cells. Consequently, diagnosis of HTLV-1 infection depends on detecting anti-viral antibody. Initially, Japanese workers developed a fluorescent antibody test using HTLV-1 producing cell lines but the need to screen large number of samples has led to the near universal adoption of indirect ELISA assays as the primary screening technique.

The first generation assays have relied on disrupted virus as antigen and while these assays have a high specificity (99.3 to 99.9%), their predictive value can be low if the incidence of HTLV-1 infection is low. Positive ELISA results must therefore be repeated and confirmed by another assay like western blotting or radioimmunoprecipitation. The US Public Health Working Party recommended that a specimen must demonstrate immunoreactivity to the *gag* gene product p24 and to an *env* gene product (gp46 and /or gp61/68) to be considered positive. Sera that do not react in western blotting or radio-immunoprecipitation assays to any viral protein are considered negative, while those that react with one or more proteins but do not fulfil the criteria of a positive sample are classed as indeterminate.

Indeterminate results are cause of considerable concern as appropriate counselling must be given to patients. At present the gold standard assay would be the demonstration of either HTLV-1 or II genomes in peripheral blood cells by PCR. HTLV-II genomes have been detected in some individuals with indeterminate serology and sera from 80% of individuals with HTLV-II infection react with HTLV-I *gag* and *env* proteins in western blots or radioimmunoprecipitation assays.[30] However HTLV-II infection is unlikely to account for the majority of these results. Other explanations include a phased reactivity to viral proteins during seroconversion, with p24 reactivity both preceding and in one instance lagging p19 reactivity by 10 months.[31]

An interesting hypothesis is that the antigen may be encoded by an endogenous retrovirus. The HRES-1 endogenous provirus contains an open reading frame that could encode for a protein with partial homology to both p19 and p24 of HTLV-1.[32] A 28-kDa protein encoded by the HRES-I genome is expressed in the H9 lymphoid cell line and this may be the same protein recognized in choriocarcinoma cell lines by certain monoclonal antibodies to HTLV-I p19. HRES antibody responses were detected in 19 out of 65 patients with multiple sclerosis 4 out of 17 (23%) with systemic sclerosis, 4 out of 19 (21%) with systemic lupus erythematosus and 2 out of 19 (10%) with Sjogren's syndrome. Nine of 30 of these HRES seropositive patients showed reactivity with HTLV-*gag* p24.

In certain regions particular Africa and Papua New Guinea, the frequency of indeterminate results is high and it has been suggested that this could be related to immune complexes or autoantibodies in the sera but this is not supported by reactivities observed in sera from patients with autoimmune disease.[33] An alternative explanation is cross reactivity with other antigens particularly those of *P. falciparum* but, in the case of the sera from Papua New Guinea, it is likely that these activities are due to a response to the HTLV-I variant recently detected in populations within this region.[34]

In the last few years, a large number of prototype tests based on recombinant proteins or peptide ELISAs have been developed. It is likely that these will replace the first generation disrupted virus systems as they offer the capacity to discriminate between HTLV-I and II infections. Discrimination between type I and II infection is important as the prognosis following infection by the latter virus is probably more favourable.

Transmission of HTLV-I HTLV-I infections are characterized by the concomitant presence of anti-viral antibodies; the temporal pattern of seroconversion providing clues to the transmission routes. The major routes are from mother to child, possibly *in utero* but particularly through breast feeding. Sexual transmission is the other major route, with male to female transmission predominating. Successful transmission of the virus may require the passage of infected lymphocytes in the semen or milk.

In endemic regions there is a low seropositivity rate in children with males and females equally represented. After the age of 20 there is a rise in seropositivity with a higher incidence in woman than men.[35,36] The time taken for seroconversion to occur is not fully resolved. An unusual serological pattern observed in Japanese migrants to Hawaii, suggested that early infection may not always be associated with early seroconversion.[37] In this study, an age dependent rise in seropositivity of children of seropositive parents was observed but no such pattern was seen in the children of seronegative parents. These data could also suggest that arthropod vectors might be involved in transmission but the bulk of the evidence is strongly against this explanation, although arthropod vectors are involved in the transmission of the closely related bovine leukaemia virus. This conclusion is supported by the failure to observe a rising incidence of infection in childhood in most surveys and by the divergent incidence of infection in different ethnic populations within the same area.

Sexual transmission of HTLV-I is central to the maintenance of the virus in populations. Up to 60% of spouses of infected men may seroconvert in a 10 year period but only 6% of males will seroconvert in the reciprocal situation.[38] There is evidence to suggest that the probability of infection will increase in males that have antibody to a non-structural regulatory protein of the virus called TAX. This may reflect an increased replication of the virus within the host.

Mother to child transmission appears to occur predominantly through infected milk. In a recent survey in Japan the seroprevalance of HTLV-1 in children born to seropositive mothers was 6.1%.[39] The copy number of the provirus in the lymphocytes of carrier mothers was a significant factor in determining the frequency of transmission. The titre of antibody to HTLV-I in the mothers and the duration of breast feeding did not appear to be important factors, although there was some suggestion that seroconversion was higher in mothers who had antibody to TAX.

Transmission by whole blood is an efficient route of transmission and emphasizes the need to screen blood donors. Until recently it was estimated that 2,800 people a year were being infected in the USA through blood transfusion.[40] Recipients of 1–2 units of seropositive blood have an 60% chance of becoming infected. Intravenous drug abuse is now playing an important part in the transmission in western countries with HTLV-II being the predominant virus transmitted by this route.

Epidemiology The epidemiology of HTLV-I reflects the familial pattern of transmission. Foci of high micro-endemnicity in isolated populations are often found in regions with a relatively low overall incidence of seropositivity. The virus is widely distributed in tropical and subtropical regions, the most intensively studied regions being Southern Japan and the Caribbean. In Japan, a million people are estimated to be infected out of a population of 121 million.[41] However, there is pronounced regional variation, 25 to 35% of the population of Okinawa and 8 to 10% of the population of the southern island of Kyushu being seropositive. In contrast, serpositivity on Honshu is limited to a few locations, while on the northern island of Hokkaido, infection is restricted to the aboriginal populations, the Ainu and Ryukuans who have seropositivity rates of 30 to 45%. It has been suggested that the virus may have been brought to the Japanese islands by the Joman settlers, the ancestors of the Ainu and Ryukuans,[42] who migrated to Japan several hundred years before the major ethnic population, the Wajins. Others have suggested HTLV-1 and the simian virus STLV, found in Japanese macaques, may have been brought from Africa by Portuguese traders.[43] However HTLV-I endemic areas are not those where wild STLV infected macaques are found.

Recent molecular epidemiological studies have indicated the low level of genetic drift in the HTLV-I genome so that the microsequence variation that exists is reflected in the geographical origin of the virus.[44,45] These minor strain variations can be used to monitor population movements. For instance, HTLV infection in the Caribbean is largely restricted to persons of African descent while the Indian population has a low incidence of infection, despite sharing the same environment for at least a century. Among the Afro-Caribbean population, isolates from the French West Indies are closely related to those in West African countries but distinct from those in Zaire, suggesting that the these strains were introduced to the Americas through the slave trade.[44] Recently a new HTLV variant has been isolated from a member of the Hagahai, a remote tribe in Papua new Guinea. Sequence analysis of this virus indicates a marked heterogeneity from the prototype strain (7%)[34] a feature that may also be reflected in the serological responses of Papua New Guineans to prototype HTLV-I.[46]

Until recently the origin of HTLV-II was enigmatic despite having a high incidence amongst drug abusers in some western countries. The virus has now been found to be endemic among certain peoples of Central and Northern America including the Guayami Indians of Panama and the Seminole Indians of Florida.[47]

Replication of HTLV-I HTLV-I has a distinct genetic structure and pattern of replication compared to FeLV and MuLV. In addition to the *gag*, *pol* and *env* genes, the genome contains an additional region termed *px* that encodes several proteins involved in the replication of HTLV-I (Fig. 4). The target cells for infection are predominantly mature CD4+ T-cells. In vivo the vast majority of infected cells are latently infected. Activation of these cells by mitogenic stimuli in vitro and possibly in vivo can initiate productive replication. The early events in HTLV-I replication are dominated by two proteins encoded in the *px* region, p40 Tax and p27 Rex. The major mRNA species encoding Tax and Rex are generated from a double splicing event in which the first splice picks up separate ATG initiation codons for Tax and Rex and the second links these with open reading frames in the *px* region[48,49] (Fig. 4).

Tax is a transactivator that upregulates expression of the HTLV provirus. Two classes of sequence within the LTR, the TRE-1 and 2 elements are responsible for conferring responsiveness to Tax. A 21 base pair repeat element forms the core of the TRE-1 elements (Fig. 5).[50] One or two of these elements confer Tax responsiveness to a heterologous promoter independently of their orientation. The TRE-1 elements can interact with a wide range of cellular transcription factors belonging to the CREB/ATF family.[51,52] In addition, a 180 kDa protein and the HEB1 and TAF factors also interact with TRE-1.[53] The latter two proteins are of particular interest as Tax does

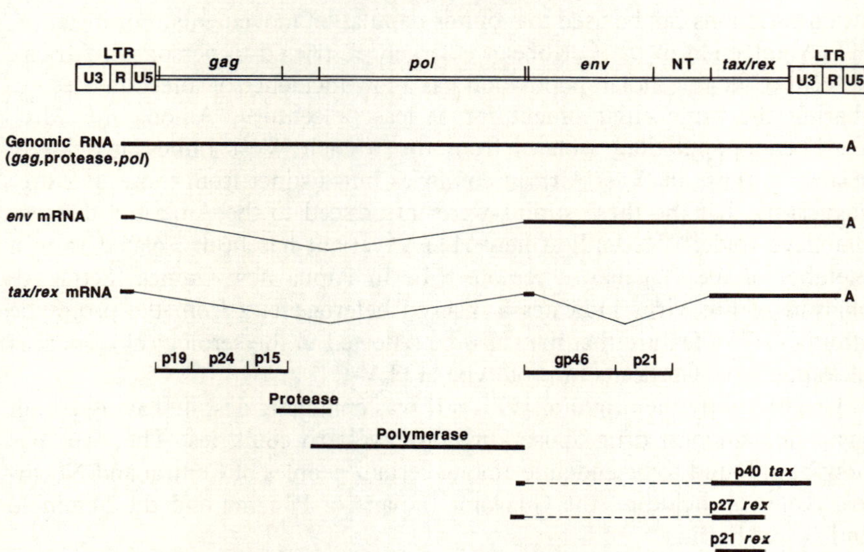

Fig. 4. The HTLV provirus contains a *px* region in addition to *gag, pol* and *env* genes. Double-spliced message encodes the p40 *tax* and p27 *rex* regulatory proteins. The accumulation of REX protein favours the production of singly spliced and unspliced messages encoding the structural proteins.

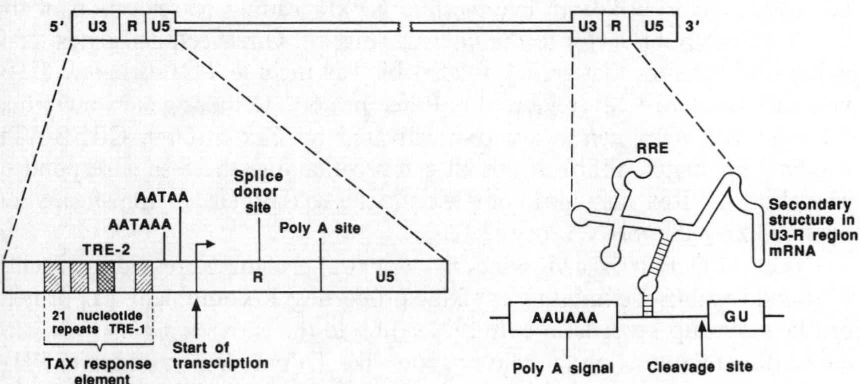

Fig. 5. Location of the Tax and Rex response elements.

not bind to DNA directly but interacts with TRE-1 indirectly, by association with HEB1 and TAF.

Similarly the TRE-2 element has binding sites for SP1, Ets1, *myb* and TIF-1, transcription factors. Tax interaction with TRE-2 is mediated by complex formation with TIF-1.[54] These data suggest that Tax may act as an activator protein, forming protein–protein interactions with TRE binding proteins and at the same time activating basal transcriptional proteins to facilitate transcription. The effect of Tax transactivation is to act as a positive feedback loop increasing transcription, but at this stage the predominant transcripts are double spliced mRNAs encoding Tax and Rex.

Rex functions as a switch in the replication cycle, favouring the production of singly spliced or unspliced messages encoding structural proteins. The Rex protein is localized in the nucleolus and the first 19 amino acids of this protein function as nucleolar targeting sequence.[55] Mutation of this region affects both nucleolar targeting and the ability of Rex to favour the accumulation of singly spliced RNAs. The effects of Rex are mediated post-transcriptionally through a Rex response element (RRE) located in a region of complex secondary structure encoded in the R region of the LTR (Fig. 5). The full mechanisms of Rex action are not understood but the protein may affect both the cytoplasmic transport and stability of mRNAs.[56]

Pathogenesis of HTLV associated diseases When HTLV-1 infects resting cord blood lymphocytes in vitro, it induces expression of interleukin-2 (IL-2) and the interleukin-2 receptor alpha chain (IL-2R) so that a polyclonal proliferation is initiated and maintained through an autocrine loop. The upregulation of IL-2 and IL-2R expression occurs through activation of the NFκB family of DNA binding proteins.[59] The mechanism leading to induction NFκB is not resolved. One possibility is that it may promote the dissociation of the inhibitory factor IxB from cytoplasmic NFxB leading to relocation of the active transcription factor to the nucleus (Fig. 6). Other cellular genes, containing NFxB sites that are stimulated by Tax include TNF-β, c-*myc* IL-6, vimentin and GM-CSF (reviewed in Reference 60). Cellular genes, including the c-*fos* and *Krox* genes, are transactivated by Tax through CREB/ATF response elements, although not all genes containing these sites respond to Tax (Fig. 6). Rex may also complement the role of Tax in transformation by stabilizing the mRNA for the IL-2R.

Tax also functions as a virokine, *i.e.* as a viral protein expressed extracellularly and capable of exhibiting cytokine properties. Recombinant Tax protein can be taken up by cells in culture, leading to the activation of NFxB with concomitant stimulation of cellular genes like TNF-β. When added to PHA stimulated lymphocytes Tax maintains the proliferation of lymphocytes and prolongs the sensitivity to IL-2.[61] In addition HTLV-1 infected cells appear to be able to stimulate the activation of non-infected T-cells through interaction with the CD2 pathway.[62] These mechanisms may be important in the pathogenesis of tropical spastic paraparesis. In TSP the number of infected cells and the antibody titres are higher than in healthy carriers.[63] In particular about one in every 5000 cells has a high expression of Tax and Rex.[64] Moreover T-cells in HAM/TSP patients show an upregulation of transcription of

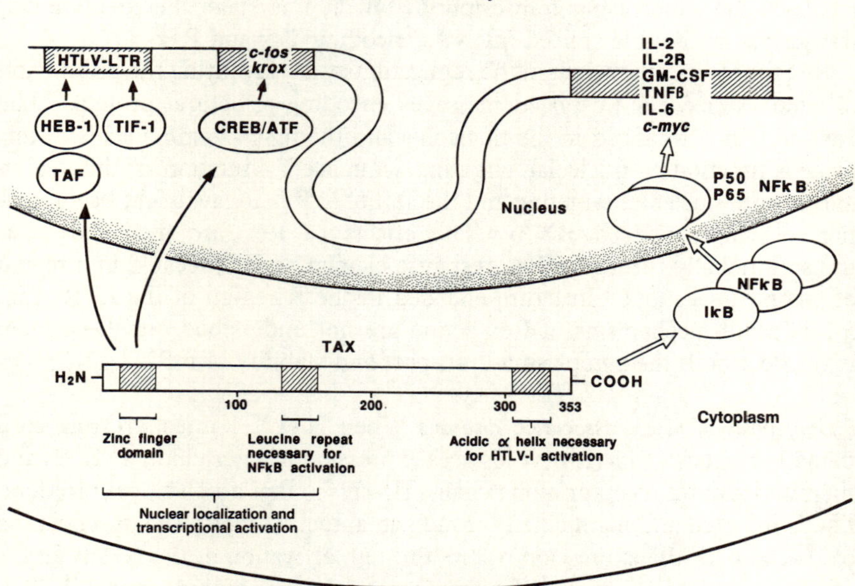

Fig. 6. Functional domains of the Tax protein and possible routes of action of Tax.

TNF-α, IL-1β and IFN-γ suggesting that T-cell activation may initiate an inflammatory cascade leading to immune destruction of the central nervous system.[65]

Given this range of cellular gene activation it is not entirely surprising that Tax can transform Rat-1 cells in vitro and that the continued expression of Tax is necessary for the maintenance of the transformed phenotype.[66] When expressed as at transgene, Tax induces tumours of mesenchymal origin including neurofibromas.[67] So far, Tax transgenic mice have not been shown to develop lymphomas. This is also true in a transgenic mouse line where the transgene's expression was targeted to the T-cell compartment by a CD3ε enhancer. However, lymphoma induction is significantly accelerated on superinfection with MuLV (Campbel et al. unpublished). Since Tax expression is not observed in the lymphomas but is present in the mesenchymal tumours that develop concurrently, it is possible that the acceleration is due to soluble Tax.

The early observations on the transformation mediated by Tax suggested that this might be the mechanism of transformation in vivo but, in primary ATLL cells, expression of Tax and Rex has not been convincingly demonstrated. However, recent PCR cDNA analysis of transcripts in the uncultured lymphocytes of HTLV-1 infected persons has revealed new transcripts associated with the pX region.[68,69] Among these were singly spliced mRNAs for a cytoplasmic product p21 *Rex* previously identified with antipeptide antisera. Additional mRNAs developed by alternative splicing patterns in open reading frames I and II of the *px* region could encode three additional proteins $p12^I$, $p13^{II}$ and $p30^{II}$ (Fig. 7). The $p30^{II}$ and $p13^{II}$ proteins synthesized from *orf II* are arginine and serine rich and located in the nucleolus and nucleus respectively. Of most interest is highly hydrophobic $p12^I$ protein which bears homology to the E5 transforming protein of bovine papillomavirus. The latter protein is known to interact with the vacuolar H+-ATPase and can bind to the PDGF receptor via its hydrophobic membrane associating domain.[70] These data suggest that both BPV-1 E5 and the HTLV-1I $p12^I$ may be involved in ligand independent activation of cell surface receptors. The development of transgenic mice expressing $p12^I$ may help to resolve the transforming potential of this protein. Many of the features of transformation by HTLV-I resemble those seen in DNA transforming viruses. It will be of interest to see if HTLV-I also has proteins that interact with tumour supressor genes, a factor that is a common theme in DNA virus mediated transformation.

Herpesviruses

Herpesviruses are a large group of viruses associated with a wide range of diseases in man and animals. A characteristic feature of this group is their capacity to remain as latent infections in either ganglionic tissue or peripheral

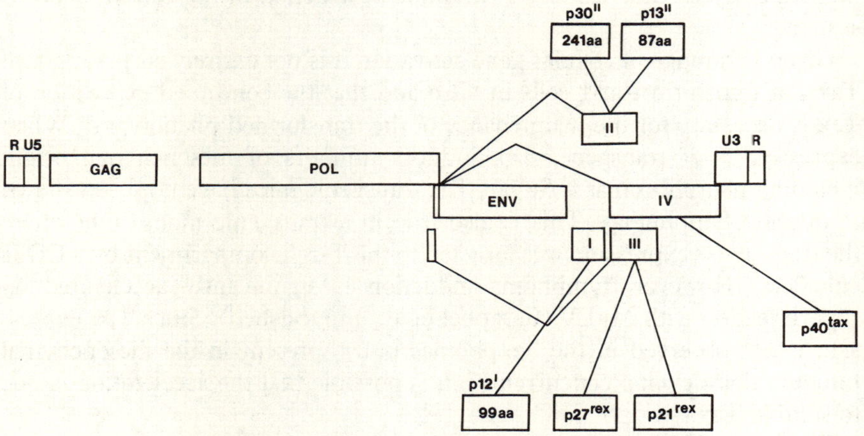

Fig. 7. Open reading frames identified by PCR cDNA analysis of transcripts (references 68,69).

blood mononuclear cells. In man, 7 distinct herpesviruses are recognized, two of which, Epstein–Barr virus and human herpes virus 6, have been associated with lymphomas, although only for the former virus is there, strong evidence for an aetiological association.

Epstein–Barr virus (EBV) like other members of this family is large and structurally complex. The genome consists of 172kb of double stranded DNA enclosed in an icosahedral capsid that in turn is surrounded by an envelope derived from the nuclear membrane. Between the capsid and the envelope is an amorphous layer known as the tegument. The envelope contains predominantly one glycoprotein, the gp350/220, which is a principal target for the neutralizing antibody response.

Infection by Epstein–Barr virus is ubiquitous in populations throughout the world but, in marked contrast to retrovirus infections, the probability of any given individual developing an EBV associated neoplasia is very low. One of the features of EBV is its capacity to infect and immortalize B-cells in vitro, an aspect of its biology which draws attention to its possible role in lymphomagenesis. Originally EBV was isolated from cells derived from a case of Burkitt's lymphoma and it probably plays a role in the aetiology of that condition. Since then it has been implicated in the aetiology of several oncogenic and nononcogenic conditions including, infectious mononucleosis, B-cell lymphomas arising in immunosuppressed individuals, some T-cell lymphomas, nasopharyngeal carcinoma and a subset of Hodgkin's disease.

Transmission and replication

EBV is primarily transmitted through saliva and, since the virus is fragile, oral contact is probably required for transmission. The virus can also be transmitted by blood transfusions and in tissue transplants. The site of replication of the virus and the source of infection for B-cells was thought to be in the epithelium of the oropharynx. Recent data has cast doubt on this since, in bone marrow transplant patients the EBV in the circulation and the oropharynx may be replaced with the donor's virus. Once infected, most individuals continue to shed virus in the saliva for life and they harbour it as a latent infection in circulating B-cells and possibly in other cells within the bone marrow.

The temporal pattern of infection varies in different communities. In lower socio-economic groups infection usually occurs in the first few years of life so that a survey in Ghana indicated that 82% of children were seropositive by 18 months of age. In contrast in some Western populations only 40% of children were found to be seropositive by the age of six.[71,72] Usually infections at this young age are asymptomatic but infection in later life, possibly by large amounts of virus, can result in the onset of infectious mononucleosis.

Two biotypes of EBV are recognized based on variable sequences within the genome. Type-1 has a worldwide distribution and is the predominant virus isolated in Western countries while type-2 has appears to be the commonest type in parts of Africa and new Guinea. The type-2 virus is less efficient at immortalizing B-cells and this could lead to an under-representation of this virus when isolation is used as part of the detection technique. In a PCR survey of persons in Tennessee 22% had EBV DNA sequences detectable in the saliva and of these 50% were type-1, 41% type-2 and 9% of samples contained both types.[73] Within a biotype fine microheterogeneity in the EBNA-2 genes of different strains enables their transmission to be followed. Common strains are often found within family members. In 7 families examined, a total 33 individuals were assayed for EBV strain type: the same strain was found in two members of five families, three members of the sixth and five members of the seventh.[74]

The virus host cell relationship

Immortalization of cells in vitro The receptor for EBV on B-cells is the CD21 molecule[75] but cells not expressing CD21, including lymphoid cells at a stage of differentiation before antigen receptor rearrangement, are also susceptible to infection. T-cells may be infected but the stage at which this occurs and receptor involved are not yet known.

The interaction between the viral envelope glycoprotein gp350/220 and the CD21 receptor activates a resting B-cell to leave the G_o stage and enter G_1 but further progression through the cell cycle requires the expression of non-structural latent viral genes. The latent genes encode six proteins detectable as nuclear antigens EBNAs 1, 2, 3a, 3b and 3c and leader protein (LP) (Fig. 8). A different nomenclature refers to 3b as EBNA 4, leader protein as EBNA 5 and EBNA 3c as EBNA 6. All of these genes are transcribed in the same direction from two promoters either Cp or Wp and

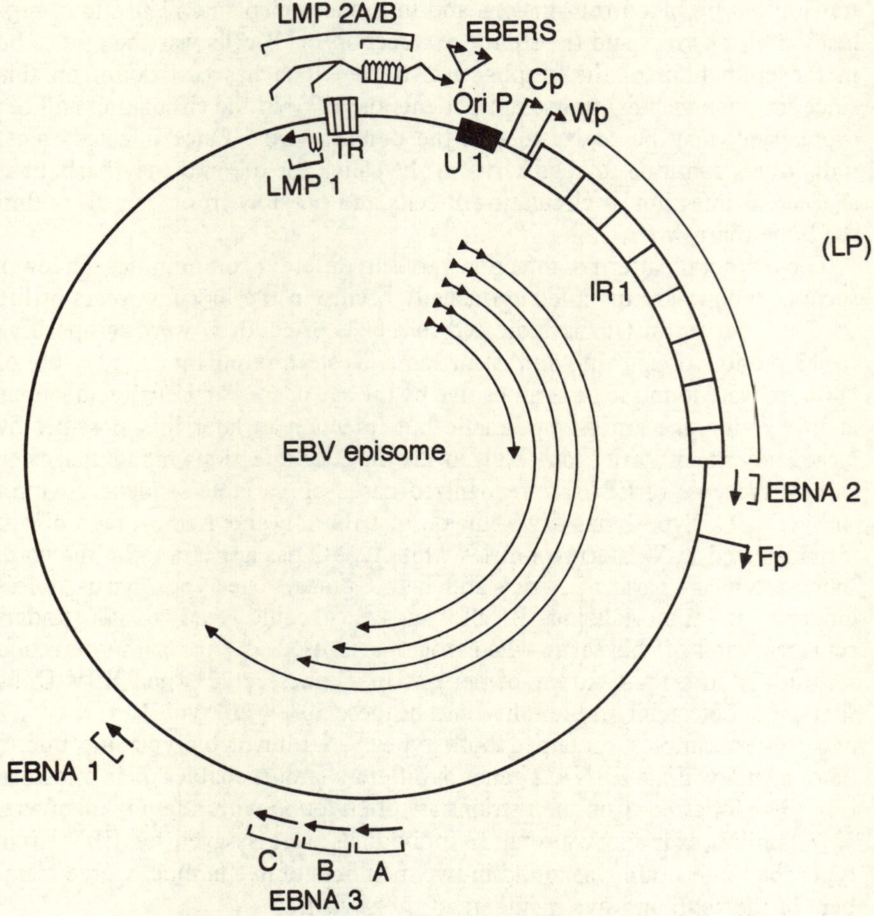

Fig. 8. Structure of EBV episome. Transcripts from Cp and Wp shown internally to the episome. LMP1 transcript shown internally, LMP2a and EBER transcripts shown outside the episome.

the transcripts are differentially spliced to produce the individual messages.[76] Initially after infection the genome is linear but it soon circularizes and during this procedure a variable number of terminal repeats (TR) are generated. Since each infected cell will contain a different number of repeats, it enables the clonality of infection to be determined from the size of the repeat region. The unintegrated viral episome may initially be amplified but eventually replication of the episome proceeds in step with cellular DNA replication and each daughter cell receives the same number of EBV episomes. The maintenance of the EBV as an unintegrated genome in dividing cells is dependent on the expression of EBNA-1 which binds to the *oriP* origin of replication. Once the genome is circularized other latent proteins LMP1, 2a and 2b can be expressed. The products of these genes are membrane spanning proteins. LMP2a is associated with a tyrosine kinase and colocalizes with LMP-1.

EBNA2 is obligatory for transformation of B-cells in vitro and has the property of a transactivator regulating the expression of both viral and cellular genes.[77] One cellular target is the CD23 gene which is upregulated from around 300 copies on uninfected cells to over 10^5 on EBV lymphoblastoid cells. CD23 is shed from the cell surface and after proteolytic cleavage can serve as an autocrine growth factor for B-cells. Recently, new EBV induced molecules have been detected by subtractive hybridization of cDNA libraries. These include two G protein-coupled membrane proteins EBI 1 and EBI 2, that are likely to be receptors for polypeptide cytokines.[79]

LMP-1 is also upregulated by EBNA2 and this protein may be involved in the immortalization process as it is known to be capable of transforming Rat-1 cells in vitro.[80] In turn LMP 1 induces the expression of vimentin, various cellular activation markers and adhesion molecules as well as *bcl-2*. The induction of *bcl-2* may spare infected centroblasts from undergoing apoptosis allowing the virus infected cell to transit towards becoming a long lived circulating B-cell. In lymphoblastoid cell lines all the EBNAs and LMP proteins are expressed as well as a number of cellular activation markers and adhesion molecules, a pattern of infection now referred to as type III latency (Fig. 9). As discussed below, the latent infection within circulating B-cells may involve a much more restricted pattern of gene expression and cells that express the full range of EBNAs may be rapidly eliminated by the immune response.

The immune response to EBV

The humoral response The importance of immune surveillance against EBV infected cells is shown by the high incidence of EBV associated lymphomas that can develop in certain immunosuppressive states. In an infected person the most important component of this surveillance process is cell mediated, while protection from reinfection is probably dependent on the presence of neutralizing antibody to the gp350/220.

The antibody response to a structurally complex virus like EBV involves many structural and nonstructural antigens. These can be divided into a number of functional groups. Early antigens (EA) are regulatory proteins expressed at the start of the replication cycle. The presence of antibody to this complex indicates recent infection or widespread reactivation of virus into the lytic cycle. The majority of latently infected persons do not have detectable antibody to EA while they do have antibody to the virus capsid antigens (VCA). Antibody to the VCA p160 becomes detectable soon after

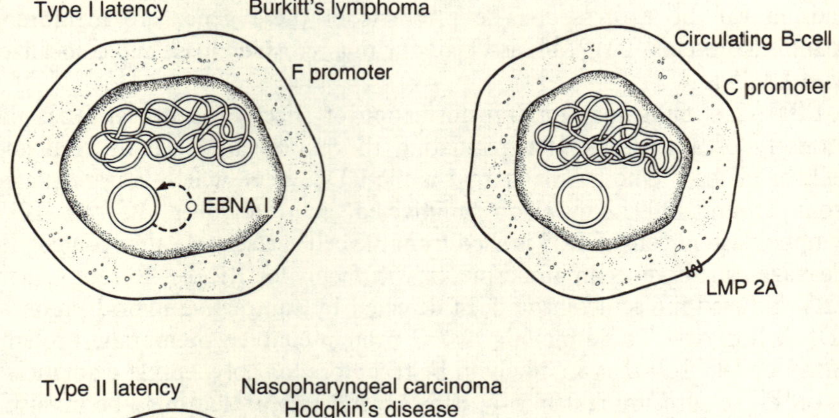

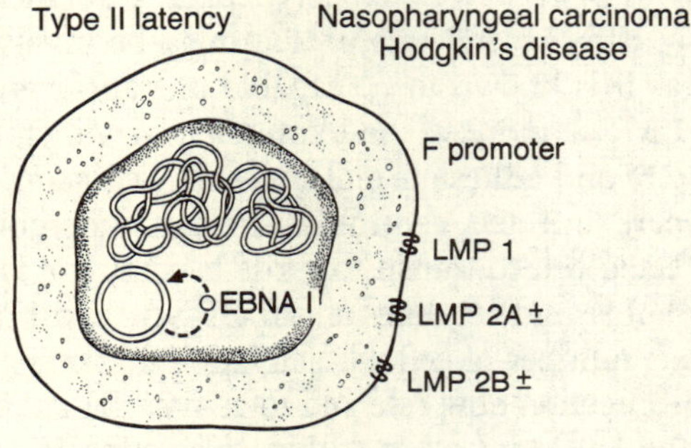

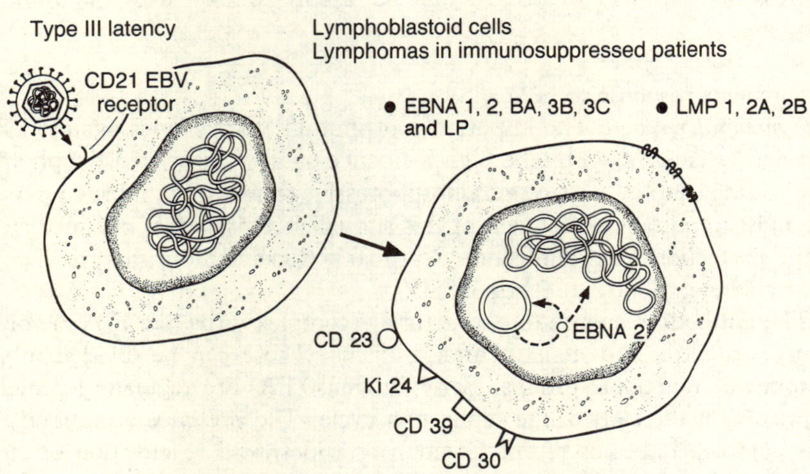

Fig. 9. Patterns of EBV latency. The pattern of gene expression in infected circulating B-cells of clinically normal persons is not fully resolved.

infection and persists for life and can therefore be used as the primary serological marker of infection.

Antibodies to the EBV Nuclear Antigens (EBNAs) are detectable later than VCA antibodies, at about 4 weeks postinfection but like VCA antibodies they persist for life.

The EA antibody response is classically defined by immunofluoresence assays and the immunofluorescence pattern is divided into restricted (R) component in which the antigens are destroyed by methanol fixation and a diffuse (D) pattern which is resistant to this fixative. In childhood infections, the R component is easily observed while in infectious mononucleosis it is the D pattern that predominates.

The proteins responsible for these D and R responses have been partially identified. The D component consists of two transactivating proteins BMRF-1 and BMLF-1.[81,82] Part of the R early antigen response is directed at the BORF2, a protein that may represent the ribonucleotide reductase found in all herpesviruses and BHRF-1, a protein that has homology with the *bcl-2* protooncogene.[83,84]

The cell mediated response Recognition of virus infected cells by cytotoxic T-cells requires the presentation of viral peptides, usually by class I major histocompatibility molecules (MHC). These peptides are derived from viral proteins through degradation by cytoplasmic proteases of the proteasome complex and are then transported to the endoplasmic reticulum by an ATP binding protein. Peptides around 9 amino acids in length and of the right 'fit' may then be bound in the antigen binding groove of the class I molecule. The MHC-I molecule consists of two chains, β-2 microglobulin forming the light chain while the heavy chain is encoded by an allele at one of three loci HLA-A, -B or -C.

The major clinical effects in IM may be related to a vigorous T-cell response to a large EBV challenge. In formative studies carried out by Rickinson and his colleagues this cytotoxic response was shown to involve both an HLA restricted component and non-HLA restricted cytotoxic activity.[85]

In latently infected persons, the frequency of cytotoxic precursor cells appears to be very high, of the order of 1 in 10^{-3} T-cells.[86] The major targets for these cytotoxic T-cells are the EBV latent proteins and most persons respond to several but not all of these. About half of the targets recognized by cytotoxic T-cells are encoded by the EBNA 3 complex whilst, remarkably, no recognition of EBNA 1 has been recorded. For LMP1, HLA-A24, B8, B40 and B51 predominate as presenting molecules whereas for LMP2a only A2.1 appears to be effective at inducing a cytotoxic response. These HLA molecules might be predicted to be protective against the development of EBV associated conditions like Hodgkin's disease, where these proteins are expressed in the absence of most other EBNAs. The dominance of particular epitopes in evoking a response can pose a selection pressure on the virus to produce variants that cannot be effectively presented by particular MHC types. The response to peptide 416 to 424 of EBNA 3b predominates in the cytotoxic response to EBV in Northern Europeans who carry the HLA-A11 allele. About 12% of Northern Europeans express HLA-11 but up to 50% of certain populations in Papua New Guinea are HLA-A11 positive. EBV isolated from Papua New Guinea usually have a lysine to threonine mutation in this epitope so that it does not induce a cytotoxic response when presented by HLA-A11 suggesting that the virus is an escape mutant selected by the immune response.[87] In a wider context, the interaction of the immune response with particular EBNAs may be an important factor governing the EBV disease patterns observed in different populations.

Diseases associations of EBV

Burkitt's lymphoma and type I latency

Although EBV was originally isolated from Burkitt's lymphoma (BL) and there is strong epidemiological evidence for an association between EBV and endemic BL, the role of the virus in the pathogenesis of the disease has been hard to resolve. Burkitt's lymphoma occurs throughout the world but, in areas where malaria is holoendemic, it is the commonest childhood cancer, with annual incidence rates of up to 30 cases per 100 000 persons. EBV infection precedes disease onset and case controlled studies have identified EBV as a risk factor in the development of BL.

Both EBV positive, endemic Burkitt's lymphoma and the sporadic non-EBV associated disease are characterized by a translocation of the c-*myc* gene into an immunoglobulin locus. The most frequently observed pattern is a reciprocal translocation t(8q24, 14q32) between c-*myc* on the long arm of chromosome 8 and the immunoglobulin heavy chain locus on the long arm of chromosome 14. In about 25% of cases other translocations involving *myc* are observed including reciprocal rearrangement with the kappa (2p11) or lambda (22q11) light chain loci. The end result is to subvert the normal transcriptional control of the *myc* gene placing it under the control of immunoglobulin gene enhancers. Within this common theme there are subtle differences in the rearrangements observed between endemic and sporadic BL.[88] In endemic BL the first noncoding exon of *myc* is retained whereas it is usually deleted in the sporadic nonEBV associated form. The first exon of *myc* contains transcriptional regulatory sequences and perhaps the interaction between EBV and this exon favours its retention.

The curious feature of BL is that while the EBV genome is retained as an unintegrated episome it is only expressing EBNA1 which is transcribed from a uniquely spliced message driven by the F promoter.[89] Possibly other viral genes, expressed early in infection, influence the pathogenesis of the disease. A relevant factor may be the ability of EBV infected cells to bypass apopotosis.[90] A potential target for infection, the proliferating centroblasts, are undergoing hypermutation of their immunoglobulin variable genes and their progeny centrocytes will undergo apoptosis unless they are stimulated by a cognate antigen. EBV infected cells can transactivate *bcl*-2 permitting their survival. This process might apply to cells that have already undergone a c-*myc* rearrangement. Concomitant malarial infection promotes a florid B-cell response, heightening the probability of developing a cell containing the a *myc* translocation. Such cells would be susceptible to programmed cell death but EBV infection might rescue them from this fate through transient activation of *bcl*-2.

A further possibility is that EBNA 1 has some direct transforming activity and recent data indicating that a line of EBNA 1 transgenic mice develop lymphomas is of importance (J. Wilson personal communication). If confirmed with further lines it will require a reappraisal of the function of EBNA 1. Whatever the role of EBNA 1, the restricted pattern of gene expression in BL cells may enable them to escape immune surveillance by cytotoxic T-cells.

Until recently it was assumed that the latent pattern of most circulating B-cells would resemble that seen in BL. However matters may be more complex than this. Qu and Rowe have recently analysed the transcripts in infected B-cells from healthy carriers.[91] They always detected transcripts to LMP2a; the C promoter was often active but there was no evidence for the 3' ends of EBNA gene transcripts normally driven by this promoter. It is not clear whether this reflects technical problems or whether novel 3' ends to these transcripts exist. The absence of a functional EBNA 1 transcript might appear surprising but, in a non-dividing cell, EBNA 1 would not be required to maintain EBV as an unintegrated episome.

Lymphomas in immunosuppressed persons

EBV associated lymphomas are a feature of a number of immunosuppressed states whether genetic, iatrogenic or infectious in origin. Patients with X-linked lymphoproliferative syndrome (XPLS) develop either a proliferative disease with lymphoma formation or a degenerative condition characterized by a hypocellular marrow and haemophagocytosis.[92,93] The underlying lesion in XPLS involves a deficient natural killer and cytotoxic T-cell response to EBV but not to other antigens.[94] However, B-cells from XPLS patients are resistant to killing by HLA matched cytotoxic T-cells, suggesting other factors might be important in the escape from surveillance.[95]

In the early days of transplant surgery, the vigorous immunosuppression employed resulted in a significant minority of patients developing EBV associated lymphomas. These tumours usually resemble cells in lymphoblastoid cell lines, expressing all the latent proteins. The persistence of cells with this phenotype is a testament to the capacity of the normal immune response to control EBV infections. Often these tumours have been described as being clonal but usually if cells from different sites are examined a multiclonal pattern is revealed.[96]

Lymphoma development is one of the defining features of AIDS and the lymphomas that develop in HIV infected persons are usually EBV associated extranodal tumours involving the gut or central nervous system. Such tumours usually exhibit a type III latency pattern but BL and EBV negative lymphomas are also observed in AIDS patients. HIV infection is associated with other unusual manifestations of EBV infection. Lymphocytic interstitial pneumonitis (LIP) is a polyclonal condition associated with increased EBV replication and an associated increase in antibodies to replicative antigens but low or undetectable antibody levels to the EBNAs.[97] In another HIV associated condition, hairy oral leukoplakia, there appears to be vigorous replication of EBV in the epithelium of the tongue leading to the development acanthotic lesions.

T-Cell EBV associated lymphomas

Classically EBV infection is associated with B-cells but it is now clear that under certain circumstances, EBV can infect T-cells as has been shown for the CD4+ T-cells in patient with Kawasaki's disease.[98] In EBV associated T-cell disease there is usual evidence for a chronic active EBV infection with high levels of anti-VCA and anti-EA antibody but low levels of anti-EBNA antibody.

EBV genomes have been detected in clonal CD4+ CD8− lymphomas developing some years after a chronic IM like disease[99] and in CD8+ CD4− lymphomas progressing from angioimmunoblastic lymphadenopathy and lethal midline granulomas.[100] In the latter case it has been possible to show that the lymphoma cells expressed LMP and EBNA-2. None of these tumours expressed a CD21 EBV receptor. Whether an alternative viral receptor is used or whether the virus employs a CD21 like molecule expressed during thymic differentiation is open to question.

EBV and Hodgkin's disease

One of the most exciting developments in EBV research has been the establishment of an association between the presence of the virus genome and Hodgkin's disease.[101–103] Hodgkin's disease (HD) poses a particular challenge for determining a viral association because of the rarity of the putative neoplastic cells, the Reed–Sternberg (RS) and Hodgkin cells, within tumours. Nevertheless, using probes to reiterated sequences within the virus it has been possible to detect EBV in HD.[104–108] In contrast EBV is only rarely detected, using the same techniques, in reactive nodes and NHLs of nonimmunosuppressed persons.[106,108] Moreover, several studies have shown that the cells bearing EBV have arisen by clonal expansion of one infected cell and, in one study, clonality was demonstrable in 25 out of 26 cases.[108]

In situ hybridization techniques have localized the EBV infection to the RS cell population and enabled criteria for defining EBV associated Hodgkin's disease cases to be established.[109–111] The most sensitive technique for detecting EBV genomes in RS cells is in situ hybridization for EBER-1, the nonpolyadenylated EBV RNA[111]. Most RS cells also display a surprising pattern of EBV gene expression. The LMP-1 protein is abundantly expressed, perhaps more than in other EBV associated tumours, suggesting that EBV is probably playing some role in the transformation process.[111–113] However, EBNA 2 expression has not been detected; a pattern of latent gene expression resembling that seen in nasopharyngeal carcinoma and now referred to as type II latency. Recent data on the transcription pattern of EBV within Hodgkin's tumours have confirmed this pattern.[114] In summary there is downregulation of the C and W promoters and their associated RNAs while EBNA 1 is expressed from the F promoter. LMP1 and usually LMP2a and 2b transcripts can be detected as well as a novel transcript from the BamHI A fragment also found in nasopharyngeal carcinoma.

One of the features that led to early scepticism of the role of EBV in Hodgkin's disease was that less than half, typically between 33 and 45%, of unselected cases were positive.[111] This situation is reminiscent of early studies of FeLV induced tumours or Burkitt's lymphoma where only a proportion of histologically similar tumours have a viral aetiology. On the basis of epidemiological data MacMahon proposed that the three distinct age groups 0–14 years, 15–34 years and >49 years had distinct aetiological patterns.[115] One of the first studies indicated that there may be an age association between EBV and HD, with the virus predominating in the paediatric and older age groups.[108] This has been confirmed by recent work which show a remarkably high incidence of EBV association in paediatric HD cases.[116] Consequently when examining the frequency of EBV by histological subtype, account must be made of this age association as mixed cellularity cases are more frequently observed in childhood and elderly cases than in the young adult peak. Intriguingly the young adult peak of nodular sclerosing cases observed in Western populations shows evidence of local clustering yet these do not appear to be EBV associated.[117] The exciting possibility is that there is another virus associated with this subtype of HD.

Future prospects

The role of EBV in HD exemplifies the problems in attributing a viral aetiology to a common virus when only a proportion of tumours contain the genome. Tumour induction by a virus is in a sense an accident, an unusual consequence of the replication or latent state of the virus. The associations between a virus and a tumour that have made are those where at least a

63

significant proportion of tumours contain the genome. It is possible that other structurally complex human viruses like herpesviruses and adenoviruses can on occasions transform cells. One such candidate is HHV–6, a ubiquitous virus[118,119] whose genome has been identified in the DNA of Sjogren's associated and other lymphomas.[120,121] Determination of a role for a virus in the aetiology of a disease will be far more difficult if other modes of action exist. For instance the genome might not have to persist in the cells (hit and run models) or a virus could have an indirect effect by perturbing the immune system or haemopoietic stem cell environment.

The association of a virus with a neoplastic disease offers a unique ability to intervene in its development. For HTLV–1 the transmission of the virus can be partially controlled by bottle feeding babies of seropositive mothers. In Burkitt's lymphoma an indirect approach has been possible by instituting malarial control programmes. Clinical trials of prophylactic vaccines for EBV and HTLV–1 will soon be underway. The first vaccines for EBV will be based on inducing a protective response to the viral glycoprotein gp350220[122] while a wider range of targets is being considered for HTLV–1. The rapid developments in the molecular biology of viruses infections opens out the prospect of a new range of therapeutic vaccines and antivirals that will expand the clinical armamentum against these virus-induced cancers.

References

(1) Jarrett O Retroviruses In: Porterfield JS ed. *Andrew's viruses of vertebrates*, London: Baillière Tindall, 1989: 166–213.

(2) Coffin JM Retroviridae and their replication. In: Fields BN ed. *Virology Vol 2*, Raven Press, 1990: 1437–1500.

(3) Gardner MB. Naturally occurring leukaemia viruses in wild mice: how good a model for humans? In: Onions DE, Jarrett O eds. *Cancer surveys Volume 6*, Oxford University Press, 1987: 55–71.

(4) Neil JC, Fulton R, Rigby M, Stewart M. Feline leukaemia virus: generation of pathogenic and oncogenic variants. In: Kung H-J, Vogt PK eds. *Current topics in microbiology and immunology 171, retroviral insertion and oncogene activation*, Springer-Verlag, 1991: 67–93.

(5) Stewart MA, Warnock M, Wheeler A, Wilkie N, Mullins JI, Onions DE, Neil JC. Nucleotide sequence of a feline leukaemia virus subgroup A envelope gene and long terminal repeat and evidence for the recombinational origin of subgroup B viruses. *J Virol* 1986; 58: 825–34.

(6) Li JP, D'Andrea AD, Lodish HF, Baltimore D. Activation of cell growth by binding of Friend spleen-focus-forming virus gp55 to the erythropoietin receptor. *Nature* 1990; 343:762–4.

(7) Onions D, Jarrett O, Testa N, Frassoni F, Toth S. Selective effect of feline leukaemia virus on early erythroid precursors. *Nature* 1982; 296: 156–8.

(8) Larrson, E, Kato N, Cohen M. Human endogenous proviruses. *Curr Top Microbiol Immunol* 1989; 148: 115–32.

(9) Kung H-J, Vogt PK. eds. *Current topics in microbiology and immunology 171. retroviral insertion and oncogene activation*, Springer-Verlag, 1991.

(10) Hosie MJ, Robertson C, Jarrett O. Prevalance of feline leukaemia virus and antibodies to feline immunodeficiency virus in cats in the United Kingdom. *Vet Rec*. 198; 128: 293–7.

(11) Hoover EA, Olsen RG, Hardy WD Jr et al. Feline leukemia virus infection: age related variation in response of cats to experimental infection. *J Natl Cancer Inst* 1976; 57: 365–9.

(12) Hardy WD Jr, Hess PW, MacEwen EG et al. Biology of feline leukaemia virus in the natural environment. *Cancer Res* 1976; 36: 582–8.

(13) Bishop JM, Varmus H. Functions and origins of retroviral transforming genes. In: Weiss R, Teich N, Varmus H, CoffinJ eds. *RNA tumor viruses*. Cold Spring Harbor, 1982: 999–1108.

(14) Neil JC, Hughes R, McFarlane R et al. Transduction and rearrangenment of the *myc* gene by feline leukaemia virus in naturally occurring T cell leukaemias. *Nature* 1983; 208: 814–20.

(15) Shen-Ong GLC, Morse HC III, Potter M, Mushinsky F. Two modes of c-*myb* activation in virus induced mouse myeloid tumours. *Mol Cell Biol* 1986; 6; 380–92.

(16) Shaw G, Kamen R. A conserved AU sequence from the 3′ untranslated region of GM-CSFmRNA mediates selective mRNA degradation. *Cell* 1986; 46: 659–67.

(17) Onions D, Lees G, Forrest D, Neil J. Recombinant viruses containing the myc gene rapidly produce clonal tumours expressing T-cell antigen gene transcripts. *Int J Cancer* 1987; 40: 40–5

(18) Tsujimoto H, Fulton R, Nishigaki K et al. A common proviral integration site *fit*-1 in T-cell tumours induced by *myc* containing feline leukaemia virus. *Virology* 1993; in press.

(19) Fulton R, Forrest D, Mcfarlane R, Onions D, Neil JC. Retroviral transduction of T-cell antigen receptor -chain and *myc* genes. *Nature* 1987; 326: 190–4.

(20) Adams JM, Harris AW, Pinkert LM et al. The c-*myc* oncogene driven by immunoglobulin enhancers induces lymphoid malignancy in transgenic mice. *Nature* 1985; 318: 533–8.

(21) Berns A, Breuer M, Verbeek S, van Lohuizen M. Transgenic mice as a means to study synergism between oncogenes. *Int J Cancer* 1989; 54: 22–5.

(22) Stewart M, Cameron E, Campbell M et al. Conditional expression and oncogenicity of c-*myc* linked to a CD2 dominant control region. *Int J Cancer* 1993; 53: 1023–30.

(23) Poiesz BJ, Ruscetti FW, Gazdar AF et al. Detection and isolation of type-C retrovirus particles from fresh and cultured lymphocytes of patients with cutaneous T-cell lymphoma. *Proc Natl Acad Sci USA* 1980; 77: 7415–9. 30: 780–6.

(24) Takkatsuki K, Uchiyama T, Ueshima y et al. Adult T-cell leukaemia: further clinical observations and cytogenetic and functional studies of leukaemic cells. *Jpn J Clin Oncol* 1979; 9 (suppl): 317–24.

(25) Catovsky D, Rosa M, Goolden AWG et al. Adult T-cell leukaemia in blacks from the West Indies. *Lancet* 1982; i: 639–43.

(26) The T- and B-Cell Malignancy Study Group. Statistical analyses of clinopathological, virological and epidemiological data on lymphoid cell

leukaemia/lymphoma: a report on the second nationwide study of Japan. *Am J Clin Oncol* 1985; 15: 635–9.

(27) Yamaguchi K, Nishimura H, Kohrogi H et al. A proposal for smouldering adult T-cell leukaemia: a clinicopathological study of five cases. *Blood* 1983; 62: 758–66.

(28) Gessain A, Barin F, Vernant J et al. Antibodies to human lymphotropic virus type I in patients with tropical spastic paraparesis. *Lancet* 1985; ii: 407–9.

(29) Sugimoto MM. Pathogenesis of T-lymphocyte alveolits associated with HTLV-1 infection. *Nippon-Kyobu-Shikkan-Gakkai-Zasshi* 1992; 30: 780–6

(30) Lee H, Swandon P, Shorty RS et al. High rate of HTLV-II infection in seropositive i.v. drug abusers in New Orleans. *Science* 1989; 244: 471–5.

(31) Gout O, Baulac M, Gessain A et al. Rapid development of myelopathy after HTLV-I infection aquired during cardiac transplantation. *N Engl J Med* 1990; 322: 383–8.

(32) Banki K, Maceda J, Hurley E et. al. Human T-cell lymphotropic virus (HTLV)-related endogenous sequence, HRES-1 encodes a 28-kDa protein; a possible autoantigen for HTLV-1 *gag*-reactive autoantibodies. *Proc Natl Acad Sci USA* 1992; 89: 1939–43

(33) Starkebaum G, Loughran VS, Kalyanaraman VS et al. Serum reactivity to human T-cell leukemia/lymphoma virus type I in patients with large granular lymphocytic leukemia. *Lancet* 1987; i; 596–9.

(34) Sherman MP, Saksena NK, Dube DK, Yanagihara R, Poiesz BJ. Evolutionary insights on the origin of human T-cell lymphoma/leukaemia virus type i (HTLV-I) derived from sequence analysis of new HTLV-I variant from Papua New Guinea. *J Virol* 1992; 66: 2556–63.

(35) Cark JW, Saxinger C, Sibbs WN et al. seroepidemiological studies of human T-cell leukaemia/lymphoma virus type 1 in Jamaica. *Int J Cancer* 1985; 36: 37–41.

(36) Hinuma Y, Komada H, Chosa T et al. Antibodies to adult T-cell leukaemia virus antigen (ATLA) in sera from patients with ATL and controls in Japan. A nationwide seroepidemiological study. *Int J Cancer* 1982; 29: 631–5.

(37) Blattner WA, Nomura A, Clark JN et al. Modes of transmission and evidence for viral latency from studies of HTLV-1 in Japanese migrant populations in Hawaii. *Proc Natl Acad Sci USA* 1966; 83: 4895–8.

(38) Kajiyama W, Kashiwagi S, Ikematsa H et al. Intrafamilial transmission of adult T-cell leukaemia virus. *J Infec Dis* 1986; 154: 851–7.

(39) Maehama T, Nakayama M, Nagamine M, Nakashima Y, Takei H, Nakachi H. Studies on factor affecting mother-to-child HTLV-I transmission *Nippon-Kyobu-Shikkan-Gakkai-Zasshi* 1992; 44: 215–22.

(40) Williams AE, Fang CY, Slamon DJ. Seroprevalence and and epidemiological correlates in of HTLV-I infection in American blood donors. *Science* 1988; 240: 643–6.

(41) Hinuma Y. Seroepidemiology of adult T-cell leukaemia virus (HTLV-1/ATLV): origin of virus carriers in Japan. *AIDS Res* 1986; 2: 517–22

(42) Ishida T, Hinuma Y. The origin of Japanese HTLV-I. *Nature* 1986; 322: 504.

(43) Gallo RC, Sliski A, Wong-Staal F. Origin of human T-cell leukaemia-lymphoma virus. *Lancet* 1983; ii: 962–3.

(44) Gessain A, Gllo RC, Franchini G. Low degree of human T-cell leukaemia-lymphoma virus type I genetic drift in vivo as a means of monitoring viral transmission and movement of ancient human populations. *J Virol* 1992; 66: 2288–95.

(45) Komurian-Pradel F, Pelloquin F, Sonada S, Osame M, de Thé G. Geographical subtypes defined by RFLP following PCR in the LTR region of HTLV-1. *AIDS Res Hum Retroviruses* 1992; 8: 527–32.

(46) Gledhill S. The involvement of viruses in the aetiology of human leukaemias and lymphomas. [Ph.D dissertation] The University of Glasgow. 1991.

(47) Anon. Human T-lymphotropic type II among Guaymi Indians, Panama. *Morbidity Mortality Weekly Rep* 1992; 41: 209–11.

(48) Yoshida M, Inoue J-I, Fujisawa J-I et al. *Trans*-regulation of HTLV-gene expression. In: Franza N, Cullen BR, Wong-Staal F, eds. *The control of human retro virus gene expression*. Cold Spring Harbor, 1988: 251–3.

(49) Nagashima KL, Yoshida M, Seiki M. A single species of pX mRNA of human T-cell leukaemia virus type 1 encodes transactivator p40^x and two other phosphoproteins. *J Virol* 1986; 60: 394.

(50) Brady J, Jeang K-T, Duvall J. Khoury G. Identification of p40x-responsive regulatory sequences within the human T-cell leukaemia virus type I long terminal repeat. *J Virol* 1987; 61: 2175–81.

(51) Yoshimura T, Fujisawa J-I, Yoshida M. Multiple cDNA clones encoding nuclear proteins that bind to the tax dependent enhancer of HTLV-1: all contain a leucine zipper structure and basic amino acid domain. *EMBO J* 1990; 9: 2537–42.

(52) Tsujimoto A, Nyunoya H, Morita T, Sato T, Shimotohno K. Isolation of cDNAs for DNA-binding proteins which specifically bind to a *tax*-responsive enhancer element in the long terminal repeat of human T-cell leukaemia virus type I. *J Virol* 1991; 65; 1420–6.

(53) Beraud C, Lombard-Platet G, Michal Y, Jalinot P. Binding of the HTLV-I Tax$_1$ transactivator to the inducible 21bp enhancer is mediated by the cellular factor HEB1. *EMBO J* 1991; 10: 3795–3803.

(54) Marriott SJ, Lindholm PF, Brown KM et al. A 36-kilodalton transcription factor mediates an indirect interaction of human T-cell leukaemia virus type I tax$_1$ with a response element in the long terminal repeat. *Mol Cell Biol* 1990; 10: 4192–201.

(55) Siomi H, Shidu H, Nam SH et al. Sequence requirements for nuclear localization of human T-cell leukaemia virus type 1 px protein which regulates viral RNA processing. *Cell* 1988; 55; 197–209.

(56) Ahmed YF, Gilmartin GM, Hanly SM et al. The HTLV-1 *rex* response element mediates a novel form of mRNA processing. *Cell* 1991; 54: 727–737.

(59) Leung K, Nabel GJ. HTLV-1 transactivator induces interleukin-2 receptor expression through an NF-kB like factor. *Nature* 1988; 333: 776–8.

(60) Lindholm F, Kashanchi F, Brady JN. Transcriptional regulation in the human retrovirus HTLV-1. *Seminars Virol* 1993; 4: 53–60.

(61) Marriott SJ, Lindholm PF, Reid RL, Brady JN. Soluble HTLV-1 Tax 1 protein stimulates proliferation of human peripheral blood lymphocytes. *New Biol* 1991; 3: 678–86.

(62) Wucherpfennig KW, Hollsberg P, Richardson JH, Benjamin D, Hafler DA. T-cell activation by autologous human T-cell leukaemia virus type I-infected T-cell clones. *Proc Natl Acad Sci USA* 1992: 89: 2110–4.

(63) Gessain A, Saal F, Gout O. High human T-cell lymphotropic virus type 1 proviral DNA load with polyclonal integration in peripheral blood mononuclear cells of French, West Indian, Guianese and African patients with tropical spastic paraparesis. *Blood* 1990; 75: 428–33

(64) Gessain A, Louie A, Gout O et al. Human T-cell leukaemia-lymphoma virus type 1 (HTLV-1) expression in fresh peripheral blood mononuclear cells from patients with tropical spastic paraparesis /HTLV-1 associated myelopathy. *J Virol* 1991; 65: 1628–33.

(65) Tendler CL, Greenberg SJ, Burton JD et al. Cytokine induction in HTLV-1 associated myelopathy and adult T-cell leukaemia: alternate molecular mechanisms underlying pathogenesis. *J Cell Biochem* 1991; 46: 302–11.

(66) Yamaoka S, Tobe T, Hatanaka M. Tax protein of T-cell leukaemia virus type-I is required for maintenance of the transformed phenotype. *Oncogene* 1992; 7: 433–7.

(67) Nernberg M, Hinrisch SH, Reynolds RK, Khoury G, Jay G. The *tat* gene of human T-lymphotropic type 1 induces mesenchymal tumors in transgenic mice. *Science* 1987; 237: 1324–1329.

(68) Korainik IJ, Gessain A, Klotman ME, Monico AL, Berneman ZN, Franchini G. Protein isoforms encoded by the *pX* region of human T-cell leukaemia/lymphotropic virus type I. *Proc Natl Acad Sci USA* 1992; 89: 8813–7.

(69) Ciminale V, Pavlakis GN, Derse D, Cunningham CP, Felber B. Complex splicing in the human T-cell leukaemia virus (HTLV) family of retroviruses: novel mRNAs and proteins produced by HTLV type I. *J Virol* 1992; 66: 1737–45.

(70) Goldstein DJ, Andresson T, Sparkowski J, Schlegel R. The BPV protein, the 16 kDa membrane pore forming protein and the PDGF receptor exist in a complex that is dependent on hydrophobic transmembrane interactions. *EMBO J* 1992; 13: 4851–9.

(71) Biggar R, Henle W, Fleisher G et al. Primary Epstein–Barr virus infection in African infants. Decline of maternal antibodies and time of infection. *Int J Cancer* 1978; 22: 239–43.

(72) Evans AS. The transmission of EB viral infections. In: Hooks J, Jordan G eds. *Viral infections in oral medicine*. New York, Elsevier North Holland 1982: 211–25.

(73) Sixeby JW, Shirley P, Chesney PJ et al. Detection of a second widespread strain of Epstein–Barr virus. *Lancet* 1989; ii: 761–5.

(74) Gratma JW, Oosterveer MAP, Klein G et al. EBNA size polymorphisms can be used to trace Epstein–Barr virus spread within families. *J Virol* 1990; 64: 4703–8.

(75) Fingeroth JD, Weiss JJ, Tedder TF et al. Epstein–Barr virus receptor of human B-lymphocytes in the C3d receptor CR2. *Proc Natl Acad Sci USA* 1984; 81: 4510–6.

(76) Speck SH, Strominger JL. Transcription of Epstein–Barr virus in latently infected, growth-transformed lymphocytes. *Adv Viral Oncol* 1989; 8: 133.

(77) Knutson JC, Sugden B. In: Klein G ed. *Advances in viral oncology vol 8*. 1989; New York, 1989: Raven Press 151–72.

(78) Rabson M, Gradoville L, Heston L et al. Non-immortalizing P3J-HR-1 Epstein–Barr virus: a deletion mutant of its transforming parent. *J Virol* 1982; 44: 834–44.

(79) Birkenbach M, Josefsen K, Yalamanchili R, Lenoir G, Kieff E. Epstein–Barr virus-induced genes: first lymphocyte-specific G protein-coupled peptide receptors. *J Virol* 1993; 67: 2209–20.

(80) Wang D, Liebowitz D, Kiett E. An EBV membrane protein expressed in immortalized lymphocytes transforms established rodent cells. *Cell* 1985; 43: 831–40.

(81) Liebermann PM, O'hare P Hayward GS et al. Promiscuous transactivation of gene expression by an Epstein–Barr virus encoded early protein. *J Virol* 1986; 60: 140–8.

(82) Wong K-M, Levine AJ. Identification and mapping of Epstein–Barr virus early antigens and demonstration of a viral gene activater that functions in *trans*. *J Virol* 1986.; 58: 748–56.

(83) Luka J, Miller G, Jornvall H *et al*. Characterisation of the restricted component of Epstein–Barr virus early antigens as a cytoplasmic filamentous protein. *J Virol* 1986; 58: 748–56.

(84) Pearson GR, Luka J, Petti L et al. Identification of an Epstei–Barr virus early gene encoding a second component of the restricted early antigen complex. *Virology* 1987; 160: 151–61.

(85) Straing G, Rickinson AB. Multiple HLA class-I dependent cytotoxicities constitute the non-HLA restricted response in infectious mononucleosis. *Eur J Immunol* 1987; 17: 1007–13.

(86) Rickinson AB, Moss DJ, Wallace LE et al. Long term T cell-mediated immunity to Epstein–Barr virus. *Cancer Res* 1981; 41: 4216–21.

(87) De Campos-Lima P-O, Gavioli R, Zhang Q-J et al. HLA-A11 epitope loss isolates of Epstein–Barr virus from a highly A11+population. *Science* 1993; 260: 98–100.

(88) Pelicci PG, Knowles DM, Magrath I et al. Chromosomal breakpoint and structural alternative of the *c-myc* locus differ in endemic and sporadic forms of Burkitt's lymphoma. *Proc Natl Acad Sci USA* 1986; 83: 2986–8.

(89) Schaffer BC, Woisetschlaeger M, Strominger JL, Speck SH. Exclusive expression of Epstein–Barr virus nuclear antigen 1 in Burkitt lymphoma arises from a third promoter, distinct from the promoters used in latently infected lymphocytes. *Proc Natl Acad Sci USA* 1991; 88: 6650–4.

(90) Gregory CD, Dive C, Henderson S et al. Activation of Epstein–Barr virus latent genes protects human B-cells from death by apoptosis. *Nature* 1991; 349: 612–4.

(91) Qu I, Rowe DT. Epstein–Barr virus latent gene expression in uncultured peripheral blood lymphocytes. *J Virol* 1992; 66: 3715–24.

(92) Purtilo DT, De Florio D, Hutt LM et al. Variable phenotypic expression of an X-linked recessive lymphoproliferative syndrome. *N Engl J Med* 1977; 297 1077–81.

(93) Mroczek EC, Weisenburger DD, Grierson HL et al. Fatal infectious

mononucleosis and virus associated haemophagocytic syndrome. *Arch Pathol Lab Med* 1987; 111:530–5.

(94) Argov S, Johnson DR, Collins M et al. Defective natural killing activity but retention of lymphocyte-mediated antibody-dependent cellular cytotoxicity in patients with x-linked lymphoprolifertive syndrome. *Cell Immunol* 1986; 100: 1–9.

(95) Ando I, Morgan G, Levinsky RJ et al. A family study of the X-linked lymphoprolifertive syndrome: evidence for a B-cell defect contributing to the immunodeficiency. *Clin Exp Immunol* 1986; 63: 271–9.

(96) Cleary ML, Nalesnik MA, Shearer WT et al. *Clonal origins of lymphoproliferative disease induced by Epstein–Barr virus. Blood* 1988; 72: 349–2.

(97) Andiman WA, Eastman R, Martin K. Opportunistic lymphoproliferation associated with Epstein–Barr viral DNA in infants and children with AIDS. *Lancet* 1985; ii: 1390–3.

(98) Kikuta H, Taguchi Y, Tomizawa k et al. Epstein–Barr virus genome positive T-lymphocytes with chronic active EBV infection associated with Kawasaki-like disease. *Nature* 1988; 333: 455–7.

(99) Jones JF, Shurin S, Abramowsky C et al. T-cell lymphomas containing Epstein–Barr viral DNA in patients with chronic Epstein–Barr virus infection. *N Engl J Med* 1998; 318: 733–40.

(100) Harabuchi Y, Yamanaka N, Akikatsu K et al. Epstein–Barr virus in nasal T-cell lymphomas in patients with lethal midline granuloma. *Lancet* 1990; i: 128–30.

(101) Jarrett R, Onions D. Viruses and Hodgkin's disease. *Leukaemia* 1992; 6 Suppl. 1: 14–7.

(102) Jarrett RF. Viral involvement in Hodgkin's disease. *Int J Cell Cloning.* 1992 10: 315–22.

(103) Herbst, H Pallensen G, Weiss LM et al. *Ann Oncol* 1992; 3 Suppl. 4: 27–30.

(104) Weiss LM, Movahede LA, Warnke RA, Sklar J. Detection of Epstein–Barr virus genomes in Reed–Sternberg cells of Hodgkin's disease. *N Engl J Med* 1989; 320: 502–6.

(105) Anagnostopoulos I, Herbst H, Niedobitek G, Stein H. Demonstration of monoclonal EBV genomes in in Hodgkin's disease and Ki-1 positive anaplastic large cell lymphoma by combined Southern blot and in situ hybridisation. *Blood* 1989; 74; 810–6.

(106) Staal SP, Ambinder R, Beschorner WE, Hayward GS, Mann R. A survey of Epstein-Barr virus DNA in lymphoid tissue. Frequent detection in Hodgkin's disease. *Am J Clin Pathol.* 189; 91: 1–5.

(107) Gledhill S, Gallagher A, Jones D et al. Viral involvement in Hodgkin's disease: detection of clonal A genomes in tumour samples. *Br J Cancer* 1991; 64: 227–32.

(108) Jarrett RF, Gallagher A, Jones DB et al. Detection of EBV genomes in Hodgkin's disease: association with age. *J Clin Pathol* 1991; 44: 844–8.

(109) Weiss LM, Chen Y-Y, Liu X-F, Shibata D. A correlative in situ hybridization and polymerase reaction study. *Am J Pathol* 1991; 139: 1259–65.

(110) Wu T, Mann RB, Charache P et al. Detection of EBV gene expression in Reed-Sternberg cells of Hodgkin's disease. *Int J Cancer* 1990; 46: 801–4.

(111) Armstrong AA, Weiss LM, Gallagher A et al. Criteria for the definition of Epstein–Barr virus association in Hodgkin's disease. *Leukaemia* 1992; 6: 869–74.

(112) Pallensen G, Hamilton-Dutoit SJ, Rowe M, Young LS. Expression of Epstein–Barr virus latent gene products in tumour cells of Hodgkin's disease. *Lancet* 1991; 64: 227–32.

(113) Herbst H, Dallenbach F, Hummel M et al. Epstein–Barr virus latent membrane protein expression in Hodgkin and Reed–Sternberg cells. *Proc Natl Acad Sci USA* 1991; 88: 4766–70.

(114) Deacon EM, Pallensen G, Niedobitek G et al. Epstein–Barr virus and Hodgkin's disease: transcriptional analysis of virus latency in the malignant cell. *J Exp Med* 1993; 177: 339–49.

(115) MacMahon B. Epidemiology of Hodgkin's disease. *Cancer Res* 1966; 26: 1189–200.

(116) Armstrong AA, Alexander FE, Pinto Paes R et al. Association of Epstein–Barr virus with paediatric Hodgkin's disease. *Am J Pathol* 1993 (in press).

(117) Alexander FE, McKinney PA, Williams J et al. Epidemiological evidence for the 'two disease hypothesis' in Hodgkin's disease. *Int J Epidemiol* 1991; 202: 354–61.

(118) Jarrett RF, Clark DA, Josephs SF, Onions DE. Detection of human herpesvirus-6 DNA in peripheral blood and saliva. *J Med Virol* 1990; 32: 73–6.

(119) Levine PH, Jarrett R, Clark DA. The epidemiology of human herpesvirus-6. In: Ablashi, Krueger, Salahuddin, eds. *Human Herpesvirus-6*. Elsevier Science, 1992: 9–23.

(120) Jarrett RF, Gledhill S, Qureshi F et al. Identification of human herpesvirus-6 specific DNA sequences in two patients with non-Hodgkin's lymphoma. *Leukaemia* 1988; 2: 496–502.

(121) Josephs SF, Buchbinder A, streicher HZ. Detection of human B-lymphotropic virus (human herpesvirus-6) sequences in B-cell lymphoma tissues of three patients. *Leukaemia* 1988; 2: 132–5.

(122) Morgan AJ, Finerty S, Lovgren K et al. Prevention of Epstein-Barr virus-induced lymphoma in cottontop tamarins by vaccination with EB virus envelope glycoprotein gp340 incorporated into immune stimulating complexes. *J Gen Virol* 1988; 69: 2093–6.

The bone marrow stromal microenvironment

M Y GORDON

Introduction

Bone marrow stroma is the tissue that supports haemopoiesis in vivo and is reproduced in the long-term bone marrow culture system in vitro. In vivo, it is not a morphologically predominant component of the marrow because the spaces between the stromal cells are packed with haemopoietic cells. In vitro, it can be cultured as a major cellular component and forms a complex layer of different cell types which can be studied in detail. These studies have shown that the stroma and the extracellular matrix it produces can support haemopoietic stem cell activity, organize spatial relationships with haemopoietic cells via adhesive interactions, regulate the access of haemopoietic growth factors to their target cells and modulate cell function. In the near future we can expect to learn more about the ways in which stromal cells and their associated extracellular matrix direct gene expression by haemopoietic cells. The stroma appears to be capable of physiological and pathophysiological responses to haemopoietic requirements and abnormalities, but little is known about this level of haemopoietic cell regulation.

Composition of the stromal microenvironment

The cellular component of the haemopoietic stromal microenvironment consists of fibroblasts, adipocytes, reticular adventitial cells and macrophages. In vivo, the sinus endothelium forms a barrier between the marrow microenvironment and the peripheral circulation. There is no satisfactory classification of the stromal cells that grow in long-term cultures in vitro and they have been defined mostly on morphological grounds. The stromal cells produce a complex extracellular matrix consisting of collagen, fibronectin and proteoglycans.[1,2]

All correspondence to: Dr MY Gordon, Leukaemia Research Fund Centre, Institute of Cancer Research, 237 Fulham Road, London SW3 6JB, UK.

Cambridge Medical Reviews: Haematological Oncology Volume 3
Cambridge University Press 1994

In long-term cultures, human stromal layers consisting of a heterogeneous mixture of cells, including flat angular cells, fat cells, fibroblastoid spindle shaped cells, endothelial cells and macrophages, have been described. The haemopoietic functions of the different cell types are not well defined and the derivation of the different cellular elements has not been completely resolved. Stromal layers have been grown from mononuclear cells and from CD34-positive cell fractions.[3] The macrophage component is ultimately derived from the pluripotent haemopoietic stem cell.

Charbord et al[4] used two monoclonal antibodies to characterize stromal cells in human long-term marrow cultures. These antibodies, which stain smooth muscle actin, reacted strongly with most of the flat and spindle-shaped cells in the stromal layer, indicating that the fibroblastoid cells in long-term cultures are a unique population. Simmons and Torok-Storb[5] studied an antibody called STRO-1 which reacts with stromal elements in vivo and in vitro but which does not react with haemopoietic progenitor cells. Cells expressing the STRO-1 antigen can form fibroblast colonies in the CFU-F assay and can generate fibroblasts, smooth muscle actin-containing cells and adipocytes but not macrophages or endothelial cells. These stromal layers grew for an extended period and, in terms of haemopoietic support function, appeared to be superior to stromal layers grown from unseparated marrow cells. These observations indicate that STRO-1 positive cells comprise a lineage distinct from endothelial cells and macrophages and that an absence of endothelial cells and macrophages might improve haemopoiesis in association with cultured stromal layers. Hasthorpe et al[6] identified large thin cells, overlying macrophages in murine long-term cultures, as endothelial cells using a monoclonal antibody H51E3 and equated them with the 'blanket' cells that had previously been described. The cells contain rough endoplasmic reticulum and active Golgi apparatus indicative of protein synthesis and display gap junctions with macrophages and microvilli indicative of cell–cell interactions. An antibody, KM16, is a marker of stromal cells restricted to areas of interaction with lymphoid cells suggesting that it identifies a microenvironment for B lymphopoiesis.[7]

Extracellular matrix

The extracellular matrix produced by the stromal cells in long-term cultures is a complex mixture of proteins and glycoproteins, including collagen, fibronectin, laminin and proteoglycans. Collagenous proteins are major components of all extracellular matrices and, in vertebrates, at least 15 types of collagen occur with unique tissue-specific patterns.[8] Type I and to a lesser extent type III collagens are produced by fibroblasts in long-term marrow cultures whilst type IV collagen, a product of endothelial cells, has sometimes been found.[2]

Fibronectin is a well-characterized protein found in a variety of extracellular matrices that can exist in a number of forms as a result of alternative splicing of mRNA transcribed from a single gene.[9] Each fibronectin polypeptide chain consists of a series of structural and functional domains. Each contains at least 6 peptide sites capable of mediating cell adhesion and a heparin-binding domain. The best known cell binding sequence is 'RGD' (Arg – Gly – Asp) which provides the attachment motif for the integrin class of cell adhesion molecules. Fibronectin is universally present in long-term cultures and can bind cells, growth factors and other components of the ECM.

The presence of laminin is an indicator of the presence of endothelial cells and it has been found in long-term cultures. Laminin can contain several subunits linked together to form a molecule of up to 10^6 Daltons.[9] The best known isoform of laminin is a cross-shaped molecule with three short arms and one long arm. Laminin provides binding sites for cells, heparin and collagen and cell proliferation by EGF receptor-expressing cells can be stimulated using laminin fragments with EGF-like repeats. It is possible, therefore, that laminin degradation could release growth factor activity.

The proteoglycans (PGs) are complex macromolecules consisting of a protein core to which glycosaminoglycan (GAG) side chains are attached. Some of the protein cores have now been cloned and shown to be complex structures with adhesion molecule, receptor and growth factor-like domains amongst others. The GAG side chains are linear polymers of repeating dissacharides that can present a wide variety of structures. According to the conformation of the GAG side chains, the proteoglycans are classified as heparan sulphate, keratan sulphate, dermatan sulphate and chondroitin sulphate. Hyaluronic acid is also a GAG but does not exist bound to a protein core.[10]

The production of proteoglycans by stromal cells in vivo is difficult to study but chondroitin sulphate has been demonstrated in rabbit bone marrow. Also, studies in starving humans led to the idea that accumulation of proteoglycans suppresses haemopoiesis. Wight and coworkers[11] characterized proteoglycans in the cell layer and medium of human long-term marrow cultures. They detected substantial amounts of chondroitin sulphate and hyaluronic acid but heparan sulphate amounted to only about 10% of the total proteoglycan. The heparan sulphate in human bone marrow stromal cultures has been studied by Morris et al[12] who showed that the molecular structure of the GAG depended on the stromal culture conditions. Heparan sulphate from stroma grown with methylprednisolone (MP+) was more highly sulphated, and therefore had a greater negative charge, than heparan sulphate from stroma grown without methylprednisolone (MP−). Similar findings were made by Siczkowski et al[13] who showed, in addition, that multiple heparan sulphate proteoglycans could be resolved by gel electrophoresis and that more bands were resolved from MP+ cultures than from MP− cultures.

Regulation of haemopoiesis by the stromal microenvironment
Cells
Haemopoiesis in long-term cultures is sustained by the adherent stromal layer and weekly feeding with medium containing serum and glucocorticoid: no exo-

genous growth factors are added. This implies that the necessary growth factors are provided by the stromal cells but it has been difficult to demonstrate the production of biologically relevant quantities by adherent stromal layers. There are several possible explanations for this finding: (a) haemopoiesis in long-term cultures is stimulated by molecules that have not yet been discovered; (b) molecules that are individually present in biologically undetectable amounts interact synergistically to stimulate haemopoiesis; (c) haemopoietic progenitor cells in the context of a stromal microevironment and those in semi-solid cultures respond differently to haemopoietic growth factors; or (d) stimulatory molecules are highly concentrated locally by the extracellular matrix or expressed as stromal cell surface molecules (see below).

Studies have shown that haemopoietic activity in long-term cultures reflects a balance between stimulatory and inhibitory molecules and that this balance is a function of the feeding cycle. Thus, Cashman et al[14] demonstrated that the re-entry of primitive progenitors into cycle after feeding could be elicited by PDGF, IL-1, IL-2 and TGFα and blocked by TGFβ. Toksoz et al[15] showed that medium from long-term cultures contained a stimulatory factor, capable of stimulating murine stem cells (CFU-S) into cycle, for the first few days after feeding but that this factor was not present when the cultures were next due to be fed.

The stromal layers that grow in long-term cultures are heterogeneous in terms of cellular constitution and it is difficult to discern which cell types are important for haemopoietic support capacity. This question has been addressed by selectively culturing different stromal cell populations and by cloning permanent lines of stromal cells.

Alteration of the culture conditions used to grow stromal layers has shown that their function as a haemopoietic support can also be changed. Thus, cultures grown without glucocorticoid but with 2-mercaptoethanol and fetal calf serum, support B cell differentiation.[16] Adherent layers grown in the absence of glucocorticoid consist of homogeneous fibroblastoid cells which stimulate colony formation by CFU-GM but totally inhibit colony formation by BFU-E and CFU-GEMM. Neither of these effects are exerted by heterogeneous layers grown in the presence of glucocorticoid.[17] Endothelial cells, obtained from human umbilical cord, stimulated CFU-GM but did not influence BFU-E or CFU-GEMM whilst macrophage populations, obtained by growing the cells in medium conditioned by a mixed lymphocyte reaction, reduced CFU-GM colony formation but, again, had little effect on BFU-E or CFU-GEMM.[17] These observations indicate that different components of marrow stroma can have contrasting effects on erythropoiesis and granulopoiesis and that the stromal microenvironment may regulate the expression of stem cell differentiation.

Many workers have studied the haemopoietic effects of cloned stromal cell lines.[18] Overall, these studies indicate that the major growth factor produced by the stromal cell microenvironemt is M-CSF, that GM-CSF and G-CSF production can be induced and that some stromal cell lines inhibit haemopoiesis. There is some suggestion that a lack of mRNA for IL-1 or of cell binding proteins may correlate with an inability to support haemopoiesis in vitro.

It is generally accepted that a stromal microenvironment is necessary for haemopoiesis in vivo and in long-term cultures in vitro and it is without doubt that cultured stromal cells can support the survival, proliferation and differentiation of haemopoietic stem cells. However, recent observations suggest that the function of the stromal layer can be replaced by the appropriate combinations of growth factors and that direct contact between stromal cells and haemopoietic cells in long-term cultures is not necessary for haemopoietic activity. For example, Brandt et al[19] cultured highly purified primitive haemopoietic progenitor cells (CD34+, HLA-DR−, CD15−, CD71−) in a combination of IL-3 plus IL-1α or IL-6 and were able to sustain haemopoiesis for 8 weeks by replenishing the growth factors every 48 hours. No stromal layers formed in these cultures and the authors concluded that a major function of the stroma is to provide growth factors which promote the proliferation and differentiation of primitive haemopoietic cells. In another study, Verfaillie[20] physically separated haemopoietic cells from stromal cells by inserting a microporous membrane into long-term cultures, allowing the passage of soluble factors but preventing cell–cell contact. Her results indicated that stromal cells were not necessary for the conservation of primitive progenitor cells or for their differentiation into CFU-GM. However, without contact with stromal cells, the production of CFU-GM was excessive suggesting that stromal cells were essential for regulating the later stages of mature blood cell production.

These two studies indicate that the major roles of the stromal haemopoietic microenvironment might be to provide stimulatory factors and to regulate the interactions between growth factors and their target cells (see below).

Matrix components and cellular constituents

Heparin/heparan sulphate Heparin receptors are found on a wide variety of cell types and the growth of some of them, such as endothelial cells,[21,22] is promoted whilst the growth of others, such as smooth muscle cells and epithelial cells[23,24] is inhibited. In the case of pre-B cells, heparin binds to IL-7 and, presumably, prevents IL-7 interacting with its receptor on the target cells.[25,26] Although little is known of the action of heparin in the haemopoietic system, it may regulate cell growth through unique changes in its chemical structure that occur in a density dependent fashion[27] and through its translocation to the nucleus.[28] It binds to monocytes of the U937 cell line and induces the release of two proteins (160 and 17 kD) and has been implicated in regulating the autocrine synthesis of growth factors by malignant cells,[29,30] thus indicating the potential for signal transduction by occupied heparin receptors. Nonphysiological experiments have shown that heparin can stimulate DNA replication and transcription when added to intact nuclei but inhibits replication and transcription of a naked DNA template.[31-35] These observations are consistent with the suggestion that the composition of the structural analogue of heparin, heparan sulphate, gives it the scope to act as a code polymer.[36]

The role of fibronectin in the differentiation of erythroid and granulocytic precursors has been studied in colony cultures. Fibronectin enhances the proliferation of BFU-E, CFU-E and CFU-GEMM but not of CFU-GM. This effect was mediated by the RGD binding site of fibronectin.[37] Other studies have shown that fibronectin is necessary for the differentiation of murine erythroleukaemia cells into reticulocytes.[38]

Fatty acids The bulk of the lipid in marrow fat cells in vivo and in vitro is triacylglycerol, but cultured marrow fat cells contain a much higher proportion of unsaturated fatty acids than bone marrow fat cells in vivo.[39,40] The immunosuppressive effects of unsaturated fatty acids have been appreciated for some time[41] and there is some evidence that saturated and unsaturated fatty acids have different effects on a variety of cell types in culture. Unsaturated fatty acids stimulate DNA synthesis in cultured tumour cells[42] but palmitic, linoleic, linolenic and arachidonic acids inhibit RNA synthesis by lymphocytes.[43] Szamel et al[44] have reported that linoleic and arachidonic acids potentiate IL-2 synthesis in human lymphocytes. Arachidonic acid metabolites derived from human stromal cell cultures can also potentiate the numbers of erythroid CFU-E in semisolid cultures[45] and prostaglandin E, a product of arachidonic acid metabolism, inhibits CFU-GM but stimulates BFU-E.[1] As well as acting as single agents, some fatty acids can act synergistically in combination.[46,47] Thus, fatty acids may influence haemopoietic cell proliferation and/or the production of regulatory cytokines by accessory cells. It is relevant in this context that the hypercellular marrow in CML is virtually devoid of fat cells whilst an increase in fat cells is characteristic of the marrow in aplastic anaemia.

Alterations in the proportions of saturated and unsaturated fatty acids have been associated with marrow hypocellularity but the available information is inconsistent. Tavassoli, Houchin and Jacobs[48] found that triacylglycerols in yellow marrow contained less saturated fatty acids that triacylglycerols in active red marrow. However, when Moloney, Flannery and Patt[49] studied the fat cell content and haemopoietic activity of ossicles produced by ectopic implants of marrow in rabbits they found that reduced haemopoietic cellularity was associated with an increased content of saturated fatty acids. Snyder[50] found that the post-irradiation depression of haemopoiesis in mice was accompanied by an increase in marrow triglyceride biosynthesis but that fatty acid oxidation was inhibited. This would result in an increase in the proportion of unsaturated fatty acids.

Organization of haemopoiesis by the stromal microenvironment

Long-term bone marrow cultures consist of two phases, the adherent stromal layer and an upper liquid layer. The more primitive progenitor cells are found amongst the adherent stromal cells[51] and they release their progeny into the culture supernatant from where they can be harvested weekly and assayed using semi-solid colony cultures (Fig. 1). It is thought that specific spatial relationships are maintained by the expression of cell adhesion molecules (CAMs) at the surface of the haemopoietic stem and progenitor cells and the expression of appropriate counter-receptors by cells of the stromal microenvironment.

Many studies have detailed the expression of CAMs by haemopoietic progenitor cells[52] but expression does not necessarily predict involvement of a particular CAM with stromal cells. This is for reasons of differing affinities of the CAMs, involvement of multiple adhesion molecules in particular adhesive interactions and the expression of negatively charged molecules by progenitor cells and stromal cells that counteract cell–cell adhesion.[53]

Functional studies of the binding of haemopoietic progenitor cells have revealed lineage- and stage-specific binding properties. Verfaillie, Blakolmer and McGlave[54] showed that the cells responsible for initiating haemopoiesis

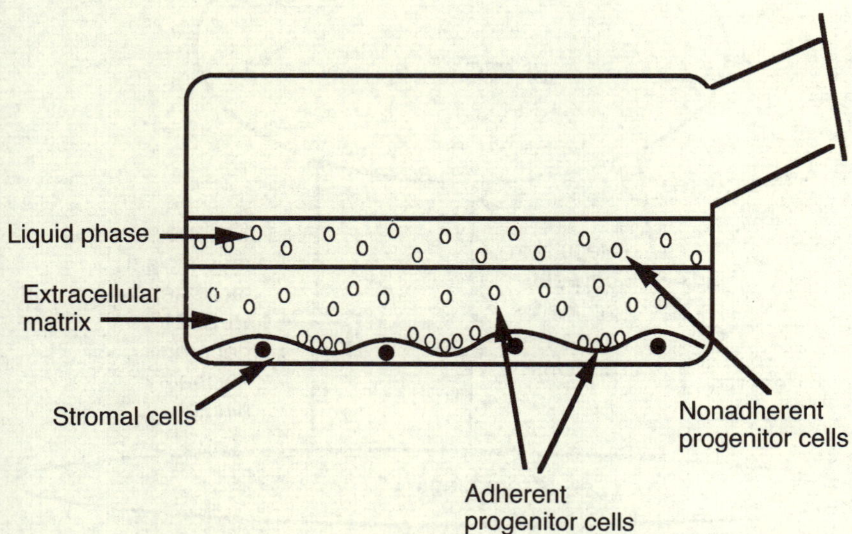

Fig. 1. Spatial arrangement of stromal and haemopoietic progenitor cells in long-term cultures.

in long-term marrow cultures adhered to stromal cells. Gordon et al[55–57] have studied the adhesive properties of a population of blast colony-forming cells (BI-CFC), that succeed long-term culture-initiating cells in haemopoietic cell development.[58] These cells bind to stroma grown in the presence of the glucocorticoid methylprednisolone but do not bind to stroma grown without methylprednisolone. The BI-CFC are progenitors of CFU-GM, BFU-E and CFU-GEMM,[59] none of which bind to stromal layers gown under either culture condition.[55]

The BI-CFC bind to stroma by a multimolecular mechanism[53] of which one component is a phosphatidylinositol (PI)-anchored CAM expressed by the BI-CFC[56,57] which binds to a specific heparan sulphate proteoglycan produced by the stromal cells in the presence of methylprednisolone.[13] Other, less specific, cell adhesion mechanisms co-operate with the PI-anchored CAM to bind the cell and the expression of negatively charged molecules, such as CD34 and leukosialin, resist nonspecific binding and thereby maintain specificity (Fig. 2). Tavassoli and colleagues[60] implicated the expression of galactosyl and mannosyl residues on the surface of haemopoietic progenitor cells, and of lectin-like molecules by the stromal cells, in binding interactions and showed that fucosyl residues were not involved. Verfaillie, McCarthy and

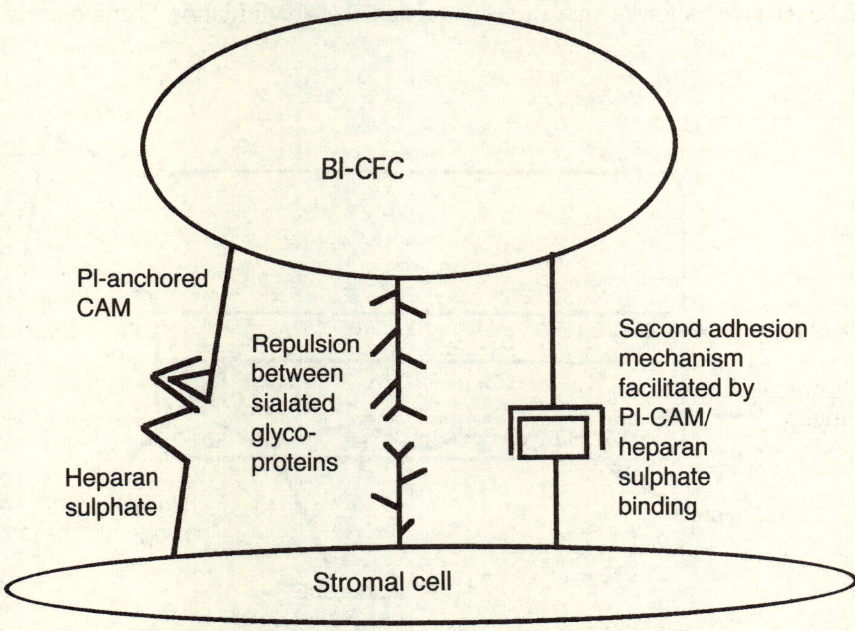

Fig. 2. A model for the binding of blast colony-forming cells (BI-CFC) to cultured stromal layers.

McGlave[61] studied the stage- and lineage-specific binding of haemopoietic progenitors to fibronectin. They showed that primitive long-term culture-initiating cells (LTCIC) and CFU-GEMM and single lineage BFU-E and CFU-GM bound to the heparin-binding domain of fibronectin. In addition, BFU-E and CFU-GM, but not LTCIC or CFU-GEMM bound to the RGD-containing fragment. They suggested that this change in adhesive properties during haemopoietic cell development might allow progenitor cells to migrate to distinct loci in the marrow microenvironment. Integrin $\alpha_4\beta_1$ is expressed by more than 90% of CD34+ positive bone marrow cells and VCAM-1, a ligand for $\alpha_4\beta_1$ is induced in stromal layers by exposure to IL-4 plus TNF. This mechanism was shown to be capable of binding haemopoietic progenitors to stromal layers by Simmons and colleagues.[62]

It has been suggested that the localization of haemopoietic progenitor cells in specific microenvironments by adhesive interactions allows them to be provided with the appropriate growth factors for their survival, proliferation and differentiation.[63] This might be accomplished by a variety of mechanisms which include the synthesis of growth factors by stromal cells which are expressed as cell surface molecules (M-CSF and c-kit ligand/stem cell factor) or are exported from the stromal cell and concentrated in the extracellular matrix. Alternatively, growth factors produced peripherally might bind to the ECM.[64] The finding that some haemopoietic growth factors can be expressed as surface molecules led to the idea that these growth factors could function as cell adhesion molecules as well as stimulators of haemopoiesis. This mechanism has been termed 'juxtacrine' by Anklesaria and colleagues.[65] It is likely that the mechanisms for binding haemopoietic cells and growth factors in the haemopoietic microenvironment exist to control the access of growth factors to their target cells since toxic effects have been observed if the growth factors are present at high concentrations and in inappropriate locations. These circumstances include retroviral or transgenic expression of growth factor genes or the chronic administration of growth factors in vivo.

Physiology and pathophysiology of the stromal microenvironment

The close link between the stromal microenvironment and haemopoiesis implies that the stromal cells might physiologically respond to changing demands for blood cell production. Alternatively, the marrow stroma might react to haemopoietic insufficiency or excess caused by haematological disease or treatment. There is some evidence that the microenvironment can be regulated by growth factors.

Aplastic anaemia

Aplastic anaemia is an extreme case of haematological insufficiency. There is evidence from bone marrow transplantation that the microenvironment is defective in a minority of cases. In other cases, microenvironmental alterations have been documented but these may reflect a physiological response to bone marrow failure rather than part of the pathophysiology of the disease. Functionally abnormal fibroblasts have been demonstrated in some aplastic patients[66] but Gordon and Gordon-Smith[67] showed that fibroblasts grown from aplastic patients' marrows had normal or supranormal ability to stimulate colony formation by normal granulocyte-macrophage colony-forming cells (CFU-GM) although their CSF-enhancing activity was reduced.[68] Gibson and colleagues (personal communication) found that marrow stromal cells grown from some aplastic patients had higher than normal levels of colony-stimulating activity and Kojima, Matsuyama and Kodera[69] demonstrated normal or elevated production of G-CSF, GM-CSF and IL-6 by marrow stromal cells from aplastic patients. Overall, these studies suggest that a stimulatory microenvironment might be 'induced' by bone marrow failure.

Marsh et al[70] assessed the function of aplastic marrow-derived stroma in long-term bone marrow cultures and concluded that stromal function was normal in the great majority of cases, although Hotta et al,[71] using a similar method, reported a stromal defect in three of the nine patients studied. Marsh et al[70] noted differences in the growth rate to confluence and the early appearance of fat cells in their glucocorticoid-supplemented long-term cultures of aplastic marrow. We have found that marrow from a proportion of aplastic patients forms fat cells in stromal cultures in the absence of glucocorticoid whereas normal marrow does not. Moreover, these aplastic stromal layers can bind blast colony-forming cells (Bl-CFC) whereas normal glucocorticoid-deprived stroma cannot (unpublished observations). Similarly, marrows from some hypoplastic patients in chemotherapy-induced remissions exhibit the same phenomenon, reinforcing the idea that the marrow microenvironment can respond to hypoplasia.

The presence of fat cells is at least compatible with haemopoiesis in the long-term bone marrow culture system and fatty atrophy of the bone marrow is characteristic of bone marrow failure in aplastic anaemia. These lines of evidence, plus the finding that there is little qualitative alteration in the fatty acid composition of the fat cells in aplastic anaemia bone marrow[40] point to a physiological compensation by the stromal microenvironment in bone marrow failure.

Chronic myeloid leukaemia

Chronic myeloid leukaemia (CML) represents the extreme of haematological excess. Generally, the marrow fibrosis that occurs in CML is thought to be a reactive process and the majority of studies suggest that fibroblast progenitors do not belong to the leukaemic clone (see 1 for references). However, Ph-positive fibroblasts have been found[72] and Singer, Keating and Fialkow[73] reported that marrow stromal cells from a glucose-6-phosphate dehydrogenase (G6PD) heterozygote with CML contained the same single isoenzyme as cells in haemopoietic colonies. In contrast to the fibroblast component of marrow stroma, stromal macrophages are likely to be members of the leukaemic population since they are derived ultimately from pluripotent haemopoietic stem cells.

Wetzler et al[74] found no difference in the constitutive or induced expression of stimulatory or inhibitory cytokines in stroma grown from the marrow of normal individuals or patients who were in the chronic phase of CML. However, spontaneous expression of cytokines normally requiring induction was found in stroma grown from the marrow of patients in blast crisis and the addition of blast crisis cells to established normal stroma induced the expression of IL-1 and IL-6.[75]

Functional studies of the capacity of CML marrow-derived stromal cells to bind normal BI-CFC have not revealed any deficiency.[76]

Myelofibrosis

The pathogenesis of myelofibrosis is that of a stem cell disorder. The haemopoietic cells are monoclonal whilst the marrow fibroblasts are polyclonal and the marrow fibrosis can be reduced by bone marrow transplantation. It has been proposed that ineffective megakaryopoiesis and intramedullary cell death result in high local concentrations of platelet-derived growth factor (PDGF) and platelet factor four, which cause excessive fibroblast proliferation and accumulation of collagen. Accordingly, PDGF stimulates fibroblast proliferation and collagen synthesis whereas platelet factor four prevents the degradation of collagen by inhibiting the activity of collagenase. The effects of the megakaryocytes may be modified by vitamin D_3. Its active metabolite $(1,25\text{-}(OH)_2\ D_3)$ inhibits fibroblast proliferation and increases collagen degradation. Thus, vitamin D_3 deficiency could contribute to the development of myelofibrosis and this notion is supported by clinical observations (Fig. 3) .[1]

Acute leukaemias

The importance of the stromal microenvironment as a spatial organiser of haemopoietic cells and growth factors has been emphasised earlier in this chapter. There is evidence that leukaemic blast cells can release factors that degrade matrix and potentially can disrupt these critical relationships. For example, HL60 and U937 myeloid leukaemia cells and neoplastic murine B cells can degrade proteoglycan.[77–79] Similar activities have been widely associated with the metastatic behavior of malignant cells.[80] Conditioned medium from peripheral megakaryoblasts in acute megakaryoblastic leukaemia and from a megakaryoblast cell line stimulated collagen synthesis by bone marrow fibroblasts much more than medium conditioned by other types of acute

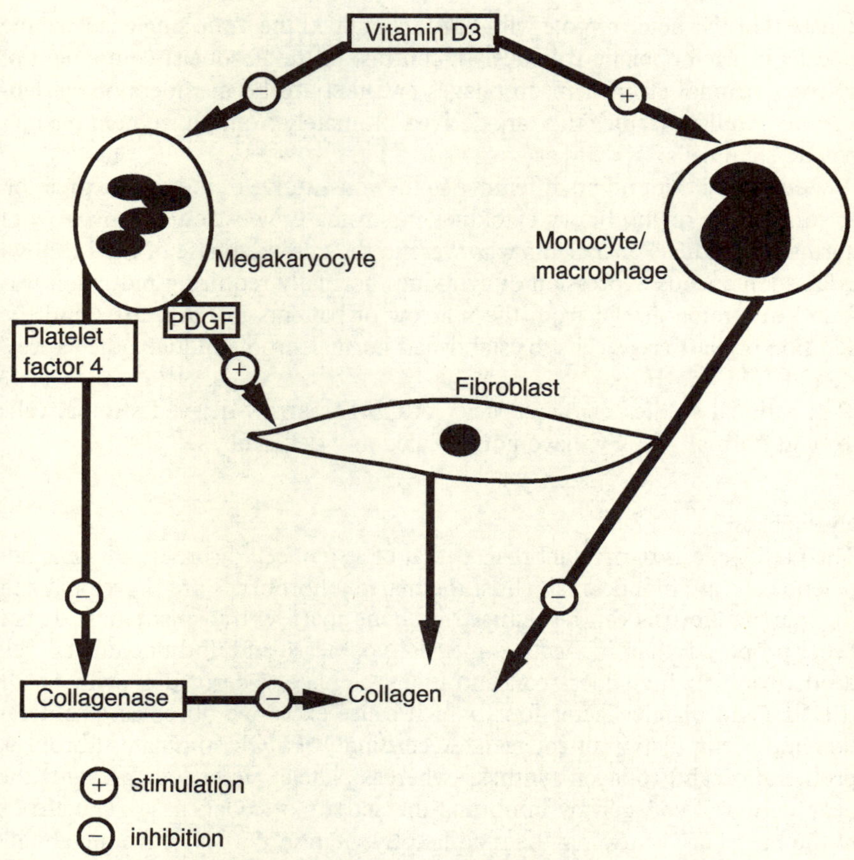

Fig 3. A model for the pathogenesis of myelofibrosis (see text for references).

leukaemia cells. This action probabaly contributes to the acute myelofibrosis that is often associated with the disease.[81]

The matrix metalloproteinases include stromelysin (transin), which degrades proteoglycans, and collagenase. They are activated by plasmin, produced from plasminogen under the agency of plasminogen activators in vivo[80] (see below) and Oliver, Keeton and Wilson[82] showed that K562 cells secrete plasminogen activator in vitro. Some growth factors, including PDGF, have positive regulatory effects on metalloproteinase gene expression. Platelet-derived growth factor is the product of the c-sis proto-oncogene and induces c-fos expression and expression of stromelysin mRNA.[83] It is of interest, therefore, that expression of c-sis, which is reciprocally translocated during the formation of the Ph chromosome, is expressed in the acute phase of CML in some patients.[84]

Mayani et al[85] investigated the composition and haemopoietic support capacity of AML marrow-derived stromal layers. In two of six AML cases investigated, the stromal layers were deficient in terms of cellular composition, produced subnormal amounts of M-CSF and exhibited poor support of haemopoiesis. Moreover, supernatants from these stromal cultures inhibited colony formation in vitro. These abnormal features were reversed by growing the stroma in the presence of M-CSF. The inhibitory activity was partially attributed to the production of TNFα and partially to other factors, including prostaglandin E. The M-CSF down-regulated TNFα production by AML stroma but increased its production by normal stroma.[86] This work indicates the presence in some cases of AML of functionally abnormal leukaemia-derived macrophages that form a component of stromal layers in vitro.

Effects of therapy

Testa, Hendry and Molineux[87] have reviewed the information concerning environmental damage incurred by treatment with cytotoxic drugs and irradiation. Busulphan and cyclophosphamide induce persistent, irreparable damage to several components of the stroma and the damage caused by BCNU therapy has been associated with an increase in sulphated glycosaminoglycan production by human bone marrow stromal cells.[88] Orazi et al[89] studied the morphology of bone marrow biopsies in patients treated with high-dose cyclophosphamide with and without GM-CSF or IL-3 to promote haematological recovery. Stromal changes in all patients included endothelial cell proliferation, increased macrophage concentration and an increase in bone marrow fibroblasts. Fibrosis occured in IL-3-treated patients but not in GM-CSF-treated patients.

The transplantability of stromal elements by the intravenous route has been a subject of considerable debate. Most components of marrow-derived stroma have been shown to be transplantable at one time or another.[90] However, the weight of evidence is against colonization of recipients marrows by infused fibroblast precursors (FCFC). Donor-derived endothelial cells have been detected in marrow transplant recipients and the macrophages of the bone marrow microenvironment are produced by donor stem cells, as might be expected from the replacement of tissue macrophages by donor cells following bone marrow transplantation.

Effects of hormones and growth factors

In vitro manipulations alter the properties of cultured stroma. For example, treatment with glucocorticoids induces efficient fat cell formation, alters sulphation levels on heparan sulphate proteoglycan[12,13] induces the capacity to bind early progenitor cells[55] and modifies the growth factor profile (Gooding, personal communication). Activated T cells release soluble products that facilitate the growth of macrophages at the expense of fibroblasts.[91]

Platelet-derived growth factor (PDGF), epidermal growth factor (EGF) and transforming growth factor α (TGFα) stimulate the growth of passaged fibroblasts and fibroblast colony-forming cells.[92] Transforming growth factor α (TGFα) and EGF stimulate the formation of osteoclast-like cells in human long-term marrow cultures and may, therefore, stimulate bone resorption in vivo.[93]

Transforming growth factor β is a potent regulator of the expression of extracellular matrix components, including fibronectin, collagen and proteoglycans.[94–97] Interleukin-1 stimulates glycosaminoglycan synthesis in cultured dermal fibroblasts[98] but induces loss of proteoglycan in synovial joints.[99] Interferon alpha modifies the adhesive properties of stroma vis-a-vis early progenitor cells in CML.[100]

The role of growth factors in regulating stromelysin gene expression and plasminogen activator activity is particularly interesting because these molecules have the potential to degrade binding sites for haemopoietic cells and growth factors. These relationships are summarized in Fig.4.

According to this scheme, TGFβ-mediated inhibition of stromelysin gene expression is mediated by a complex of fos protein and TGFβ inhibitory element binding protein (TIEbp) to TIE in a promoter region upstream of the stromelysin gene. This inhibits the action of the AP-1 site and suppresses

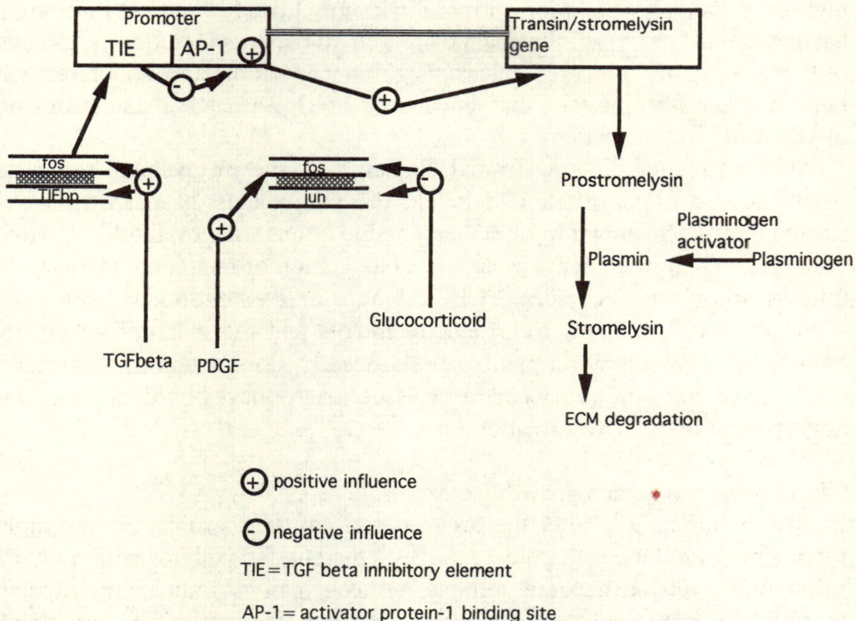

Fig 4. The potential influence of TGF beta, PDGF and glucocorticoid on the degradation of the extracellular matrix.

stromelysin gene expression.[80,101] Platelet-derived growth factor (PDGF)-mediated stimulation occurs via fos-jun binding to the AP-1 site. This stimulatory pathway is inhibited by glucocorticoid.[102–105] The enzyme is secreted in a latent form and its activation involves plasmin, derived by the action of plasminogen activator on plasminogen. Saksela, Moscatelli and Rifkin[105] demonstrated that plasminogen activator is inhibited by TGFβ and that this effect is counteracted by basic fibroblast growth factor (bFGF) but Hannocks et al[106], found that IL-1β, FGF and TGFβ stimulated the production of plasminogen activator, suggesting that the generation of plasmin might be involved in regulating the precise composition of specific micro-environments. In addition to its activities on ECM, stromelysin can 'super-activate' collagenase.[80]

Fat cell formation by stromal cells is antagonised by tumour necrosis factor (TNF), interleukin-1 (IL-1) and transforming growth factor β (TGFβ). These factors are produced within the bone marrow stroma and the addition of TGFβ to long-term cultures inhibits haemopoiesis as well as adipogenesis.[108] It seems likely, therefore, that the differentiation of stromal cells can be regulated by autocrine and paracrine mechanisms involving growth factors produced locally and growth factors produced by circulating blood cells. Granulocyte-CSF has no effect on the development of stromal layers but GM-CSF and IL-3 enhanced the development of the stromal layers and reduced fat cell formation.[109] Similarly, M-CSF[110] IL-1, IL-6, IL-11, TNF and LIF inhibit adipogenesis[111] It is, however, unclear how these effects might contribute to the control of haemopoiesis.

It will be clear to readers of this review that much remains to be learnt about the complex interrelationships between haemopoietic cells and stromal cells that are responsible for regulating haemopoiesis. Studies of the biochemistry of the extracellular matrix and its function in the genetic regulation of haemopoiesis will be of fundamental importance to the further understanding of the physiology and pathophysiology of this complex and elegantly regulated system.

References

(1) Gordon MY, Barrett AJ. *Bone marrow disorders: the biological basis of clinical problems*. Oxford, UK: Blackwell Scientific Publications, 1985.

(2) Gordon MY. Annotation: Extracellular matrix of the marrow micro-environment. *Br J Haematol* 1988; 70: 1–4.

(3) Simmons PJ, Torok-Storb B. CD34 expression by stromal precursors in normal human bone marrow. *Blood* 1991; 78: 2848–53.

(4) Charbord P, Gown AM, Keating A, Singer JW. CGA-7 and HHF, two monoclonal antibodies that recognise muscle actin and react with adherent cells in human long-term marrow cultures. *Blood* 1985; 66: 1138–42.

(5) Simmons PJ, Torok-Storb B. Identification of stromal cell precursors in human bone marrow by a novel monoclonal antibody, STRO-1. *Blood* 1991; 78: 55–62.

(6) Hasthorpe S, Bogdanovski M, Rogerson J, Radley JM. Characterisation of endothelial cells in murine long-term marrow culture. Implication for hemopoietic regulation. *Exp Hematol* 1992; 20: 478–81.

(7) Jacobsen K, Miyake K, Kincade PW, Osmond DG. Highly restricted expression of a stromal cell determinant of mouse bone marrow in vivo. *J Exp Med* 1992; 176: 927–35.

(8) Linsenmeyer TF. Collagen. In: ED Hay, ed. *Cell biology of extracellular matrix 2nd ed*. New York: Plenum Press, 1991: 7–44.

(9) Yamada KH. Fibronectin and other interactive glycoproteins. In: ED Hay, ed. *Cell biology of extracellular matrix 2nd ed*. New York: Plenum Press, 1991: 111–46.

(10) Wight TN, Heinegard DK, Hascall VC. Proteoglycans: structure and function. In: ED Hay, ed. *Cell biology of extracellular matrix 2nd ed*. New York: Plenum Press, 1991: 45–78.

(11) Wight TN, Kinsella MG, Keating A, Singer JW. Proteoglycans in human long-term marrow cultures: Biochemical and structural analyses. *Blood* 1986; 67: 1333–43.

(12) Morris AJ, Turnbull JE, Riley GP, Gordon MY, Gallagher JT. Production of heparan sulphate proteoglycans by human bone marrow stromal cells. *J Cell Sci* 1991; 99: 149–56.

(13) Siczkowsi M, Clarke D, Gordon MY. Binding of primitive hematopoietic progenitor cells to marrow stromal cells involves heparan sulfate. *Blood* 1992; 80: 912–9.

(14) Cashman JD, Eaves AC, Raines EW, Ross R, Eaves CJ. Mechanisms that regulate the cell cycle status of very primitive hematopoietic cells in long-term human marrow cultures. I. Stimulatory role of a variety of mesenchymal cell activators and inhibitory role of TGFβ. *Blood* 1990; 75: 96–101.

(15) Toksoz D, Dexter TM, Lord BI. The regulation of hematopoiesis in long-term marrow culture. II. Stimulation and inhibition of stem cell proliferation. *Blood* 1980; 55: 931–6.

(16) Whitlock CA, Robertson D, Witte ON. Murine B cell lymphopoiesis in long-term culture. *J Immunol Methods* 1984; 67: 353–69.

(17) Gordon MY, Kearney LU, Hibbin JA. Effects of human marrow stromal cells on proliferation by human granulocytic (GM-CFC), erythroid (BFU-E) and mixed (mix-CFC) colony-forming cells *Br J Haematol* 1983; 53: 317–25.

(18) Greenberger JS. The hematopoietic microenvironment. *Critical reviews in oncology/hematology* 1991; 11: 65–84.

(19) Brandt J, Srour EF, van Besien K, Bridell RA, Hoffman R. Cytokine-dependent long-term culture of highly enriched precursors of hematopoietic progenitor cells from human bone marrow. *J Clin Invest* 1990; 86: 932–41.

(20) Verfaillie CM. Direct contact between human primitive hematopoietic progenitors and bone marrow stroma is not required for long-term in vitro hematopoiesis. *Blood* 1992; 79: 2821–6.

(21) Folkman J, Klagsbrun M. Angiogenic factors. *Science* 1987; 235: 442–7.

(22) Ulrich S, Lagente O, Choay J, Lenfant M. Structure activity relationship in

heparin: stimulation of non-vascular cells by a synthetic heparin pentasaccharide in co-operation with human acidic fibroblast growth factor. *Biochem Biophys Res Commun* 1986; 139: 728–32.

(23) Wright TC, Johnston TV, Castellot JJ, Karnovsky MJ. Inhibition of rat corneal epithelial cell growth by heparin and its reversal by EGF. *J Cell Physiol* 1985; 125; 499–508.

(24) Castellot JJ, Choay J, Lormeau J-C, Petitou M, Sache F, Karnovsky MJ. Structural determinants of the capacity of heparin to inhibit the proliferation of vascular smooth muscle cells. II. Evidence for a pentasaccharide sequence that contains a 3.0 sulphate group. *J Cell Biol* 1986;102: 1979–84.

(25) Kimura K, Matsubaru H, Sagoh S et al. Role of glycosaminoglycans in the regulation of T cell proliferation induced by thymic stroma-derived T cell growth factor. *J Immunol* 1991; 146: 2618–24.

(26) Clarke D, Katoh O, Siczkowski M, Griffiths S, Gordon MY. The interaction of IL-7 with glycosaminoglycans and its relevance to biological systems. Submitted for publication. 1992.

(27) Fedarko NS, Conrad HE. A unique heparan sulphate in the nuclei of hepatocytes: structural changes with the growth state of the cells. *J Cell Biol* 1986; 103: 587–99.

(28) Ishihara M, Fedarko NS, Conrad HE. Transport of heparan sulfate into the nuclei of hepatocytes. *J Biol Chem* 1986; 261: 13575–80.

(29) Leung L, Saigo K, Grant D. Heparin binds to human monocytes and modulates their procoagulant activities and secretory phenotypes. *Blood* 1989; 73; 177–84.

(30) Zvibel I, Halay E, Reid LM. heparin and hormonal regulation of mRNA synthesis and abundance of autocrine growth factor: relevance to clonal growth of tumors. *Mol Cell Biol* 1991; 11: 108–16.

(31) Arnold EA, Yawn DH, Brown DG, Wyllie RC, Coffrey DS. Structural alterations in rat liver nuclei after removal of template restrictions by polyanions. *J Cell Biol* 1992; 53: 737–57.

(32) Dynan J, Burgess RR. In vitro transcription by wheatgerm RNA polymerase II: effects of heparin and role of template integrity. *Biochemistry* 1981; 18; 4581–8.

(33) Furukawa K, Bharanandan VP. Influence of anionic polysaccharides on DNA synthesis in isolated nuclei and by DNA polymerase alpha: correlations of observed effects with properties of polysaccharides. *Biochim Biophys Acta* 1983; 740: 466–74.

(34) Kovacs J, Frei A, Seifert KH. Activation of transcription complexes of RNA polymerase B by the polyanion heparin. *Biochem Int* 1981; 3: 645–53.

(35) Kraemer RJ, Coffey DS. The interaction of natural and synthetic polyanions with mammalian nuclei. I. DNA synthesis. *Biochim Biophys Acta* 1970; 224: 553–67.

(36) Keating A, Gordon MY. Hierarchical organisation of hematopoietic micro-environments: role of proteoglycans. *Leukemia* 1988; 2: 766–9.

(37) Weinstein R, Riordan MA, Wenc K, Kreczka S, Zhou M, Dainiak N. Dual role of fibronectin in hematopoietic differentiation. *Blood* 1989; 73: 111–6.

(38) Patel VP, Lodish HF. A fibronectin matrix is necessary for the differentiation of murine erythroleukaemia cells into reticulocytes. *J Cell Biol* 1987: 105: 3105–318.

(39) Lund PK, Abadi DM, Mathies JC. Lipid composition of normal human bone marrow as determined by column chromatography. *J Lipid Res* 1962; 3: 95–8.

(40) Malik FM, Gordon MY, Goldman JM, Gordon-Smith EC. Comparison of the composition of fat cells obtained from the marrow of normal individuals or of subjects with aplastic anemia and from bone marrow cultures. *Exp Hematol* 1984; 12: 191–7.

(41) McCormick JN, Neill WA, Simm AK. Immunosuppressive effects of linoleic acid. *Lancet* 1977; ii: 508.

(42) Holley RW, Baldwin JH, Kiernan JA. Control of growth of a tumor cell line by linoleic acid. *Proc Natl Acad Sci USA* 1974; 71: 3976–8.

(43) Kageyama K, Nagesawa T, Kimura S, Kobayashi T, Kinoshita Y. Cytotoxic activity of unsaturated fatty acids to lymphocytes. *Canad J Biochem* 1980; 58: 504–8.

(44) Szamel M, Retterman B, Krebs B, Kurrle R, Resche K. Activation signals in human lymphocytes: Incorporation of polyunsaturated fatty acids into plasma membrane phospholipids regulates IL-2 synthesis via sustained activation of protein kinase C. *J Immunol* 1989; 143: 2806–13.

(45) Abraham NG, Feldman E, Falck JR, Lutton JD, Schwartzman ML. Modulation of erythropoiesis by novel human bone marrow cytochrome p450–dependent metabolites of arachidonic acid. *Blood* 1991; 78: 1461–6.

(46) Yoshida K, Asaoka Y, Nishizuka Y. Platelet activation by simultaneous actions of diacyglycerol and unsaturated fatty acids. *Proc Natl Acad Sci USA* 1992; 89: 6443–6.

(47) Seifert R, Schachtele C, Schultze G. Activation of protein kinase C by cis- and transoctadecadienoic acids in intact human platelets and its potentiation by diacylglycerol. *Biochem Biophys Res Commun* 1987; 149: 762–8.

(48) Tavassoli M, Houchin DN, Jacobs P. Fatty acid composition of adipose cells in red and yellow marrow: a possible determinant of haemopoietic potential. *Scand J Haematol* 1977; 18: 47–53.

(49) Maloney MA, Flannery ML, Patt HM. Fat content of ectopic marrow implants and cellularity of resulting ossicles. *Proc Soc Exp Biol Med* 1980; 165: 309–12.

(50) Snyder F. Fatty acid oxidation in irradiated bone marrow cells. *Nature* 1965; 206: 733–75.

(51) Coulombel L, Eaves AC, Eaves CJ. Enzymatic treatment of long-term human marrow cultures reveals the preferential location of primitive hemopoietic progenitors in the adherent layer. *Blood* 1983; 62: 291–7.

(52) Clarke BR, Gallagher JT, Dexter TM. Cell adhesion in the stromal regulation of haemopoiesis. *Baillière's Clin Haematol* 1992; 5: 619–52.

(53) Siczkowsi M, Dowding CR, Gordon MY. Stromal regulation of haemopoiesis. In: Abraham NG, Konwalinka G, Marks P, Sachs L, Tavassoli M. *Molecular biology of haematopoiesis volume 2*. Andover, Hants: Intercept Ltd, 1992: 263–76.

(54) Verfaillie C, Blakolmer K, McGlave P. Purified primitive hematopoietic progenitor cells with long-term in vitro repopulating ability adhere selectively to irradiated bone marrow stroma. *J Exp Med* 1990; 172: 509–20.

(55) Gordon MY, Hibbin JA, Dowding C, Gordon-Smith EC, Goldman JM.

Separation of human blast progenitors from granulocytic, erythroid, megakaryocytic and mixed colony-forming cells by 'panning' on cultured marrow-derived stromal layers. *Exp Hematol* 1985; 13: 937–40.

(56) Gordon MY, Clarke D, Atkinson J, Greaves MF. Haemopoietic progenitor cell-binding to the stromal microenvironment in vitro. *Exp Hematol* 1990; 18: 837–42.

(57) Gordon MY, Atkinson J, Clarke D et al. Deficiency of a phosphatidylinositol-anchored cell adhesion molecule influences haemopoietic progenitor binding to marrow stroma in chronic myeloid leukaemia. *Leukemia* 1991; 5: 693–8.

(58) Dowding CR, Gordon MY. Physical, phenotypic and cytochemical characterisation of stroma-adherent blast colony-forming cells. *Leukemia* 1992; 6: 347–51.

(59) Gordon MY, Dowding CR, Riley GP, Greaves MF. Characterization of stroma dependent blast colony-forming cells in human marrow. *J Cell Physiol* 1987; 130: 150–6.

(60) Aizawa S, Tavassoli M. Molecular basis of the recognition of intravenously transplanted hemopoietic cells by bone marrow stroma. *Proc Natl Acad Sci USA* 1988; 85: 3180–3.

(61) Verfaillie CM, McCarthy JB, McGlave PB. Differentiation of primitive human multipotent hematopoietic progenitors into single lineage clonogenic progenitors is accompanied by alterations in their interaction with fibronectin. *J Exp Med* 1991; 174: 693–703.

(62) Simmons PJ, Masinovsky B, Longenecker BM, Berenson R, Torok-Storb B, Gallatin WM. Vascular cell adhesion molecule-1 expressed by bone marrow stromal cells mediates the binding of hematopoietic progenitor cells. *Blood* 1992; 80: 388–95.

(63) Gordon MY, Greaves MF. Physiological mechanisms of stem cell regulation in bone marrow transplantation and haemopoiesis. *Bone Marrow Transpl* 1989; 4: 335–8.

(64) Gordon MY. Hemopoietic growth factors: bound and free. *Cancer Cells* 1991; 3: 127–33.

(65) Anklesaria P, Teixido J, Laiho M, Pierce JH, Greenberger JS, Massague J. Cell-cell adhesion mediated by binding of membrane-anchored transforming growth factor α to epidermal growth factor receptors promotes cell proliferation. *Proc Natl Acad Sci USA* 1990; 87: 3289–93.

(66) Juneja HS, Gardner FH. Functionally abnormal marrow stromal cells in aplastic anaemia. *Exp Hemat* 1985; 13: 194–9.

(67) Gordon MY, Gordon-Smith EC. Bone marrow fibroblast colony-forming cells (F-CFC) in aplastic anaemia: colony growth and stimulation of granulocyte-macrophage colony-forming cells (GM-CFC). *Br J Haematol* 1981; 49: 465–77.

(68) Gordon MY, Gordon-Smith EC. Bone marrow fibroblast function in relation to granulopoiesis in aplastic anaemia. *Br J Haematol* 1983; 53: 483–8.

(69) Kojima S, Matsuyama T, Kodera Y. Hematopoietic growth factors released by marrow stromal cells from patients with aplastic anemia. *Blood* 1992; 79: 2256–61.

(70) Marsh JCW, Chang J, Testa NG, Hows JM, Dexter TM. The hematopoietic

defect in aplastic anemia assessed by long-term marrow culture. *Blood* 1990; 76: 1748–57.

(71) Hotta T, Kato T, Maeda H, Yameo H, Yamada H, Saito H. Functional changes in marrow stromal cells in aplastic anaemia. *Acta Hematol* 1985; 74: 65–9.

(72) Hentel J, Hirshhorn K. The origin of some bone marrow fibroblasts. *Blood* 1983; 38: 81–7.

(73) Singer JW, Keating A, Fialkow PJ. Evidence suggesting a common progenitor for hematopoietic and marrow stromal cells. *Exp Hematol* 1983; 11 (Suppl 14): 4 (abstract).

(74) Wetzler M, Kurzrock R, Taylor K et al. Constitutive and induced expression of growth factors in normal and chronic phase chronic myelogenous leukemia Ph' bone marrow stroma. *Cancer Res* 1990; 50: 5801–5.

(75) Wetzler M, Kurzrock R, Lowe DG, Kantarjian H, Gutterman JM, Talpaz M. Alteration in bone marrow adherent layer growth factor expression: a novel mechanism of chronic myelogenous leukaemia progression. *Blood* 1991; 78: 2400–6.

(76) Dowding CR. PhD Thesis 1991, University of London.

(77) Luikart SD. Degradation of cartilage proteoglycans by myeloid leukemia cells. *Exp Hematol* 1988; 16: 102–5.

(78) Yahalom J, Fibach E, Bar-Tana R, Fuks Z, Vlodavsky I. Differentiating human leukemia cells express heparanase that degrades heparan sulphate in subendothelial extracellular matrix. *Leuk Res* 1988;12: 711–7.

(79) Laskov R, Michaeli R-I, Sharir H, Yefenof E, Vlodavsky I. Production of heparanase by normal and neoplastic murine B lymphocytes. *Int J Cancer* 1991; 47: 92–8.

(80) Matrisian LM. Metalloproteinases and their inhibitors in matrix remodelling. *Trends Genet* 1990; 6: 121–5.

(81) Terui T, Niitsu Y, Mahara K et al. The production of transforming growth factor-β in acute megakaryoblastic leukemia and its possible implications in myelofibrosis. *Blood* 1990; 75: 1540–8.

(82) Oliver LJ, Keeton M, Wilson EL. Regulation and secretion of plasminogen activators and their inhibitors in a human leukemic cell line (K562). *Blood* 1989; 74: 1321–7.

(83) Kerr LD, Holt JD, Matrisian LM. Growth factors regulate transin gene expression by c-fos-dependent and c-fos-independent pathways. *Science* 1988; 242: 1424–7.

(84) Romero P, Blick M, Talpaz M, Murphy E, Hester J, Gutterman J. C-sis and c-abl expression in chronic myelogenous leukemia and other hematologic malignancies. *Blood* 1986; 67: 839–41.

(85) Mayani H, Guillbert LJ, Clarke SC, Belch AR, Janowska-Wieczorek A. Composition and functional integrity of the in vitro hemopoietic microenvironment in acute myelogenous leukemia: Effect of macrophage colony-stimulating factor. *Exp Hematol* 1992; 20: 1077–84.

(86) Mayani H, Guillbert LJ, Sych I, Janowska-Wieczorek A. Production of tumor necrosis factor α in human long-term marrow cultures from normal subjects and patients with acute myelogenous leukemia: Effect of recombinant macrophage colony-stimulating factor. *Leukemia* 1992; 6: 1148–54.

(87) Testa NG, Hendry JH, Molineux G. Long-term bone marrow damage after

cytotoxic treatment. In: NG Testa and RP Gale, eds. *Hematopoiesis: long-term effects of chemotherapy and radiation*. New York: Marcel Dekker Inc, 1988: 75–91.

(88) Ogle KM, Luikart SD. BCNU-induced increase in sulfated glycosaminoglycan production by human bone marrow stromal cells. *Exp Hemat* 1988; 16: 636–40.

(89) Orazi A, Cattoretti G, Schiro R et al. Recombinant human interleukin-3 and recombinant human granulocyte-macrophage colony-stimulating factor administered in vivo after high-dose cyclophosphamide cancer chemotherapy: Effect on hematopoiesis and microenvironment in human bone marrow. *Blood* 1992; 79: 2610–9.

(90) Gordon MY. The origin of stromal cells in patients treated by bone marrow transplantation. *Bone Marrow Transpl* 1988; 3: 247–51.

(91) Gordon MY, Aguado M, Grennan D. Human marrow stromal cells in culture: changes induced by T lymphocytes. *Blut* 1982; 44: 131–9.

(92) Kimura A, Katoh O, Kuramoto A. Effects of platelet derived growth factor, epidermal growth factor and transforming growth factor β on the growth of human bone marrow fibroblasts. *Br J Haematol* 1988; 69: 9–12.

(93) Takahashi N, MacDonald BR, Hon J et al. Recombinant human transforming growth factor-alpha stimulates the formation of osteoclast-like cells in long-term human marrow cultures. *J Clin Invest* 1988; 78: 894–8.

(94) Ignotz RA, Massague J. Transforming growth factor beta stimulates the expression of fibronectin and collagen and their incorporation into the extracellular matrix. *J Biol Chem* 1986; 261: 4337–45.

(95) Bassols A, Massague J. Transforming growth factor β regulates the expression and structure of extracellular matrix chondroitin/dermatan sulphate proteoglycans. *J Biol Chem* 1988; 263: 3039–45.

(96) Newton LK, Yung WKA, Pettigrew LC, Steck PA. Growth regulatory activities of endothelial extracellular matrix: mediation by transforming growth factor-β. *Exp Cell Res* 1990; 190: 127–32.

(97) Chen J-K, Hoshi H, McKeehan WL. Transforming growth factor type β specifically stimulates synthesis of proteoglycan in human arterial smooth muscle cells. *Proc Natl Acad Sci USA* 1987; 84: 5287–91.

(98) Postlethwaite AE, Smith GN, Lachman LB et al. Stimulation of glycosaminoglycan synthesis in cultured dermal fibroblast by interleukin-1. *J Clin Invest* 1989; 83: 629–36.

(99) Pettifer ER, Higgs GA, Henderson B. Interleukin-1 induces leukocyte infiltration and cartilage proteoglycan degradation in the synovial joint. *Proc Natl Acad Sci USA* 1986; 83: 8749–53.

(100) Dowding C, Guo A-P, Siczkowski M, Osterholz J, Goldman J, Gordon M. Interferon α overrides the deficient adhesion of CML primitive progenitor cells to bone marrow microenvironmental cells. *Blood* 1991; 78: 499–505.

(101) Kerr LD, Miller DB, Matrisian LM. TGFβ inhibition of transin/stromelysin gene expression is mediated through a Fos binding sequence. *Cell* 1990; 61: 267–78.

(102) Jonat C, Rahmsdorf HJ, Park K-K, Cato ACB, Gebel S, Ponta H, Herrlich P. Antitumor promotion and antiinflamation: Downmodulation of AP-1 (Fos/Jun) activity by glucocorticoid hormone. *Cell* 1990; 62: 1189–204.

(103) Schule R, Rangarajan P, Kliewer S et al. Functional antagonism between oncoprotein c-jun and the glucocorticoid receptor. *Cell* 1990; 62: 1217–26.

(104) Yang-Yen H-S, Chambard J-C, Sun Y-L et al. Transcriptional interface between c-jun and the glucocorticoid receptor. *Cell* 1990; 62: 1205–15.

(105) Saksela O, Moscatelli D, Rifkin DB. The opposing effects of basic fibroblast growth factor and transforming growth factor beta on the regulation of plasminogen activator activity in capillary endothelial cells. *J Cell Biol* 1987; 105: 957–67.

(106) Hannocks MJ, Oliver L, Gabrilove JL, Wilson EL. Regulation of proteolytic activity in human bone marrow stromal cells by basic fibroblast growth factor, interleukin-1 and TGFβ. *Blood* 1992; 79: 1178–84.

(107) Gimble JM. The function of adipocytes in the bone marrow stroma. *New Biol* 1990; 2: 304–12.

(108) Cashman JD, Eaves AC, Raines EW, Ross R, Eaves CJ. Mechanisms that regulate the cell cycle of very primitive hemopoietic cells in long-term human marrow cultures.I. Stimulatory role of a variety of mesenchymal cell activators and inhibitory role of TGF-beta. *Blood* 1990; 75: 96–101.

(109) Coutinho LH, Will A, Radford J, Schiro R, Testa NG, Dexter TM. Effects of recombinant human granulocyte colony-stimulating factor (CSF), human granulocyte macrophage CSF, and gibbon interleukin-3 on hematopoiesis in human long-term bone marrow culture. *Blood* 1990; 75: 2118–29.

(110) Mayani H, Guillbert LJ, Clarke SC, Janowska-Wieczorek A. Inhibition of hematopoiesis in normal human long-term marrow cultures treated with recombinant human macrophage colony-stimulating factor. *Blood* 1991; 78: 651–7.

(111) Clarke SC, The biology of human interleukin-11. In: Abraham NG, Konwalinka K, Marks P, Sachs L, Tavassoli M, eds. *Molecular biology of hematopoiesis volume 2*. Andover, Hants: Intercept Ltd, 1992: 65–72.

Comparing treatments for multiple myeloma: analysis in relation to the MRC trials

P WARBURTON, J A DUNN and I C M MacLENNAN

Introduction

Many different chemotherapy regimens have been used for the treatment of multiple myeloma. While treatment has prolonged survival, a curative regimen has not been identified. In general, there is uncertainty or disagreement about which, if any, of the available treatments is best. This has arisen largely due to lack of information from controlled trials which have studied sufficiently large numbers of patients. Furthermore, relatively few of the small trials have compared similar treatments. Even when there are several small trials addressing similar questions, such as the use of interferon-α for maintaining stable responses, these have not been subjected to a comprehensive overview of all the available data. Such an overview has been successful in identifying the real benefits of adjuvant therapy in early breast cancer.[1,2] There is clearly a need for a properly conducted overview of therapy in multiple myeloma. Although we may be confident that curative therapies have not been missed, it is possible that we have failed to identify treatments which are capable of significantly prolonging survival compared with others which are frequently used.

The MRC myelomatosis trials

Since 1964 the MRC Working Party on Leukaemia in Adults has conducted six prospective randomized trials with large numbers of patients with multiple myeloma. The aim of these trials has been to test those treatments which appear most likely on the basis of existing data to prolong survival. The more recent trials have investigated the following:

All correspondence to: Professor ICM MacLennan, MRC Myelomatosis Trials Office, PO BOX 1894, Vincent Drive, Edgbaston, Birmingham B15 2SZ, UK.

1. Does the addition of vincristine as a bolus injection to intermittent melphalan and prednisone therapy prolong survival? (IVth trial)
2. Does the addition of an anthracycline and nitrosourea to the widely used alkylating agents melphalan and cyclophosphamide (ABCM) offer advantages over intermittent melphalan therapy? (Vth trial)
3. Does the addition of cytoreductive doses of prednisolone, which produce faster and greater serological responses, increase survival when added to the ABCM regimen? (VIth trial)
4. Is it useful to continue first-line therapy after patients have reached plateau phase? (IIIrd and IVth trials)
5. Does the administration of interferon-α during first plateau phase prolong plateau or survival? (current interferon-α trial)

The importance of staging only using factors which are of independent prognostic significance

Each MRC myeloma trial has collected data on presentation factors and these have been reviewed on several occasions with respect to their usefulness as prognostic factors. Analysis of these prognostic factors has allowed recognition of the heterogeneity of disease behaviour in multiple myeloma. It has also highlighted the difficulty of comparing treatments in different studies in which the spectrum of patients, as defined by reliable prognostic factors, has not been reported. If patients have been stratified by prognostic groups, it is possible to compare groups with equivalent prognoses. In the MRC trials, the rates of entry and the proportions of patients with good and poor prognoses have varied. This effect is likely to be much greater when comparing treatments given by different trial organizations for reasons which will be discussed later. Stratifying for prognostic factors will not account for all the differences between trials. Treatment may not be given equally well in different centres, especially with intensive regimens. This is exemplified by the marked improvement in the prognosis of AML that resulted from advances in supportive care for these patients, even though the drugs used had altered little. This is probably not a major factor with conventional low dose chemotherapy and similar treatments given in sequential MRC trials have yielded reproducible results when comparable prognostic groups are analysed (Tables 1 and 2).[3]

Staging systems

Data collected on patients entered in the MRC IIIrd myelomatosis trial were used to develop a prognostic classification which has become known as the Cuzick Index.[4] Presentation clinical and laboratory data were analysed on 485 patients. Three factors were identified as being of far greater importance than any others: a measure of post rehydration renal function (either blood urea concentration or serum creatinine), haemoglobin level and performance

Table 1. *Comparative survival for different treatment regimens stratified by presentation serum β2 microglobulin*

Serum β2 microglobulin	Treatment	Trial	No*	Months to percentile of survival†		
				75th	50th (median)	25th
≤4 mg/l	MP or MVP	IV	158	18.8	38.5	70.8
	M7	V	45	18.1	39.1	64.4
	ABCM	V	50	41.6	58.3	>84.0
	ABCM	VI	87	24.2	43.9	>69.0
	ABCMP	VI	94	18.7	41.1	63.7
>4–≤8 mg/l	MP or MVP	IV	186	11.1	28.0	52.2
	M7	V	123	13.7	30.5	46.1
	ABCM	V	130	17.7	36.4	60.0
	ABCM	VI	148	17.2	33.0	>69.0
	ABCMP	VI	133	15.9	36.6	59.5
>8 mg/l	MP or MVP	IV	156	1.8	13.5	29.0
	M7	V	132	5.7	14.5	33.3
	ABCM	V	114	6.3	19.0	41.8
	ABCM	VI	103	7.4	23.0	46.6
	ABCMP	VI	109	2.4	12.8	40.8

* number of patients in each treatment arm.
† indicates number of months from entry to trial when percentage of patients shown remained alive.

Table 2. *Cross-trial analysis of comparative survival in the IVth, Vth and VIth trial treatment groups after stratification for prognostic factors*

Prognostic factor	Trial and treatment*	χ^2	P
Serum β2 microglobulin	V M7<IV MVP<IV MP	0.3	0.9
	V ABCM>V M7	8.8	0.003
	V ABCM<VI ABCM	0.2	0.7
Cuzick Index	V M7<IV MVP<IV MP	5.0	0.08
	V ABCM>V M7	11.2	0.0008
	V ABCM<VI ABCM	1.8	0.18

* number of patients on each therapy: IV MP-262; IV MVP-266; V M7–316; V ABCM-314; VI ABCM-317.

status (Table 3). These had independent prognostic significance while other factors, although of prognostic importance when considered alone, did not add to the prognostic information obtained using the Cuzick index. This index divides patients into three groups, which have significantly different

Table 3. *Prognostic groupings of the Cuzick Index*

Group	Criteria	Percentage* of patients	2 Year* Survival (%)
I. Good	BUC†≤8 mM *and* Hb≥10.0 g/dl *and* no or minimal symptoms	22	76
II. Intermediate	belonging to neither groups I or II	56	50
III. Poor	either BUC≥10 mM or Hb≤7.5 g/dl *and* restricted activity	22	9

* blood urea concentration.

† percentage and 2 year survival in each strata for patients in the MRC IIIrd trial.

survival durations (χ^2=117.1, p<0.0001 for the IIIrd trial). To verify the independent predictive power of the prognostic groups, they were applied to patients in the MRC Ist and IInd trials. In both of these trials the three groups had significantly different survivals (χ^2=53.0, p<0.001 for Ist trial; χ^2=44.9, p<0.0001 for IInd trial). The application of the index in subsequent trials has continued to show its usefulness not just in trials of melphalan-based regimens[5] but also in those of combination chemotherapy regimens[3] (χ^2=36.31, p<0.0001 for IVth trial; χ^2=46.6, p<0.0001 for Vth trial). Since the introduction of routine continued high fluid intake in patients with renal failure in the IVth trial and all patients in subsequent trials, the blood urea concentration has less predictive power but it still remains an important prognostic factor (χ^2=102, p<0.0001 for IIIrd trial compared to χ^2=46.6, p>0.0001 for IVth trial).[4,5] This measure considerably reduces the mortality and morbidity associated with renal failure, dehydration and hypercalcaemia.[6]

Two other major staging systems were developed at approximately the same time. The Durie and Salmon staging system (DS) was devised to reflect myeloma cell mass.[7] Patients were divided into three stages on the basis of haemoglobin, serum calcium, extent of radiological bone disease and the paraprotein level with serum creatinine used to divide each stage into A and B. The Merlini–Waldenström–Jayakar staging system (MWJ) divided patients into three groups on the basis of serum creatinine, serum calcium and bone marrow plasma cell percentage for IgG and Bence-Jones only myeloma and haemoglobin, serum calcium and serum paraprotein level for IgA myeloma.[8] Both of these systems were based on the analysis of possible prognostic factors in smaller groups of patients than that used by the MRC study: 71 for the DS and 123 for the MWJ. In studies which have compared these three staging systems, the Cuzick Index was superior in three studies [9–11] and the DS in one.[12] These staging systems have been criticized for various reasons. First, all three staging systems contain a variable which can be considered at least partially subjective: the assessment of the extent of lytic bone lesions in the DS, performance status in the Cuzick Index and the percentage of bone marrow plasma cells in the MWJ.[12] Secondly, the MWJ and DS systems contain variables which have been identified in other studies as having either no or limited prognostic import. The serum paraprotein level, which is used in both systems, had no prognostic significance for IgG myelomas in either the MRC II[13] or III[4] myelomatosis trials. For IgA myelomas it was not significant in the MRC II trial but did attain significance in the IIIrd trial (p=0.004). However the χ^2 value was low at 8.43 and it did not retain significance after correction for the three most important prognostic factors in this trial. The extent of osteolytic bone lesions, which is used in the DS system, has been analysed as a single variable for the MRC IV and V trials and the SWOG M8229 trial.[14] The presence of osteolytic lesions was only weakly associated with a poor prognosis, approaching statistical significance only in MRC IV (χ^2=3.84, p=0.05 for MRC IV; χ^2=4.05, p=0.13 for MRC V; χ^2=4.61, p=0.1 for SWOG M8229). Furthermore, in the DS system the emphasis on the presence of lytic bone lesions is such that it is responsible for the allocation of the majority of patients, at least in large multicentre trials, to Stage III, the group with worst prognosis. In each of the three trials mentioned above, at least 78% of patients were in DS stage III, whereas the patient numbers were more evenly distributed between the three groups of the Cuzick Index. The Cuzick Index gave a better discrimination between the groups in terms of prognosis with a χ^2=50 compared to χ^2=18 for the DS system.[14] Other factors, particularly serum β2 microglobulin, which have been identified in the last 15 years, are capable of identifying prognostic groups within the DS stage III patients.

Serum β2 microglobulin

β2 microglobulin (β2m) is the invariant β polypeptide chain of HLA Class I molecules which are present on almost all nucleated cells in the body. β2m is present in the serum as a result of membrane turnover. It is freely filtered by the renal glomeruli and normally is catabolized by the tubules.[15,16] Serum levels of β2m (sβ2m) rise when the glomerular filtration rate decreases and there is a strong correlation with serum creatinine.[17–19] In disease sβ2m is a balance between the production rate and its clearance from the blood by glomerular filtration. Both of these factors can be abnormal in myelomatosis and both contribute to the strong prognostic value of this analyte.

In the MRC IVth myelomatosis trial 476 of 530 patients entered had available presentation information for sβ2m, blood urea concentration, serum creatinine, haemoglobin and performance status.[5] Serum β2 microglobulin, not corrected for serum creatinine, was the single most powerful prognostic variable (χ^2=58.21, df=4, p<0.0001) (Fig. 1). Uncorrected sβ2m was more powerful than the corrected value because the contribution due to renal failure is an important element of the prognostic value of sβ2m. On multivariate analysis of sβ2m, creatinine, haemoglobin and performance status, only the haemoglobin value provided some additional information to that provided by sβ2m. Serum β2m adds to the prognostic value of serum creatinine but the opposite is not the case, reflecting a prognostic component to sβ2m which is independent of renal failure. In both this trial[5] and a cross-trial analysis of later MRC and SWOG trials,[14] sβ2m was also of greater predictive value for survival than the prognostic groups based on the Cuzick Index, which in turn was more powerful than the DS staging system.

Other studies of prognostic factors in myeloma have also concluded that sβ2m at diagnosis is a prognostic factor for survival[18–20] and frequently it has been identified as the single most important factor.[11,12,21–24] Serum β2m as a continuous variable has been found to be better than either the Cuzick, DS or MWJ staging systems and it has been suggested that it may be useful to combine sβ2m and the Cuzick Index.[11]

The role of sβ2m for monitoring disease activity in myeloma has been disputed. One group has reported that it was of no value[25] but most groups have reported that sβ2m is useful for monitoring disease activity in patients with normal renal function.[5,22,26–28]

Plasma cell labelling index
The other important prognostic variables identified during the last decade were measures of the proliferative activity of the myeloma cells. The most

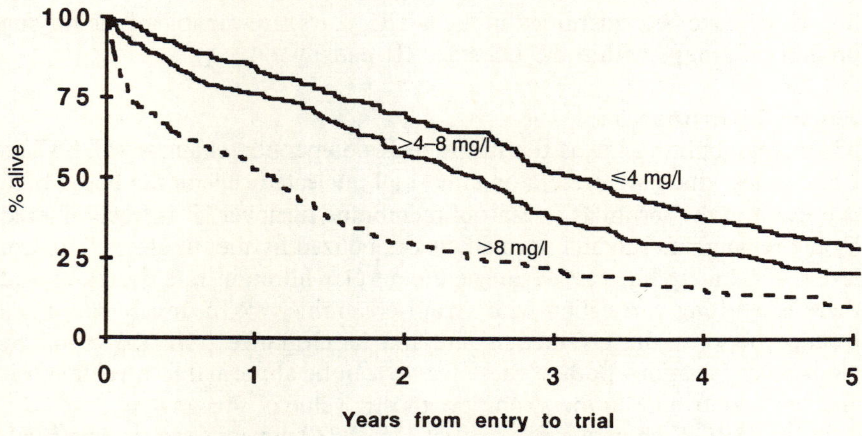

Fig. 1. Survival after stratification by presentation serum β2 microglobulin for the IVth trial.

$$(\chi^2=51.34, df=2, p<0.0001)$$

100

commonly used of such variables is the plasma cell labelling index (Ll), which measures the percentage of cells in S-phase of the cell cycle. There are several methods available, including the use of tritiated thymidine autoradiography or immunofluorescence methods using antibodies to 5-bromo-2-deoxyuridine.[29,30] The Ll has found several roles in assessing myeloma patients. First, it is predictive of survival at diagnosis[19,31-33] and adds independent prognostic information to that provided by sβ2m. Secondly, it can be used during plateau to monitor for the onset of disease progression.[20,34,35] Thirdly, it helps to distinguish patients with monoclonal gammopathy of uncertain significance or smouldering multiple myeloma from patients with active myeloma requiring therapy.[20,31,34-37] The Ll has not been assessed in any MRC trials only because it is not easily applied in a reliable way to large multicentre trials.

Treatment of multiple myeloma

Introduction

Prior to the introduction of melphalan in 1958, the median and mean survivals from the time of diagnosis for patients with multiple myeloma were 3.5 and 11.2 months, respectively.[38] The reported median survival using melphalan with or without prednisone ranges from 19 months upwards[39,40] with 2–4% of patients being alive 10 years after diagnosis.[41,42] Whether the introduction of various combination chemotherapy regimens has improved prognosis further has been a contentious issue for the last decade and the focus of numerous trials. When the literature is reviewed, there have been few large prospective randomised trials comparing combination chemotherapy regimens with single alkylating agents with or without steroids. A recent review of 18 prospective randomized trials of a broad range of different combination chemotherapies versus melphalan plus prednisone (MP) highlighted the problems of interpreting the literature on this subject.[43]★ Only 7 of these trials had more than 100 patients in each arm of the trial. The median survival times for both MP and combination regimens were notable for their wide range: being, respectively, 19–50 months and 24–45 months. It is improbable that the details of administration of low dose melphalan-based regimens or the available supportive care varied sufficiently between the centres entering patients to different trials to explain the differences in survival obtained with MP. It is far more plausible that like is not being compared to like. In some trials different eligibility criteria may result in patients with smouldering multiple myeloma, who do well when not given chemotherapy,[46,47] being included. In multicentre trials physicians' attitudes and

★ Problems with the methods used in this overview of trials have been discussed in detail.[44,45] Consequently its conclusions about the relative value of MP and combination regimens are not cited.

perceptions of a given trial may influence the spectrum of patients entered into the trial. These points can be illustrated by experience in the IVth, Vth and VIth trials (Table 1). When patients were divided into prognostic groups based on sβ2m levels, the proportion of patients in the best prognostic group in the Vth trial was 16% compared to 32% in the IVth trial and the rate of entry into the Vth trial was lower. It is plausible that this reflects an unwillingness in 1982 of the physicians to enter good prognosis patients into a trial testing a combination regimen that was perceived to be more intensive and hazardous than MP. By 1986, when the VIth trial started, ABCM was no longer thought to be hard to give and physicians again started to enter more good prognosis patients.

Addition of an anthracycline and nitrosourea to alkylating agents

The Vth MRC myelomatosis trial was a large prospective randomized trial comparing melphalan to a combination of two alkylating agents plus adriamycin and BCNU.[3] The doses of adriamycin and BCNU used in the Vth trial had been shown to be effective for treating both relapsed patients and those progressing on first-line therapy with melphalan-based regimens by Alberts et al[48] and this was subsequently confirmed in MRC trials.[49] Over 600 patients were randomized into the Vth trial: 316 to receive intermittent oral melphalan (M7) and 314 to receive ABCM (adriamycin, BCNU, cyclophosphamide and melphalan). The actuarial survival was significantly longer for patients receiving ABCM (p=0.0003). The 75th, median and 25th percentile survival times were 7, 24 and 42 months for M7 and 10, 32 and 56 months for ABCM. The difference in survival time in the two treatment groups remained significant after correction for the presentation prognostic factors sβ2m, serum creatinine, haemoglobin, Cuzick Index, Durie–Salmon stage and age.[3]

The number and degree of serological responses were similar for both therapies but the proportion of patients achieving plateau was significantly higher with ABCM (61%) than M7 (49%) (χ^2=8.1, p=0.004) (Table 4). Plateau phase is a state of disease stability when patients have no more than minimal symptoms attributable to active disease, no transfusion requirement and serological stability. Attainment of plateau is now recognised as being more important than the degree of serological response. Several studies have demonstrated that survival does not correlate with the attainment of response as defined by either SWOG or the Chronic Leukemia–Myeloma Task Force criteria.[50,51] The actual percentage fall in paraprotein also fails to correlate with duration of plateau or survival.[52,53] Consequently patients cannot be considered to have progressive disease requiring an alternative chemotherapy regimen solely on the basis of the absence of a fall in paraprotein although this is still done in some trials. Such patients do not have a survival different to those who have an obvious serological response followed by plateau phase.[53] These findings have been confirmed in the Vth and VIth trials.

Table 4. *Response to treatment in Vth MRC trial*

	M7		ABCM	
Response*	Number†	Plateau (%)‡	Number	Plateau (%)
Complete	27	89	25	96
Partial	159	67	167	80
Stable	38	58	46	61
Progression	17	0	9	0
Nonsecretor	4	75	2	0
Early death	57	0	44	0
Inadequate data	11	9	12	42
Major treatment deviation	3	–	9	–
Total	316	49	314	61

* complete-total loss of serum and urine paraprotein; partial-reduction of serum paraprotein by >25% or reduction in urinary light chain output by >50%; stable-stable
disease or decrease in paraprotein level or light chain output less than that required
for partial response; early death-death before first follow-up at 3 months
† number of patients
‡ percentage of patients reaching plateau in each response group

Patients treated with ABCM who did not achieve a defined serological
response but did not have progressive disease *ab initio* (nonresponders) did
not have a significantly different survival from those who had either a com-
plete or objective serological response ($\chi^2=2.95$, p=0.23 for Vth trial; $\chi^2=0.49$, p=0.78 for VIth trial). Patients who became asymptomatic but were
serologically nonresponders were considered to have reached plateau and
their survival from reaching plateau was a little better than those who attained
plateau following either a complete or objective serological response (Fig. 2).

In the MRC V myelomatosis trial therapy was discontinued when plateau
was reached. The duration of first plateau phase and survival after reaching
plateau were longer in those patients receiving ABCM but did not reach the
level of significance ($\chi^2=1.5$, p=0.22 for plateau duration; $\chi^2=2.8$, p=0.09
for survival). Thus the longer survival with ABCM therapy is due to the
increased number of patients reaching plateau. ABCM was not associated
with more bone marrow depression than M7 and the other toxicities (eg
alopecia, nausea) were not excessive.[3]

One potential criticism of the MRC V trial might be that melphalan is
inferior to melphalan plus prednisone and that this resulted in combination
chemotherapy appearing to prolong survival. Trials comparing melphalan
with melphalan and prednisone are limited and the results contradictory
with only two studies suggesting a survival advantage from the addition of
prednisone. Alexanian and colleagues[54] grouped patients receiving melphalan
intermittently or continuously as a single agent and compared their survival

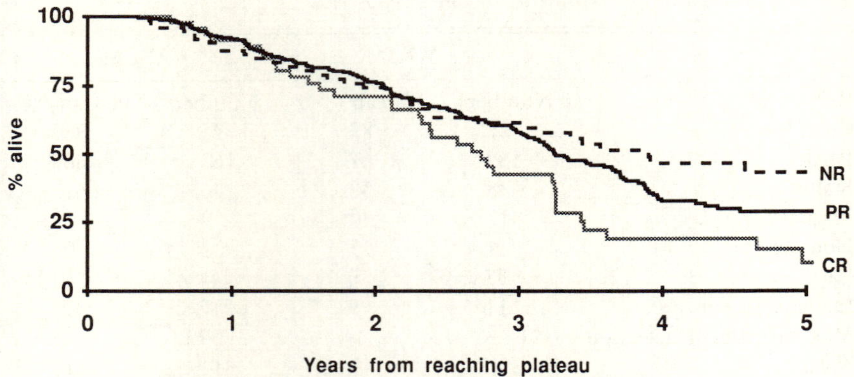

Fig. 2. Survival from reaching plateau stratified by serological response for patients treated with ABCM in the Vth and VIth trials.
Serological response groups: CR-total loss of serum and urine paraprotein; PR-reduction of serum paraprotein by >25% or reduction in urinary light chain output by >50%; NR-stable disease or decrease in paraprotein level or light chain output less than that required for partial response.

to a combined group of patients receiving melphalan and prednisone on different protocols. The patients receiving both melphalan and prednisone had a survival advantage that just reached the level of significance (p<0.05). The Cancer and Leukemia Group B studied the addition of both vincristine and prednisone (VP) at week 22 of induction chemotherapy. In an 8-way randomization of 302 patients they found significantly increased response rates and survival in patients receiving VP with melphalan but not in those receiving VP with nitrosoureas.[55] On the other hand a small randomized study (<50 patients in each arm) found no survival advantage from adding prednisone to melphalan.[56] The MRC II myelomatosis trial prospectively randomized 124 patients to daily oral cyclophosphamide, 128 to intermittent oral melphalan and 120 to intermittent oral melphalan and prednisone. There was no difference in survival between the three arms but this too was a small study.[13] Cross-trial analysis of prognostic subgroups based on sβ2m and Cuzick Index for the melphalan-based regimens in the IVth and Vth trials showed that there was little difference between the survival achieved using melphalan and prednisone with or without vincristine (MP and MVP) in the IVth trial and melphalan without steroids in the Vth trial (Tables 1 and 2).[14] Similarly the performance of ABCM within the Vth trial was equivalent to that in the VIth trial. Overall the conclusion is that ABCM is superior to melphalan with or without corticosteroids.

Role of cytoreductive doses of glucocorticoids

There has been interest in the use of intermediate or high dose glucocorticoids in myelomatosis as they are capable of inducing a rapid reduction in the size of the malignant clone. The MRC VIth myelomatosis trial investigated the role of a cytoreductive dose of steroids in addition to the combination chemotherapy regimen ABCM. In the arm randomized to receive glucocorticoids, prednisolone 60 mg/m^2/day for 5 days every 14 days was given for four courses at the commencement of treatment. This trial was closed after the entry of 683 patients as at that time patients receiving prednisolone had a significantly shorter survival (χ^2=13.2, p=0.024), even though the addition of prednisolone resulted in more rapid cytoreduction with a shorter time to reach plateau. There was an excess of deaths in the first 100 days in the group receiving prednisolone mainly due to progressive tumour with a small number due to infection or cardiac failure. With further follow-up, as early deaths have come to be a smaller proportion of total deaths, the difference in survival for these two therapies has become nonsignificant (χ^2= 1.528, p= 0.22). After correction for known prognostic factors at presentation, survival remains nonsignificant. The median time to plateau was significantly shorter for ABCMP at 5.7 months compared to 8.2 months for ABCM (χ^2=19.023, p>0.0001) (Fig. 3). For those patients reaching plateau, survival from the time of reaching plateau was similar for both treatment arms with a median of 41.2 months for ABCM and 38.6 months for ABCMP (χ^2=0.096, p= 0.76).

There have been other studies of cytoreductive doses of glucocorticoids as either a single agent or as part of a combination regimen. Intermediate dose oral prednisolone has been used in a small group of patients with refractory or relapsing multiple myeloma at a dose of 60 mg/m^2 for 5 consecutive days at fortnightly intervals.[57] Ten of 17 patients responded to this regimen and eight attained plateau. An ECOG pilot study[58] of single agent oral

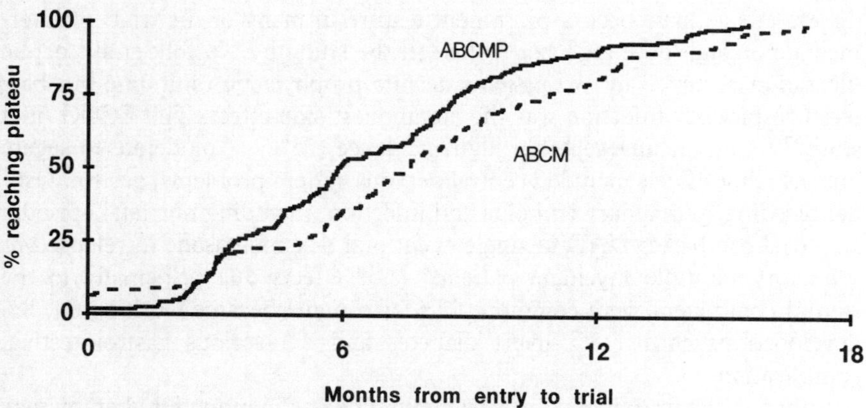

Fig. 3. Time to plateau for patients in the VIth trial.

$$(\chi^2=19.023, \ p<0.0001)$$

dexamethasone at 40 mg daily for 4 days every week for 8 weeks and then fortnightly also reported responses in refractory and relapsing patients. A phase II trial of interferon-α plus dexamethasone in patients who failed to achieve an objective response with first-line therapy resulted in further reductions in paraprotein levels in some cases.[59]

VAD comprises vincristine 0.4 mg/day and adriamycin 9 mg/m^2/day administered as a continuous infusion for 4 days every 5 weeks and oral dexamethasone 40mg daily for four days starting on days 1, 9 and 17 of each cycle. This was originally used in a small group of refractory patients and produced high response rates and survival times.[60] VAD-based regimens in previously untreated patients have subsequently been compared to melphalan and prednisone in an historical control group of patients.[61] Although the responses were more rapid with the VAD-based protocols, the response rates, remission duration and survival times were no better than with melphalan and prednisone. It was concluded that VAD-based regimens should only be used for salvage treatment except if there was a clinical indication for obtaining a rapid response in untreated patients. VAD has been compared to oral dexamethasone given as a single agent in the same doses as the VAD protocol in both patients with relapsed myeloma and in patients who had never achieved an adequate serological response to previous chemotherapy.[62] The response rates were the same for both therapies in patients who had been refractory to previous treatment but were significantly better for VAD in relapsed patients. However, the survival times were no better in any of the patient groups receiving VAD. Thus, at least in refractory patients, the effective agent in the VAD regimen would appear to be the high dose dexamethasone. The same conclusion was reached when high dose dexamethasone was administered to untreated patients and the results compared to an historical group treated with VAD.[63]

Side effects have been a prominent feature in many of the trials of intermediate or high dose glucocorticoids. In the study by Norfolk et al[57] peptic ulceration occurred in two patients despite prophylactic ranitidine but bacterial respiratory infection was the commonest side effect. The ECOG pilot study[58] found an unacceptably high incidence (55%) of moderate to severe toxicity. Side effects included central nervous system problems, gastrointestinal bleeding, pulmonary embolus and infection, including one fatal episode. In a trial comparing VAD to single agent oral dexamethasone in relapsed or refractory multiple myeloma patients[60] side effects due principally to the steroid component were common: 22% of patients became Cushingoid, 8% developed psychosis, 5% overt diabetes and 2% serious gastrointestinal complications.

Although the introduction of dexamethasone late in induction therapy may be beneficial, this is probably not the case for cytoreductive doses of corticosteroids at the beginning of therapy. The potential side effects of cytoreductive doses of glucocorticoids must be balanced against the potential benefits of rapid response in individual patients. Steroids used as a single agent or in addition to multiagent chemotherapy in these doses may be useful for specific indications such as the presence of symptomatic hyperviscosity or the need to avoid myelosuppressive agents in the small proportion of patients who present with pancytopenia. In the Vth trial which randomized 630 patients to either M7 or ABCM, there was an additional 60 patients who were not randomized but were treated with weekly intravenous cyclophosphamide as they had neutropenia ($<1.8\times10^9/1$) or thrombocytopenia ($<1.8\times10^9/1$) at presentation. Regimens such as VAD and VAMP may have a role in cytoreduction prior to intensive cytotoxic therapy with bone marrow rescue as they have the advantage of less myelotoxicity than MP or ABCM.

The role of vincristine

Vincristine is commonly included in combination chemotherapy regimens but there is very little evidence to support its use. A SWOG study in 1975 compared three regimens: melphalan and prednisone; melphalan, prednisone and procarbazine; melphalan, prednisone, procarbazine and vincristine as a bolus intravenous injection every 10–14 days. This was not a randomized study but at least 140 patients were entered into each arm. The response rates and survivals were not significantly different between arms. A subsequent nonrandomized SWOG study compared nine chemotherapy regimens including the three reported previously. In the survival analysis the 305 patients who received the three regimens containing bolus vincristine were compared to 727 patients receiving six regimens without vincristine. An assessment of this complex of trials led to the conclusion that the survival was longer in those receiving vincristine. They did not report the results obtained by comparing the chemotherapy regimens in which vincristine was the only variable. As discussed in the previous section, the Cancer and Leukemia Group B in a complex trial with eight small groups found some evidence of benefit of vincristine and prednisone added to melphalan therapy after the first 22 weeks of cytotoxic therapy.

There has only been one randomized study in which the incorporation of bolus vincristine as part of induction therapy as used by Alexanian was the only variable. In the MRC IVth myelomatosis trial 530 patients were randomized to receive either melphalan 10 mg daily and prednisone 40 mg daily for 7 days every 4 weeks or to receive these same drugs plus vincristine on day one of each cycle. The survival of patients was not improved by the addition of vincristine even after adjustment for known prognostic factors at presentation ($\chi^2=1.5$, p=0.225 uncorrected; $\chi^2=0.16$, p=0.69 after correction for presentation serum $\beta2$ microglobulin).

Vincristine has also been given as a continuous infusion and it is theoretically possible that it may be more active when administered in this way. The best known of these protocols is VAD. Recent studies have attempted to elucidate which of the component drugs are primarily responsible for the reduction of the myeloma clone with this regimen. As was discussed in the previous section, comparison of VAD versus dexamethasone suggested that most of the effect was due to high dose dexamethasone.[62,63]

Maintenance therapy of multiple myeloma
Continuing chemotherapy

Several studies have considered the optimal duration of chemotherapy in multiple myeloma. When melphalan initially became available the usual practice was to continue therapy from the time of diagnosis until death, especially as complete responses or cures were rare. In a review of the patterns of response to initial induction chemotherapy, almost half the patients had an initial response followed by stable disease (plateau phase) irrespective of the continuation of chemotherapy.[66] This raised the possibility that chemotherapy could be ceased after achieving disease stability. There are arguments in favour of limiting the duration of first-line chemotherapy. The possibility of drug resistance may be reduced, thus increasing the chance of obtaining a second response to therapy. The quality of life for the patients would be improved during the time off therapy. Reducing the total dose of alkylating agents may reduce the incidence of secondary myelodysplasia and acute leukaemia. These disorders were very rare in patients treated to plateau with melphalan containing regimens in the IVth and Vth MRC trials but were common with the continuous alkylating agent regimens used in the Ist and IInd trials.

There have been several trials of chemotherapy maintenance versus no maintenance. The criteria for and timing of randomization have varied but, despite this, none of the trials demonstrated a survival advantage for continuing chemotherapy.[67,69,70–75] Two of the six studies which analysed remission duration found an advantage for maintenance but there was no difference in survival as these patients responded to the reintroduction of chemotherapy.[73,75] In one of these studies[75] it is possible that many patients, although responding, were not stable as they had received only 6 months of therapy prior to randomization. The median time to plateau as assessed within studies is approximately nine months[3,53] but there is marked variability in the time taken to reach plateau.[53] For patients treated with ABCM in the VIth trial, the range was 0–23 months with 25% of patients reaching plateau in 5.5 months, 75% in 11.5 months and 95% in 18 months (Fig. 3). The IVth trial analysed the outcome in patients reaching plateau rapidly. This group has a significantly shorter survival than slow responders (χ^2=5.9, p=0.015) to but this was not due to them receiving less chemotherapy. For fast responders who were randomized to continue treatment during plateau, there was a trend towards shorter survival compared to those who ceased therapy.[49]

108

Interferon-α

Recently attention has been focussed on the use of interferon-α as a maintenance agent. Similar to the trials of continuing chemotherapy, the randomization criteria have varied: some based principally on the requirement for a defined serological response[59,76,77] and others on the attainment of plateau phase disease,[78,79] (such as the current MRC interferon-α trial). The former criteria may allow the randomization of patients who have responded but are not stable and exclude some patients with 'inadequate' response but stable disease. This latter group of patients constituted 14% of patients reaching plateau in the MRC Vth myelomatosis trial.[3] Only 2 studies have enrolled more than 200 patients.[59] The other trials contain ≤120 patients. This may present a problem in analysing the results as myeloma is very heterogeneous in terms of disease behaviour, as has already been discussed. No results have been released for the MRC trial and so far definitive results have only just been published for the Italian study[76] which enrolled 101 patients. There was a significantly longer duration of remission in patients receiving interferon (p=0.0002) and also a trend towards longer survival (p<0.06). For the 4 studies with published interim analysis, 1 has reported a significantly longer remission duration with interferon[77] and 3, including the SWOG study of 210 patients when the median follow-up was 10 months, have found no significant difference.[59,78,79] The median duration of remission has not yet been published. One of the major problems when assessing the results of these studies is the short duration of remission in the control arms. The MRC Vth and VIth trials treated 662 patients with ABCM, of whom 420 reached plateau. The median duration of unmaintained plateau was 18.9 and 19.8 months in the Vth and VIth trials respectively. The remission duration of the control groups in the interferon studies has been less than that in this group of patients in the four studies for which it has been published[76–79] and the remission duration of the interferon arm has been less in 3 of these 4 trials.[77–79] Thus the role of interferon as maintenance therapy of myeloma is not yet clear and the results of the larger randomized trials are awaited as is the outcome of formal meta-analysis, especially if only a subgroup of patients benefits from interferon.

Conclusion

The MRC trials have shown that real differences exist between commonly used treatments. There is a need for further trials to compare different regimens. Improved staging of patients using factors of independent prognostic significance will facilitate comparison of similar treatments in these trials. Factors such as sβ2m and the Cuzick Index provide a simple and reliable means of dividing patients into prognostic groups. Important new data should be available on the relative value of different treatments if there is near universal participation in overviews of comparable randomized trials.

P Warburton, J A Dunn and I C M MacLennan

References

(1) Early Breast Cancer Triallists' Collaborative Group. Systemic treatment of early breast cancer by hormonal, cytotoxic, or immune therapy. *Lancet* 1992; 339: 1–15.

(2) Early Breast Cancer Triallists' Collaborative Group. Systemic treatment of early breast cancer by hormonal, cytotoxic, or immune therapy. *Lancet* 1992; 339: 71–85.

(3) MacLennan ICM, Chapman C, Dunn J, Kelly K. Combined chemotherapy with ABCM versus melphalan for treatment of myelomatosis. *Lancet* 1992; 339: 200–5.

(4) Medical Research Council's Working Party on Leukaemia in Adults. Prognostic features in the third MRC myelomatosis trial. *Br J Cancer* 1980*b*; 42: 831–40.

(5) Cuzick J, Cooper EH, MacLennan ICM. The prognostic value of serum β2 microglobulin compared with other presentation features in myelomatosis. (A report to the Medical Research Council's Working Party on Leukaemia in Adults.) *Br J Cancer* 1985; 52: 1–6.

(6) MRC Working Party on Leukaemia in Adults. Analysis and management of renal failure in fourth MRC myelomatosis trial. *Br J Haematol* 1984: 288: 1411–6.

(7) Durie BGM, Salmon SE. A clinical staging system for multiple myeloma. Correlation of measured myeloma cell mass with presenting clinical features, response to treatment, and survival. *Cancer* 1975; 36: 842–54.

(8) Merlini G, Waldenström JG, Jayakar SD. A new improved clinical staging system for multiple myeloma based on analysis of 123 treated patients. *Blood* 1980; 55: 1011–9.

(9) Gassman W, Pralle H, Haferlach T et al. Staging systems for multiple myeloma: a comparison. *Br J Haematol* 1985; 59: 703–10.

(10) San Miguel JF, Sànchez J, Gonzalez M. Prognostic factors and classification in multiple myeloma. *Br J Cancer* 1989; 59: 113–8.

(11) Gobbi PG, Bertolini D, Grignani G et al. A plea to overcome the concept of 'staging' and related inadequacy in multiple myeloma. *Eur J Haematol* 1991; 46: 177–81.

(12) Bataille R, Durie BGM, Grenier J, Sany J. Prognostic factors and staging in multiple myeloma: a reappraisal. *J Clin Oncol* 1986; 4: 80–7.

(13) Medical Research Council's Working Party on Leukaemia in Adults. Report on the second myelomatosis trial after five years of follow-up. *Br J Cancer* 1980; 42: 813–22.

(14) Kelly KA, Durie B, MacLennan IC. Prognostic factors and staging systems for multiple myeloma: comparisons between the Medical Research Council studies in the United Kingdom and the Southwest Oncology Group studies in the United States. *Hematol Oncol* 1988; 6: 131–40.

(15) Berggärd I, Bearn AG. (1968) Isolation and properties of a low molecular weight B2-globulin occurring in human biological fluids. *J Biol Chem* 1968; 243: 4095–103.

(16) Peterson PA, Rask L, Lindblom B. Highly purified papain-solubilised HL-A antigens contain beta 2-microglobulin. *Proc Natl Acad Sci USA* 1974; 71: 35–9.

(17) Wibell L, Evrin PE, Berggärd J. Serum β_2 microglobulin in renal disease. *Nephron* 1973; 10: 320–31.

(18) Van Dobbenburgh OA, Rodenhuis S, Ockhuizen Th et al. Serum beta₂-microglobulin: a real improvement in the management of multiple myeloma? *Br J Haematol* 1985; 61: 611–20.

(19) Greipp PR, Katzmann JA, O'Fallon WM, Kyle RA. Value of β_2-microglobulin level and plasma cell labeling indices as prognostic factors in patients with newly diagnosed myeloma. *Blood* 1988; 72: 219–23.

(20) Boccadoro M, Durie BGM, Frutiger Y et al. Lack of correlation between plasma cell labelling index and serum beta-2-microglobulin in monoclonal gammopathies. *Acta Haemat* 1987; 78: 239–41.

(21) Simonsson B, Källander CFR, Brenning G et al. Biochemical markers in multiple myeloma: a multivariate analysis. *Br J Haematol* 1988; 69: 47–53.

(22) Cuzick J, De Stavola BL, Cooper EH, Chapman C, MacLennan ICM. Long-term prognostic value of serum β_2 microglobulin in myelomatosis. *Br J Haematol* 1990; 75: 506–10.

(23) Durie BG, Stock-Novack D, Salmon SE et al. Prognostic value of pretreatment serum beta 2 microglobulin in myeloma: a Southwest Oncology Group Study. *Blood* 1990; 75: 823–30.

(24) San Miguel JF, González M, Gascón A et al. Lymphoid subsets and prognostic factors in multiple myeloma. *Br J Haematol* 1992; 80: 305–9.

(25) Boccadoro M, Omedè P, Frieri R et al. Multiple myeloma: beta-2-microglobulin is not a useful follow-up parameter. *Acta Haematol* 1989; 82: 122–5.

(26) Bataille R, Grenier J, Sany J. Beta-2 microglobulin in myeloma: optimal use for staging, prognosis, and treatment: a prospective study of 160 patients. *Blood* 1984; 63: 468–76.

(27) Garewal H, Durie BGM, Kyle RA, Finley P, Bower B, Serokman R. Serum beta-2-microglobulin in the initial staging and subsequent monitoring of monoclonal plasma cell disorders. *J Clin Oncol* 1984; 2: 51–8.

(28) Brenning G, Wibell L, Bergström R. Serum $\beta2$ microglobulin at remission and relapse in patients with multiple myeloma. *Eur J Clin Invest* 1985; 15: 242–7.

(29) Gratzner HG. Monoclonal antibody to 5-bromo- and 5-iododeoxyuridine: a new reagent for detection of DNA replication. *Science* 1982; 218: 474–5.

(30) Gonchoroff NJ, Greipp PR, Kyle RA, Katzmann JA. A monoclonal antibody reactive with 5-bromo-2-deoxyuridine that does not require DNA denaturation. *Cytometry* 1985; 6: 506–12.

(31) Durie BGM, Salmon SE, Moon TE. Pretreatment tumor mass, cell kinetics, and prognosis in multiple myeloma. *Blood* 1980; 55: 364–72.

(32) Latreille J, Barlogie B, Johnston D, Drewinko B, Alexanian R. Ploidy and proliferative characteristics in monoclonal gammopathies. *Blood* 1982; 59: 43–51.

(33) Montecucco C, Riccardi A, Ucci G et al. Analysis of human myeloma cell population kinetics. *Acta Haematol* 1986; 75: 153–6.

(34) Boccadoro M, Gavarotti P, Fossati G et al. Low plasma cell 3(H) thymidine incorporation in monoclonal gammopathy of undetermined significance (MGUS), smouldering myeloma and remission phase myeloma: A reliable indicator of patients not requiring therapy. *Br J Haematol* 1984; 58: 689–96.

(35) Greipp PR, Witzig TE, Gonchoroff NJ et al. Immunofluorescence labeling indices in myeloma and related monoclonal gammopathies. *Mayo Clin Proc* 1987; 62: 969–77.

(36) Greipp PR, Kyle RA. Clinical, morphological, and cell kinetic differences among multiple myeloma, monoclonal gammopathy of undetermined significance and smoldering multiple myeloma. *Blood* 1983; 62: 166–71.

(37) Büchi G, Girotto M, Veglio M et al. Kappa/lambda ratio on peripheral blood lymphocytes and bone marrow plasma cell labelling index in monoclonal gammopathies. *Haematologica* 1990; 75: 132–36.

(38) Feinleib M, MacMahon B. Duration of survival in multiple myeloma. *J Natl Cancer Inst* 1960; 24: 1259–69.

(39) Sporn JR, McIntyre OR. Chemotherapy of previously untreated patients: an analysis of recent treatment results. *Semin Oncol* 1986; 13: 318–25.

(40) Bersagel DE. Chemotherapy of myeloma: drug combinations versus single agents, an overview, and comments on acute leukemia in myeloma. *Hematol Oncol* 1988; 6: 159–66.

(41) Alexanian R. Ten year survival in multiple myeloma. *Arch Intern Med* 1985; 145: 2073–4.

(42) Kyle R. Long-term survival in multiple myeloma. *N Engl J Med* 1983; 308: 314–6.

(43) Gregory WM, Richards MA, Malpas JS. Combination chemotherapy versus melphalan and prednisolone in the treatment of multiple myeloma: an overview of published trials. *J Clin Oncol* 1992; 10: 334–42.

(44) Bersagel DE. Myeloma, melphalan, and meta-analysis (editorial). *J Clin Oncol* 1992; 10: 178–9.

(45) Clarke M, Gray R, Dunn J, MacLennan I. Combination chemotherapy for myelomatosis (letter). *Lancet* 1992; 340: 433.

(46) Kyle RA, Greipp PR. Smoldering multiple myeloma. *N Engl J Med* 1980; 302: 1347–9.

(47) Alexanian R, Barlogie B, Dixon D. Prognosis of asymptomatic multiple myeloma. *Arch Int Med* 1988; 148: 1963–5.

(48) Alberts DS, Durie BGM, Salmon SE. Doxorubicin/BCNU chemotherapy for multiple myeloma in relapse. *Lancet* 1976; i: 926–8.

(49) MacLennan ICM, Kelly K, Crockson RA, Cooper EH, Cuzick J, Chapman C. Results of the MRC myelomatosis trials for patients entered since 1980. *Hematol Oncol* 1988; 6: 145–58.

(50) Palmer M, Belch A, Brox L, Pollock E, Koch M. Are the current criteria for response useful in the management of multiple myeloma? *J Clin Oncol* 1987; 5: 1373–7.

(51) Baldini L, Radaelli F, Chiorboli O et al. No correlation between response and survival in patients with multiple myeloma treated with vincristine, melphalan, cyclophosphamide, and prednisone. *Cancer* 1991; 68: 62–7.

(52) Palmer M, Belch A, Hanson J, Brox L. Reassessment of the relationship between M-protein decrement and survival in multiple myeloma. *Br J Cancer* 1989; 59: 110–2.

(53) Joshua DE, Snowdon L, Gibson J et al. Multiple myeloma: plateau phase revisited. *Haematol Rev* 1991; 5: 59–66.

(54) Alexanian R, Haut A, Khan AU et al. Treatment for multiple myeloma. *JAMA* 1969; 208: 1680–5.

(55) Cornwell GG, Pajak TF, Kochwa S et al. Vincristine and prednisone prolong the survival of patients receiving intravenous or oral melphalan for multiple myeloma: Cancer and Leukemia Group B experience. *J Clin Oncol* 1988; 6: 1481–90.

(56) Costa G, Engle RI, Schilling A et al. Melphalan and prednisone: an effective combination for the treatment of multiple myeloma. *Am J Med* 1973; 54: 589–99.

(57) Norfolk DR, Child JA. Pulsed high dose oral prednisolone in relapsed or refractory multiple myeloma. *Hematol Oncol* 1989; 7: 61–8.

(58) Friedenberg WR, Kyle RA, Knospe WH, Bennett JH, Tsiatis AA, Oken MM. Highdose dexamethasone for refractory or relapsing multiple myeloma. *Am J Haematol* 1991; 36: 171–5.

(59) Salmon SE, Crowley J. Impact of glucocorticoids (GC) and interferon (IFN) on outcome in multiple myeloma. *Proc ASCO* 1992; 11: 316.

(60) Barlogie B, Smith L, Alexanian R. Effective treatment of advanced multiple myeloma refractory to alkylating agents. *N Engl J Med* 1984; 310: 1353–6.

(61) Alexanian R, Barlogie B, Tucker S. VAD-based regimens as primary treatment for multiple myeloma. *Am J Haemat* 1990; 33: 86–9.

(62) Alexanian R, Barlogie B, Dixon D. High-dose glucocorticoid treatment of resistant myeloma. *Ann Intern Med* 1986; 105: 8–11.

(63) Alexanian R, Dimopoulos MA, Delasalle K, Barlogie B. Primary dexamethasone treatment of multiple myeloma. *Blood* 1992; 80: 887–90.

(64) Forgeson GV, Selby P, Lakhani S et al. Infused vincristine and adriamycin with high dose methylprednisolone (VAMP) in advanced previously treated multiple myeloma patients. *Br J Cancer* 1988; 58: 469–73.

(65) Gore ME, Selby PJ, Viner C et al. Intensive treatment of multiple myeloma and criteria for complete remission. *Lancet* 1989; ii: 879–82.

(66) Durie BGM, Russell DH, Salmon SE. Reappraisal of plateau phase in myeloma. *Lancet* 1980; ii: 65–8.

(67) Southwest Oncology Group Study. Remission maintenance therapy for multiple myeloma. *Arch Intern Med* 1975; 135: 147–52.

(68) Alexanian R, Salmon S, Bonnet J, Gehan E, Haut A, Weick J. Combination therapy for multiple myeloma. *Cancer* 1977; 40: 2765–71.

(69) Medical Research Council Working Party on Leukaemia in Adults. Objective evaluation of the role of vincristine in induction and maintenance therapy for myelomatosis. *Br J Cancer* 1985; 52: 153–58.

(70) Medical Research Council's Working Party on Leukaemia in Adults. Treatment comparisons in the third MRC myelomatosis trial. *Br J Cancer* 1980; 42: 823–30.

(71) Finnish Leukaemia Group. Aggressive combination chemotherapy in multiple myeloma. A multicentre trial. *Scand J Haematol* 1985; 35: 205–9.

(72) Cohen HJ, Bartolucci AA, Forman WB, Silberman HR. Consolidation and maintenance therapy in multiple myeloma: randomized comparison of a new approach to therapy after initial response to treatment. *J Clin Oncol* 1986; 4: 888–99.

(73) Belch A, Shelley W, Bersagel D et al. A randomized trial of maintenance *versus* no maintenance melphalan and prednisone in responding multiple myeloma patients. *Br J Cancer* 1988; 57: 94–9.

(74) Kildahl-Andersen O, Bjark P, Bondevik A et al. Multiple myeloma in central and northern Norway 1981–1982: a follow-up study of a randomized clinical trial of 5-drug combination chemotherapy versus standard therapy. *Eur J Haematol* 1988; 41: 47–51.

(75) Peest D, Deicher H, Goldewey R, Schmoll H-J, Schedel I. Induction and maintenance therapy in multiple myeloma: a multicenter trial of MP versus VCMP. *Eur J Cancer Clin Oncol* 1988; 24: 1061–7.

(76) Mandelli F, Avvisati G, Amadori S et al. Maintenance treatment with recombinant interferon alfa-2b in patients with multiple myeloma responding to conventional induction chemotherapy. *N Engl J Med* 1990; 322: 1430–4.

(77) Westin J, Cortelezzi A, Hjorth M, Rödjer S, Turesson I, Zador G. Interferon therapy during the plateau phase of multiple myeloma: an update of the Swedish study. *Eur J Cancer* 1991; 27 (suppl 4): S45–8.

(78) Ludwig H, Cohen A, Huber H et al. Interferon alfa-2b with VMCP compared to VMCP alone for induction and interferon alfa-2b compared to controls for remission maintenance in multiple myeloma: interim results. *Eur J Cancer* 1991; 27 (suppl 4): S40–5.

(79) Peest D, Deicher H, Coldeway R et al. Melphalan and prednisone (MP) versus vincristine, BCNU, adriamycin, melphalan and dexamethasone (VBAM Dex) induction chemotherapy and interferon maintenance treatment in multiple myeloma. Current results of a multicenter trial. The German Myeloma Treatment Group. *Onkologie* 1990; 13: 458–60.

Bone marrow transplantation for multiple myeloma

D SAMSON

Introduction

The treatment of multiple myeloma remains unsatisfactory; few patients survive more than 5 years, and conventional therapy fails to cure even a minority of patients. It has taken many years and a large number of randomized studies to establish that combination chemotherapy confers a statistically significant survival advantage compared with single agent oral melphalan or melphalan/prednisolone. This is because the difference in survival is small. Thus, in the recent Medical Research Council trial of ABCM (adriamycin, BCNU, cyclophosphamide and melphalan) versus melphalan alone (M7), the median survival was 32 months for ABCM compared with 24 months for M7, while the projected 5 year survival probabilities were approximately 22% for ABCM and 12% for M7.[1] Furthermore, complete remissions with conventional chemotherapy are rare, and it is reasonable to assume that complete remission (CR) is a prerequisite for cure. Alternative approaches to chemotherapy such as high dose melphalan[2] or initial treatment with VAD[3] were initially encouraging, with approximately 25% of patients entering CR. However longer follow-up demonstrated that these remissions were not durable, and in both studies the median response duration was only 18 months, even in CR patients.

Again, the early data on the use of interferon maintenance were very encouraging[4] but as the results mature and as the results of more trials are reported, it is becoming clear that not all studies are confirming an effect on response duration[5–7] and furthermore that even in studies which have demonstrated a benefit on response duration there has not been a significant survival benefit.[8,9] In this context it is not surprising that over the past few years there has been increasing interest in the use of myelo-ablative treatment for myeloma.

All correspondence to: Dr D Samson, Charing Cross Hospital, London W6 8 RF, UK.

Cambridge Medical Reviews: Haematological Oncology Volume 3
© Cambridge University Press 1994

General considerations
Myeloablative regimens

It has been clearly established that a dose–response relationship exists between melphalan dosage and remission rate in refractory myeloma. Significant increases in remission rate have been observed between doses of 70 mg/m², 100 mg/m² and 140 mg/m², with approximately 40% of refractory patients achieving remission at the highest dose.[10,11] The next logical step was further dose escalation of melphalan stem cell support, and single agent high dose melphalan (HDM) has been used for ABMT at a dose of 200 mg/m² by the Royal Marsden team[12–14] and by Barlogie and co-workers.[15,16] Most other groups have used a combination of HDM and total body irradiation (TBI); Barlogie et al showed early in their series of studies that the addition of TBI (8.5 Gy in five fractions) to HDM 140 mg/m² produced a higher response rate and longer survival than HDM alone in patients with refractory disease.[17–19] This schedule, and a variation using TBI 8 Gy in 4 fractions, has since been widely used. This dose of TBI is less than would normally be used in conditioning for an allogeneic transplant. Higher doses of TBI, eg 12 Gy in 6 fractions, have been used in combination for HDM for ABMT, particularly in some of the French studies. There are no data directly comparing regimens using different TBI dosages, but it is quite possible that differences may affect outcome.

It is perhaps surprising that the combination of HDM and TBI, which is the most widely used regimen for ABMT, has not been extensively used for allogeneic BMT. In the collected EBMT (European Bone Marrow Transplant Group) registry data,[20] only five of 90 patients received conditioning with HDM/TBI, although others received melphalan in addition to standard cyclophosphamide (Cy)/TBI. It is likely that the reason for this is largely historical, ie centres have used the regimens that they were using at the time for conditioning for patients with leukaemia. Thus cyclophosphamide and total body irradiation (Cy/TBI), which has been for many years the standard regimen for allogeneic BMT in acute and chronic leukaemias, has been to date the most widely used regimen for allogeneic BMT in myeloma. More recently, as in allogeneic BMT for leukaemias, there has been increasing use of busulphan–cyclophosphamide regimens (BuCy) in various dose combinations. Another reason that HDM with 'full-dose' TBI has not been more extensively used in allogeneic BMT may be concern over toxicity, in view of the data in AML showing significantly higher transplant-related mortality after HDM/TBI than after Cy/TBI.[21] The addition of HDM to either Cy/TBI or BuCy certainly appears to increase the toxicity of these regimens.[20,22]

The clinical results of various studies using different conditioning regimens are discussed below. Obviously it is not possible to compare except in very general terms the efficacy of a regimen used predominantly for allogeneic BMT, eg Cy/TBI, with one that is used for ABMT, eg HDM/TBI 8 Gy, because of the inherent difference in relapse risk between autologous and allogeneic BMT.

Source of stem cell support

In all haematological malignancies, the relapse risk is higher after autologous bone marrow transplantation than after allogeneic BMT, even when marrow is harvested in complete remission (CR). This is likely to be particularly the case in myeloma, because it is rare for patients to be in CR after conventional chemotherapy, and even where CR has been achieved (eg after high dose melphalan or VAD as initial treatment) early relapse is frequently observed,[2,3] indicating that clonogenic myeloma cells persist in these patients even when there is no demonstrable paraprotein and no excess of plasma cells. Barlogie has expressed the view that relapse after ABMT results from residual disease rather than reinfused myeloma cells, because there is no demonstrable relationship between degree of plasmacytosis in the reinfused marrow and relapse-free survival after ABMT.[19,23] This observation could however be equally well explained on the basis that plasma cells are not the clonogenic cells. Attempts to reduce the relapse rate by decreasing the number of reinfused myeloma cells have been made by 'in vivo purging' with high dose treatment before harvest, by in vitro purging of bone marrow, or by the use of peripheral blood stem cells (PBSC). In vivo purging has involved either administration of a cycle of high dose chemotherapy before harvest and ABMT[24] or double ABMT.[25] In vitro purging using monoclonal antibodies or chemical agents is the subject of current study in some centres, while others have focussed on the use of PBSC transplant on the basis that PBSC are less likely to be contaminated with myeloma cells than bone marrow. The theoretical problems associated with these latter approaches and the current clinical results are discussed below.

Additional therapy after BMT

Relapse is at present a major obstacle to success in BMT for myeloma, particularly after ABMT, but also after allogeneic BMT, indicating that relapse can certainly occur from residual disease even after very intensive conditioning regimens. One approach to reducing relapse rate after ABMT has been to administer maintenance interferon as soon as engraftment has occurred,[14,26,27] and interferon maintenance after allogeneic BMT is the subject of a pilot study currently being carried out by the EBMT. The use of interleukin-2 (IL-2) infusions after ABMT for myeloma has also been reported.[28,29]

Allogeneic BMT

Only a minority (<10%) of all patients with myeloma will be potential candidates for allogeneic BMT, because of age and donor availability. The number of allogeneic transplants performed is, however, increasing steadily; from 1983–1989 a total of 102 allogeneic transplants were reported to the EBMT registry, but by 1991, 65 transplants were reported in the single year. This increase probably reflects increasing awareness of the role of allogeneic BMT for myeloma and also the accumulating evidence that autologous stem cell transplant as currently performed is not curative.

Current results of allogeneic BMT

The largest reported experience is that collected by the EBMT, which opened a registry for myeloma transplants in 1983 and first published results in 1987.[30] The majority of patients transplanted in Europe are reported to this registry; between 1983 and 1989 102 transplants were reported. 90 from HLA-matched sibling donors, six from syngeneic donors, and six from alternative donors.

The results on the 90 patients transplanted from HLA-matched sibling donors between 1983 and 1989 have recently been published.[20] The median age was 42 years (range 23–55). At the time of BMT 41 patients were in remission (7 CR, 34 PR) and 49 had relapsed or refractory disease. 33 patients were transplanted after first-line treatment, 31 after two lines of treatment and the remaining 26 later in the course of the disease. Thus, most patients had late stage disease.

Eighty-one of the 90 patients received conditioning which included TBI – 33 patients received standard TBI plus cyclophosphamide (Cy/TBI), 43 patients received Cy/TBI plus other drugs (usually including melphalan) and five patients received HDM/TBI. Only nine patients were conditioned with chemotherapy alone, of whom six received BuCy.

The overall transplant-related mortality was high at approximately 40%, the major cause of death being infection. Mortality was lower in patients transplanted electively after first-line treatment, but was still of the order of 30%. GVHD did not appear to be more common or more severe than after allogeneic BMT for other haematological malignancies, in spite of the relatively high median age of the patients. 46% of evaluable patients had no GVHD and only 10% had grade III or IV.

CR was defined as disappearance of monoclonal immunoglobulin on either conventional electrophoresis or immunofixation, and less than 5% plasma cells in the bone marrow. 18 patients died before engraftment and 5 were not yet evaluable. Of the remaining 67 patients, 39 achieved CR (including 6 of 7 who were in CR pre-transplant), and 28 did not achieve CR. Thus 43% of all patients transplanted and 58% of all evaluable patients achieved CR post BMT. Factors predicting for CR post-BMT were Durie-Salmon stage at diagnosis (79% for stage I vs 37% for stages II and III), number of lines of previous treatment (61% for single line treatment vs 33% for two or more lines), and responsive rather than refractory disease (50% vs 36%).

Stage at diagnosis was more important than stage at time of BMT; this could be explained on the basis that stage at diagnosis reflects the biology of the disease better than stage at BMT which also depends on the effects of treatment. The higher CR rate in patients transplanted after first-line treatment is partly due to the lower mortality but mainly to a true difference in response. Insufficient data on newer prognostic factors such as beta-2 microglobulin, labelling index or CRP were available in this series to evaluate their relationship to outcome.

In spite of the high early mortality and a number of later deaths from transplant-related causes or progressive disease, the survival curve reaches a plateau by 3 years which is currently maintained as far out as 6 years, giving an overall projected survival probability of 40% for all patients (Fig. 1). The major factor affecting survival was whether or not patients achieved CR post-BMT. Thus, the projected survival probability for patients achieving CR is 70%, whereas very few of those failing to achieve CR survived beyond 2 years. The factors predicting for CR post-BMT therefore also predict for improved survival, ie stage I at diagnosis, one line of treatment only, and responsive disease. Age had no significant effect on survival within the age range of patients transplanted, ie there was no significant difference in survival of patients under the age of 40 years and those aged between 40 and 55 years. Thus patients up to the age of 50–55 years can be considered as candidates for allo-BMT. Neither was any correlation observed between the type of conditioning and outcome, althought the number who received chemotherapy only was too small to evaluate usefully. It appeared, however, that multidrug combinations with TBI did not increase CR rate as compared with standard Cy/TBI, and the mortality was slightly higher.

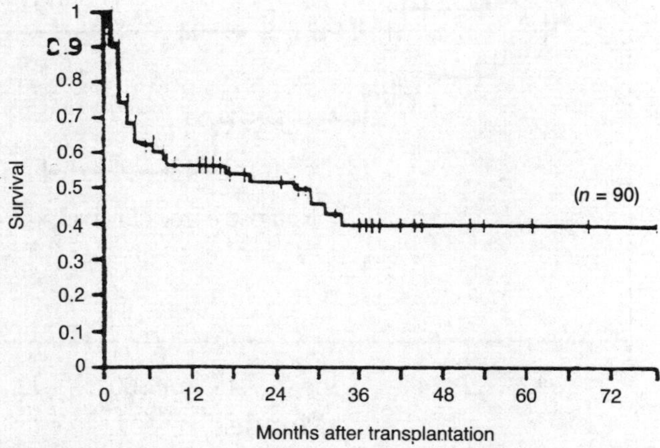

Fig. 1. Projected overall survival in 90 patients with myeloma after allogeneic BMT from HLA matched siblings: EBMT data (from Gahrton et al, 1991).[20]

D Samson

The median relapse-free survival for patients in CR post-BMT is 48 months with a projected 5 year relapse-free survival of 40% (Fig. 2). In other words, approximately 60% of CR patients who are surviving at 5 years can expect to be disease-free, while 40% will have relapsed. Relapse has been observed as late as 4 years post-BMT and as yet the relapse-free survival curve has not reached a clear plateau, so although the results are encouraging, it is not yet certain from the clinical data whether or not patients who are relapse-free at 5 years are cured. However, preliminary results of molecular evaluation of minimal residual disease, discussed below, suggest that disease eradication may occur in long-term survivors.

Within those centres reporting to the EBMT registry, the largest single-centre experience is from the Bologna transplant team, who have reported data on 34 patients allografted from matched sibling donors between 1984 and 1992. They have analysed the effect of the timing of BMT in their series.[31] Of their patients 16 had responsive disease at BMT (Group I), and 18 had refractory/relapsed disease (Group 2). Transplant-related mortality was 31% in Group 1 v 58% in Group 2. 93% of group 1 patients entered CR post-BMT compared with 13% of group 2 patients. Overall survival at 5 years was 60% for group 1 patients and 30% for group 2 patients, while median progression- free survival was 45 months and 13 months respectively. 20 of these patients received BuCy and 14 Cy/TBI (an earlier cohort). Trans-

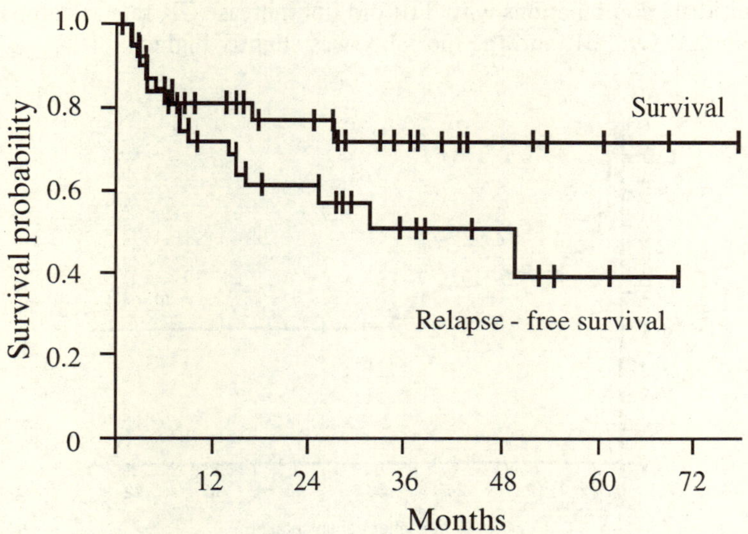

Fig. 2. Overall survival and relapse-free survival in patients in CR after allogeneic BMT (EBMT Registry data, 1991).

120

plant-related mortality was lower with BuCy: 35% v 64% with Cy/TBI, but median PFS in those who survived the transplant was somewhat shorter: 36 months compared with 45 months.

The Seattle transplant team also observed a high transplant-related mortality in their initial studies of allogeneic BMT in myeloma patients using Cy/TBI as conditioning. This led them to evaluate the use of BuCy for BMT in myeloma.

The original BuCy protocol described by Santos et al[32] comprised 16 mg/kg busulphan and 200 mg/kg cyclophosphamide. Tutschka et al[33] had modified this protocol by reducing the dose of cyclophosphamide to 120 mg/kg and this regimen had induced remission in a patient with previously refractory myeloma.[34] The Seattle team initially used the Tutschka regimen in 5 patients, but 2 of 5 patients died of regimen related toxicity, and they therefore subsequently reduced the busulphan dose to 14 mg/kg. More recently they have been exploring the potential of increasing the cylophosphamide dose, and have combined the busulphan dose of 14 mg/kg with escalating doses of cyclophosphamide, with the intention of using doses of 120, 147, 174 and 200 mg/kg. The results of this study have recently been reported.[35] Of patients 20 were transplanted, 16 from matched sibling donors, 3 from one-antigen mismatched family donors, and one from a matched unrelated donor. Severe regimen-related toxicity occurred in 2 of 5 patients who received Bu 16 mg/kg and Cy 120 mg/kg (both died), in none of four patients who received Bu 14 mg/kg and Cy 120 mg/kg, in one of eight patients who received Bu 14 mg/kg and Cy 147 mg/kg (died from sepsis and renal failure) and in two of three patients who received Bu 14 mg/kg and Cy 174 mg/kg (both died of VOD). No patient therefore received the Cy dose of 200 mg/kg which was the dose in the original Santos regimen. These results showed that the maximum tolerable dose combination for BuCy in myeloma patients was Bu 14 mg/kg and Cy 147 mg/kg.

In terms of response and relapse-free survival, five of 20 patients died within 55 days of regimen-related toxicity (three VOD and two sepsis) and response was not evaluable. 12 of the remaining 15 patients (80%) achieved CR, including six of seven who received the maximum tolerated dose of BuCy (14mg/kg and 147 mg/kg) but also three of four who received Bu 14 mg/kg and Cy 120 mg/kg. BuCy thus appears at least as effective at inducing CR as Cy/TBI. Of the 12 who achieved CR, three patients subsequently died of transplant-related causes, as did two of three who failed to achieve PR. Two of the CR patients relapsed, and seven (35% of all patients transplanted and 58% of those who achieved CR) remained alive in CR at 190 to 1271 days at the time of reporting. There was no apparent difference in CR rate according to remission status before BMT or according to whether patients had responsive or refractory disease, but the number in each group was small. Survival was clearly worse for patients with refractory or relapsed disease; with only 1 of 6 surviving beyond 170 days. The projected probabilities for survival and relapse-free survival for all patients were 36% and 32% respectively (Fig. 3).

The overall outcome of patients treated according to this protocol is very similar to that of the patients reported by the EBMT, the majority of whom received conditioning including TBI (projected overall survival 36% and 40% respectively). The relapse rate in CR patients is currently lower in the Seattle series but the follow-up is shorter. The Seattle and Bologna data certainly suggest that BuCy is as effective at inducing CR as conditioning regimens which include TBI, and may be less toxic. Further studies are needed to determine whether regimen-related toxicity is significantly less, and whether there is a difference in long-term relapse-free survival.

The Vancouver group have reported results of allogeneic BMT in 13 patients conditioned with BuCy plus additional HDM–BuCyMel.[36] Six patients were in initial PR, 2 had primary refractory disease and 5 had relapsed disease (3 sensitive, 2 resistant). Eight patients were transplanted from matched related donors, 2 from mismatched related donors, and 3 from matched unrelated donors. The median age was 42 years.[30–46] Conditioning was with BuCy (Tutschka regimen) in 10 patients, with the addition of high dose melphalan (90 mg/m^2) in 8 of these; 3 patients received standard Cy/TBI. At the time of reporting there had been 2 transplant-related deaths, 4 patients were not yet evaluable for response, 4 achieved CR and 3 PR. 2 relapses had occurred, ie 5 of 7 responding patients remained in remission at a median follow-up of 11 months. Follow-up is too short and the numbers too small to evaluate the efficacy of BuCyMel conditioning as compared with BuCy. However, the authors note that they observed significant regimen-

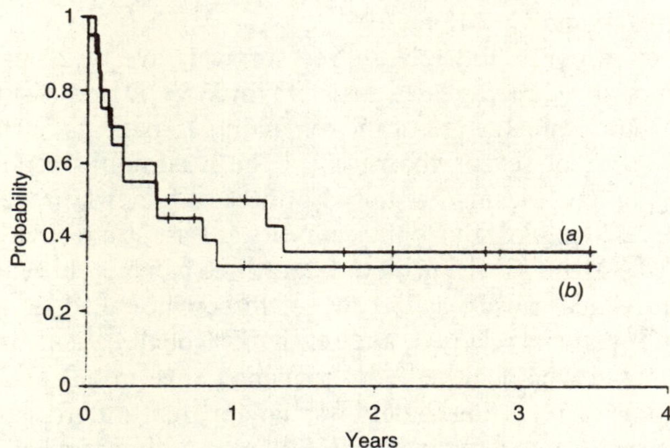

Fig. 3. Projected survival (*a*) and disease-free survival (*b*) in 20 patients after allogeneic BMT with BuCy conditioning: Seattle data (from Bensinger et al 1992).[35]

related toxicity, including 2 deaths from veno-occlusive disease, in other patients with myeloma who were not part of this series and advised caution in the use of this regimen, especially in heavily pretreated patients.

The Vancouver group have also used BuCyMel as conditioning for ABMT in myeloma and in patients with other haematological malignancies.[22] The BuCy schedule was again Bu 16 mg/kg and Cy 120 mg/kg. Melphalan could be safely added to this schedule at a dose of 90 mg/m^2 (regimen-related toxicity > grade 3 in 31%) but a dose of 135 mg/m^2 was found too toxic, with grade 3 regimen-related toxicity in 3 of 5 patients. The major toxicities were VOD and haemorrhagic cystitis. 14 patients with myeloma were then treated with BuCy and HDM 90 mg/m^2 with ABMT; 3 died due to hepatotoxicity (2 had received prior high dose cyclophosphamide). At the same time 7 patients with CML were treated; none died from toxicity. These data again illustrate the increased toxicity of high dose therapy in myeloma patients, and suggests that this type of regime should only be considered in those patients who have received little previous chemotherapy.

All these studies indicate a transplant-related toxicity higher than that observed in patients with leukaemia; even patients with myeloma in first remission have a risk of transplant-related death of at least 30%. Age is clearly one factor which could contribute; although there was no difference in the EBMT series between patients below or above 40 years, very few were below 30 years of age. Pre-existing immunosuppression may contribute to infection, which was the major cause of death in the EBMT series, and prior alkylating agent therapy may predispose to VOD. A degree of renal impairment is also common even in patients with normal serum creatinine levels. Of 10 patients recently transplanted at Charing Cross Hospital, all with normal creatinine levels (median 91 mmol/1, range 54–106), 4 had values for EDTA clearance which were less than 60% of those predicted according to height and weight (personal observations).

Syngeneic BMT

There are several reports of syngeneic BMT in myeloma, including the first two patients transplanted for this disease.[37,38] Both had advanced disease and both relapsed within three years of BMT. These patients were included in a later report from Seattle[39] of eight transplants with syngeneic donors, seven of whom were transplanted late in the course of the disease. Two patients died early, four died later, with myeloma as the main cause of death, and two were surviving – it is not clear whether or not in remission – at 4–5 years post-BMT. The EBMT registry has data on six syngeneic transplants, five of whom were stage III and three being on second or third line treatment. At the time of analysis five were alive from 3 months to 4 years post-BMT, but only one was in CR. Thus immediate transplant-related mortality appears lower than that observed using nonsyngeneic siblings, and prolonged survival may be obtained, but it appears that most patients who survive still have evidence of disease and so may ultimately relapse.

Use of alternative donors

Six patients transplanted from donors other than HLA-identical siblings were reported to the EBMT registry between 1983 and 1989. Unrelated donors were used in three cases. All these patients had advanced disease at BMT and five of six died within 100 days; at the time of reporting one patient was surviving at 200 days, not in remission.[23] The Seattle series included three patients receiving grafts from partially matched related donors. One died early and two were surviving 240 and 446 days post-BMT at the time of the report.[39] The Vancouver series[36] included five patients who were transplanted from alternative donors, but it is not clear from the report whether or not the two transplant-related deaths in their series occurred in these patients, and the follow-up was short.

Given the already high transplant-related mortality in myeloma, and the experience of using alternative donors in CML, which suggests an increase in mortality rate of around 20%,[40] it does not seem justified at present to recommend the use of other than syngeneic or matched sibling donors, except perhaps for the rare patient under 30–35 years of age. Certainly this type of transplant should not be performed in patients with advanced disease.

Effect of allogeneic BMT on bone lesions

In the majority of patients the appearance of bone lesions on X-ray is not significantly altered after BMT. Improvement in the appearance of lytic lesions was observed in only seven out of 58 evaluable patients in the EBMT study.[20] Whether persisting bone lesions harbour residual myeloma cells is unknown.

Is there a graft-versus-myeloma effect?

The information which would help to address this important question would include data on relapse risk in relation to syngeneic BMT, to T-cell depletion and to GVHD. This data is lacking for a number of reasons. Although relapse can be clearly defined in patients who achieve CR post-BMT, the total number of these patients is as yet small, and relapse is hard to define in those not achieving CR (many of whom die early after BMT) where it is very difficult to separate progressive disease and transplant-related factors as causes of morbidity and mortality. The EBMT data show a trend for improved survival in patients with grade I GVHD as compared to no GVHD, but this trend is not significant, while higher grades of GVHD are associated with a significant increase in mortality which obscures any possible effect on relapse. Data on the use of T-cell depletion or other methods of prophylaxis against GVHD are reported to the EBMT registry but have not so far been analysed for any effect on relapse risk. As discussed above, there have been a small number of reported syngeneic transplants, less than 20 worldwide, and no direct comparison of the results with those of sibling BMT has been made. The recipients of syngeneic transplants as expected have a low risk of procedure-related death, and hence a better survival probability than recipients of nonsyngeneic grafts, but only two of the reported patients survive in long-term CR, suggesting that persistent disease may be more common than in survivors of nonsyngeneic transplants. However we have observed disappearance of the specific clonal Ig gene rearrangement in one patient in CR 4.5 years after syngeneic BMT.[41] This would suggest that a graft-versus-myeloma effect is not essential for cure, but otherwise the existence of such an effect and its role remain speculative at present.

Minimal residual disease after allogeneic BMT

As discussed above, it is not yet clear from the clinical data whether patients in long-term CR after BMT are cured of their disease. Evaluation of residual disease at the molecular level might help to clarify this question. Conversely it might enable identification of a group of patients at risk of relapse, who might benefit from additional post-transplant treatment, eg with maintenance interferon.

We have used immunoglobulin gene fingerprinting, a PCR-based method first described by Deane and Norton,[42] to study serial bone marrows in five patients in CR after allogeneic BMT.[41,43] This method employs a set of variable region (VH) family-specific primers and a common joining region (JH) primer to amplify across the hypervariable region of the IgH gene. Amplification across a clonally rearranged VDJ region will generate a product of between 300 and 400 base pairs, the exact size being specific to a given rearrangement depending on V, D and J usage and 'N' nucleotide insertions and deletions at the VD and DJ junctions. A polyclonal population of plasma cells will generate a series of differently sized products, whereas a monoclonal poulation will generate a product of one particular size, specific for the particular clone. Using a radiolabelled JH primer and the appropriate VH family primer (determined by screening with the series of VH family primers), radiolabelled products are generated and can be visualized by autoradiography after separation on a high resolution sequencing gel. The specific size of the amplification product generated from the myeloma clone in an individual patient can be used to follow minimal residual disease. The level of sensitivity of this technique as shown by dilution experiments is 0.1–0.01%.

We have studied five patients in continuing CR from 10 months to 5 years after allogeneic BMT. Bone marrow samples obtained within 1 year of BMT showed persistence of the clonal rearrangement seen at diagnosis in all patients. Later samples have been studied in two of three patients who are in remission longer than one year post-BMT. One was PCR-positive at 1 year, but at 2 and at 3 years the follow-up marrow showed a normal ladder without a visible clonal band (PCR-negative). The other patient was PCR-positive at 6 months and at 2 years post-BMT, but had become PCR negative at 4.5 years (Fig. 4). It appears that, as in CML,[44] early PCR-positivity is not predictive of relapse. Analysis of more patients is required to assess whether persistent PCR-positivity is predictive of relapse ie. whether it is possible to detect a subgroup of patients who might benefit from further intervention such as interferon maintenance after allogeneic BMT. Although more patients and longer follow-up are also needed to assess the significance of negative results, the observation that two patients show no detectable disease at the molecular level suggests that long-term survivors of allogeneic BMT may be cured.

Which patients should be offered allogeneic BMT?

All the published data indicate that, if allogeneic BMT is to be performed, it should be carried out early in the course of the disease, ie after first-line

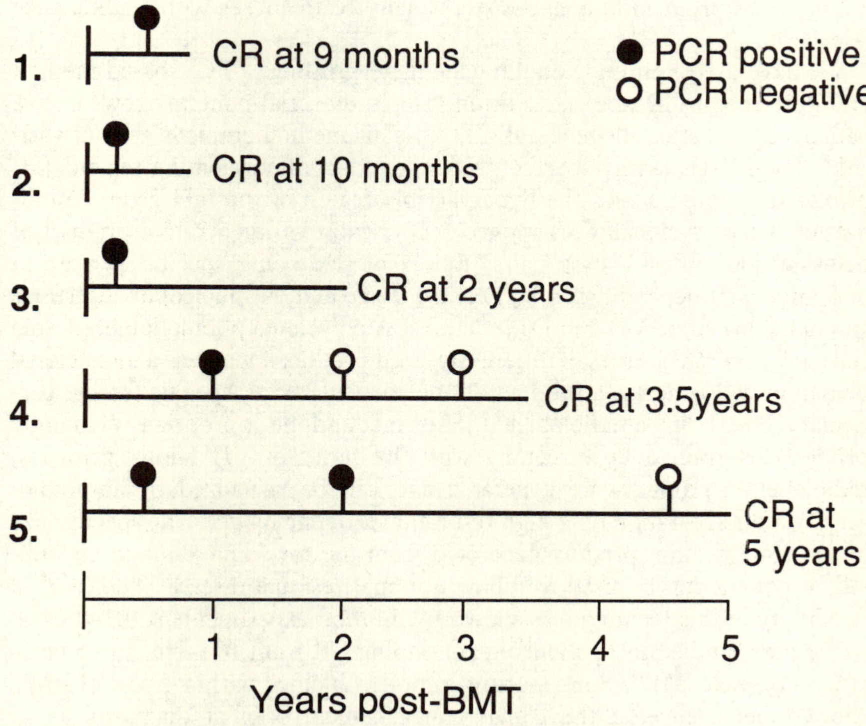

Fig. 4. Detection of minimal residual disease in patients in CR after allogeneic BMT using a PCR-based method to detect clonal IgH rearrangements (personal data).

chemotherapy. It is clearly difficult to decide whether patients with good prognostic factors, who can be predicted to have a median survival of at least 4 years with conventional chemotherapy, should be subjected to the risk of allogeneic BMT, even though these are the very patients who will have the best chance of long-term disease-free survival. However it appears reasonable to conclude that early BMT should be offered to patients with poor prognostic factors (such as high beta-2 microglobulin, high labelling index or stage III disease) and also to patients who fail to respond to first-line treatment. Patients with sensitive relapse should also be considered as candidates for allogeneic BMT, but those with resistant relapse are unlikely to benefit and have a very high risk of transplant-related death.

Autologous transplantation

Autologous transplantation is potentially applicable to many more patients, and the mortality can be expected to be small. However, it could be predicted that reinfusion of myeloma cells would represent a major obstacle to success. CR is rare after most types of induction chemotherapy, and CR is not necessarily predictive of durable remission, as shown by the data on high dose melphalan and first-line VAD.[2,3] CR after VAMP was, in fact, shown to be associated with increased numbers of clonogenic myeloma cells in the marrow, even when the marrow was in morphological CR.[45] This is consistent with several other lines of evidence indicating that the myeloma clone involves cells earlier in the B-cell lineage and possibly even myeloid progenitor cells.[46,47] The other factor which may affect relapse rate as compared with allogeneic BMT is that in many reported studies of ABMT the conditioning regimes used have been less intensive than those used for allogeneic BMT. The development of conditioning regimes for autologous transplant in myeloma has followed on from the initial use of high dose melphalan by the Marsden group, and has involved increasing the dose of melphalan or adding TBI. The most widely used regime has been high dose melphalan 140 mg/m^2 with TBI, but the dose of TBI has in many studies been less than the 12 Gy in six fractions which would be standard for allogeneic BMT.

Initial studies of ABMT in myeloma focussed on the use of ABMT as supportive therapy to allow the administration of moderately high dose treatment to patients with advanced disease. These studies, carried out at the MD Anderson Hospital in the early 1980s, showed that the mortality of intensive treatment with standard high dose melphalan (140 mg/m^2) was reduced by ABMT support. ABMT also allowed the use of the combination of high dose melphalan (70mg/m^2) and TBI (8.5 Gy), which was found to be more effective in terms of remission rate and survival.[17] However, there was no evidence of durable remission in these patients, who had advanced disease. More recently a number of groups have been assessing the role of high dose therapy and ABMT as consolidation therapy after initial induction chemotherapy. Most of the currently reported experience has involved the used of unpurged bone marrow, but there is an increasing amount of data on the use of peripheral blood stem cells (PBSC) and a few centres have been investigating the use of in vitro purging of marrow prior to ABMT.

Results of ABMT using unpurged marrow

The MD Anderson group continued to use HDM /TBI as conditioning for ABMT and extended this to the treatment of patients in first or later remission. In an updated report of 55 patients, 34 were in first or later remission.[19] Of patients, 7 were resistant to primary treatment and 14 had resistant relapse. Of the latter 14 patients, none entered CR and median survival was only seven months. In the remaining 41 patients, including those who had primary refractory disease, 27% entered CR and there was a projected survival of 82% at 4 years. In these patients, prognosis was determined mainly by pretreatment beta-2 microglobulin level and Ig isotype. Those with beta-2 levels above 2.5 mg/1 and non-IgG isotype (six pts) had a median relapse-free survival of less than 12 months, while those without these poor risk features (35 patients) had a median relapse-free survival of approximately 20 months.

In other reported studies, ABMT has been included as part of an initial treatment programme for newly diagnosed myeloma. The Royal Marsden Hospital have published data on a series of patients autografted in first remission using single agent high dose melphalan (HDM) at a dose of 200 mg/m^2.[12] After initial chemotherapy with VAMP (infused vincristine and adriamycin with high dose methyl prednisolone), patients achieving remission (<30% plasma cells in marrow) and with adequate renal function proceeded to ABMT. Patients not fulfilling these criteria received HDM at the conventional dose of 140 mg/m^2 without marrow rescue. There were 28 patients in the former group and 11 patients in the latter group. The results of both groups were combined. Approximately 50% of all patients achieved CR after VAMP plus HDM but the median remission duration even in CR patients was not more than 2 years. The mortality associated with HDM was reduced by the ABMT, but in terms of response duration these results of dose escalation to 200 mg/m^2 represented only a small improvement on their earlier results using HDM alone at a dose of 140 mg/m^2 as initial treatment, where median response duration was 18 months.[2]

The long-term results of this study and of other patients who received HDM and ABMT between 1986 and 1991 were reported at the 1993 EBMT meeting.[13] A total of 53 newly diagnosed patients had been treated with either VAMP, C-VAMP (cyclophosphamide-VAMP) or V-C-VAMP (verapamil-C-VAMP) as initial therapy, followed by ABMT with HDM 200 mg/m^2. At the time of ABMT, 9 were in CR, 38 in PR, and six had not responded. After ABMT 52 had responded with 40 entering CR (75%); there was one early death. At a median follow-up of 51 months 77% patients are alive, and median survival has not yet been reached. Comparison of the survival curves of these patients and of other patients who received HDM 140 mg/m^2 without ABMT, in whom median survival was 47 months, shows that the longer median survival in the former group is entirely due to the reduction of early deaths by marrow support. The median relapse-free survival of the ABMT group was still 23 months.

Similar results were observed in a collaborative French study of ABMT after initial chemotherapy with HDM, where suitable patients (responders with an adequate bone marrow harvest and good renal function) proceeded to ABMT using HDM alone or HDM/TBI.[48] Of patients 97 were entered into the study, of whom 53 were newly diagnosed and 44 had resistant or relapsed disease. After initial treatment with HDM (140 mg/m^2) 69 patients had responded but only 38 could proceed to BMT (3 allogeneic, 35 autologous) because of relapse, inadequate harvest, unfitness or other reasons. Of the 35 ABMT patients, 20 were newly diagnosed and 10 had initially relapsed or refractory disease. The first 18 received HDM alone at the same dose of 140 mg/m^2, and the following 17 received melphalan/TBI; the TBI dose was 12 Gy in six fractions or ten Gy single dose, ie these 17 patients received conditioning equivalent to that which would have been used for allogeneic BMT. The median duration of remission after ABMT was 28 months with no plateau on the remission duration curve. This compared with a median response duration of 20 months for the whole group of responders to initial HDM (Fig. 5). Given that the ABMT group were in a better prognostic category a priori, these data do not suggest any additional benefit of the second intensification with ABMT. It is noteworthy that there was no difference in response duration between the group who had HDM only for ABMT and those who had additional TBI.

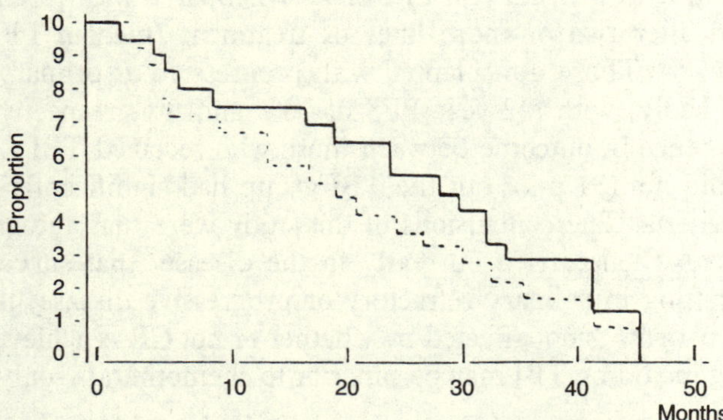

Fig. 5. Duration of remission in 69 patients treated with high dose melphalan and in a sub-group of these patients who received subsequent ABMT (from Harousseau et al 1992).[48]

D Samson

These data were included in those collected by the French Autograft Registry which has reported data on 154 autologous stem cell transplants for myeloma, including 56 PBSC transplants.[49] The median age was 52 years (range 35–66). Of patients 120 were transplanted as part of first line treatment, of whom 90 were responders to initial chemotherapy and 30 were refractory. 34 patients were transplanted after relapse (16 refractory, 18 sensitive or not tested). Conditioning included TBI in 115 cases, predominantly using melphalan 140 mg/m^2 and TBI (8–12 Gy). PFS was 42% at three years for the patients transplanted after first-line therapy and 0% for those transplanted after relapse. There was no difference in PFS between patients who entered CR after BMT and those who did not. The use of PBSC resulted in more rapid recovery of neutrophils (median 14 vs 20 days) but the relapse rate after PBSCT and ABMT was identical.

The EBMT registry has collected data on 103 patients who received autologous stem cell transplantation;[50] this series does not at present include the patients in the French Registry Study discussed above. The median age was 49 years with a range of 27–65. The majority of patients were stage III at diagnosis (60 patients), 17 patients were stage I, and 23 stage II (3 unknown). 41 patients were transplanted after first-line treatment and 62 later in the course of the disease. At the time of transplant, 75 were in remission or had stable disease and 26 had refractory or relapsed disease (2 not evaluable). Of patients 74 received bone marrow alone, 25 received PBSC alone and 4 patients received both marrow and PBSC. Eighty-four patients responded, with 39 patients achieving CR and 45 patients PR. Overall, progression-free survival (PFS) was 35% at 2 years with no evidence of a plateau and the median PFS was 12 months. There was no difference in PFS between patients in CR post-BMT and those in PR, ie patients relapsed at the same rate in both groups. Results were better in patients transplanted as part of first-line treatment, with a 2-year PFS of 40% compared with 10% for patients transplanted after two or more lines of treatment (median PFS 12 v 30 months, Fig. 6). Those transplanted with progressive or primary refractory disease did badly, with a 2-year PFS of 10% and 0%, respectively. There was no difference in outcome between those who received TBI (72 pts) and those who did not (31 pts), but the TBI group had significantly more poor prognosis criteria. The conclusions of the study were that autografting was most effective when carried out early in the disease, that survival is poor after autografting in primary refractory or progressive disease, that PFS in responding patients is not affected by whether or not CR is achieved and that conditioning including TBI may be superior to chemotherapy-only regimens.

Double intensification regimens

It is possible that relapse from reinfused myeloma cells would be reduced by intensive treatment prior to harvest, with or without stem cell rescue at

130

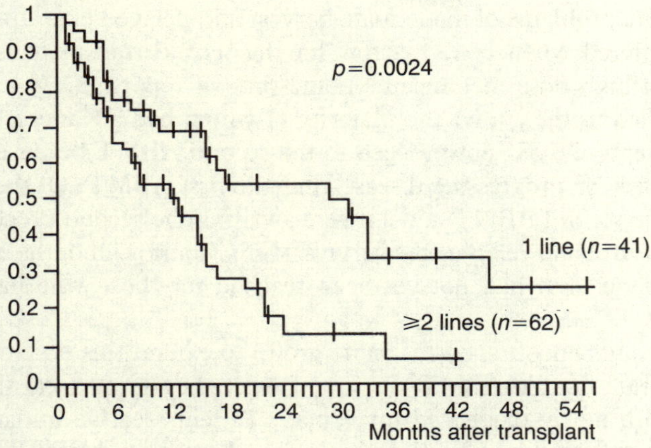

Fig. 6. Progression-free survival after ABMT for myeloma (EBMT Registry data, 1992). Outcome is better in patients transplanted after first-time treatment.

that point. The study reported by Harousseau et al,[48] where HDM was used as the initial treatment, has been discussed above. Relapse rate after ABMT was not different from that seen after the initial HDM alone, and there was a major problem in proceeding to ABMT because of toxicity of the initial treatment and inadequate yield at harvest. Similar problems have been observed in a double ABMT programme reported by Stoppa et al.[25] In this study the same initial HDM treatment (140 mg/m^2) was given with bone marrow support, followed by a second marrow collection and second ABMT using BuCy (Bu 14 mg/kg and Cy 120 mg/kg). Of patients 34 were enrolled, all with poor prognosis myeloma. Fourteen had responsive disease and 20 progressive disease. At the time of reporting, second BMT had been performed in 18 patients, including three allogeneic BMTs; 7 did not proceed to the second transplant because of toxicity, relapse or patient refusal, and the others were awaiting the second transplant. Significant toxicity was observed including delayed engraftment, related infective problems and hepatic dysfunction. At a median follow-up of 24 months, 52% of patients remained in remission but only four were in CR.

Barlogie and co-workers have reported early results of a double HDM/ABMT programme using single agent HDM 200 mg/m^2 for both procedures.[15] The difference between this programme and the two French studies is that bone marrow for both transplants was collected prior to the first transplant. Thus the first high dose treatment is designed as an additional

D Samson

treatment for disease in the patient rather than as a means of in vivo purging of the marrow prior to collection. As would be expected, they have not observed the problems of inadequate harvest and delayed engraftment which are encountered when bone marrow for the second transplant is harvested after initial high dose melphalan. At the time of reporting, 74 patients had been enrolled in the study, the majority of whom had advanced disease. Of the 74 patients, 28 did not proceed to the second ABMT because of incomplete recovery or progressive disease after the first ABMT. Of these, 33 had received the second ABMT and 13 were awaiting the second procedure. The median survival and relapse-free survival were 21 and 17 months respectively for all patients, but had not yet been reached for those who had received double ABMT.

These results encouraged the same group to extend this type of approach to incorporate double ABMT as part of what they term 'total therapy' for patients with newly diagnosed myeloma.[16] Patients receive initial treatment with VAD, followed by high dose cyclophosphamide and EDAP (etoposide, dexamethasone, ara-C and *cis*-platinum). Two courses of HDM 200 mg/m^2 are then administered 1 month apart, supported by bone marrow and peripheral blood stem cells collected prior to EDAP. Of patients 63 had been enrolled at the time of reporting, of whom 18 had to date completed the total treatment. Of patients 56% completing the treatment had entered CR compared with 2% after the initial VAD and 7% after EDAP; long term results are awaited.

ABMT using in vitro purging

Purging remission marrow in vitro is clearly an attractive idea, especially since the publication of the data from the Dana–Farber Institute[51] on purged ABMT in NHL, where the efficacy of purging (assessed by molecular markers) significantly affected relapse rate. The major problem of purging myeloma bone marrow is that the phenotype of the myeloma stem cell is not known. It is clear that the malignant clone involves the B-cell lineage as far back as pre-B cells[46,52,53] and any purging technique must therefore be directed at the whole B-cell lineage. There is also evidence that earlier stem cells may be involved, since 13% of cases express myeloid antigens and 30% show TcR rearrangement.[54,55] The second and related problem is how to assess the efficacy of purging. Phenotypic analysis can demonstrate removal of plasma cells and other McAb targeted cells but this does not necessarily mean that the putative stem cells have been removed. Clonogenic assays can be used, but most myelomas are poorly clonogenic in vitro and these assays are not therefore suitable for routine use. Identification of clone-specific Ig rearrangements would be a generally applicable and more sensitive technique, but has not yet been widely used, although Chan and Stephenson[56] have recently

132

shown that Ig gene rearrangements can be detected in purged marrow where immunocytochemistry is negative.

There is currently only a small clinical experience of ABMT using purged marrow. The Vancouver group have used pharmacologic purging with 4-HC, while the Dana–Farber and Bologna groups have used monoclonal antibodies covering the spectrum of B cells from immature cells to mature plasma cells. The use of the lectin peanut-agglutinin (PNA), which binds bone marrow plasma cells in the majority of myeloma patients without binding to normal haemopoietic progenitors, has been evaluated in vitro as a purging agent in combination with CD19 McAb,[57,58] but clinical use of this technique has not yet been reported.

Gobbi et al[59] have reported results of ABMT in 14 patients with advanced disease using an immunotoxin for in vitro purging. The monoclonal antibodies 8A and 62B1 were used, which recognize B-lineage cells from the TdT positive stage up to and including plasma cells.[60] These were coupled to a ribosome-inactivating protein called momordin to produce an immunotoxin which had been found to achieve up to 96% purging efficiency using a clonogenic assay for myeloma cells. A variety of conditioning regimes were used but 11 of 14 patients received TBI, plus either Cy, HDM, both drugs, or both drugs plus BCNU. Three patients received BuCy (2 pts) or HDM alone (1 pt). Platelet reconstitution was significantly prolonged. Three patients died of transplant-related toxicity and six of progressive disease. The remaining five patients survived from 4–18 months post-transplant at the time of reporting, but only one was in remission. This approach therefore did not result in long-term remissions and was associated with significant toxicity due to delayed engraftment.

The Dana–Farber transplant team have reported the results of purged ABMT in 11 patients with advanced but sensitive disease in whom they used a combination of monoclonal antibodies to purge the marrow.[61] All patients had stage II or III disease at diagnosis and had received at least two lines of prior therapy but were in partial remission with responsive disease at the time of ABMT. All had less than 10% plasma cells in the marrow at the time of harvest. The harvested mononuclear cells were treated with a mixture of complement-fixing antibodies directed against CD10 (CALLA), CD20 (pan-B) and PCA-1, which reacts with mature plasma cells, with the aim of targeting cells from the pre-B cell stage to mature plasma cells. Phenotypic analysis of treated cells did not detect any residual cells bearing these antigens; molecular genetic studies were not performed. Patients were conditioned with either HDM/TBI (10 pts) or Cy/TBI (1 pt). Full dose TBI (12 Gy in six fractions) was used. There was one treatment-related death associated with poor engraftment. The remaining patients engrafted satisfactorily, although rather slowly in some cases: 12–46 days to achieve neutrophils $>0.5 \times 10^9/l$ and 12–53 days to achieve platelets >20. There were seven complete responses and three partial responses. At a median follow-up of around 15 months four patients had relapsed, the projected 2-year PFS was 30% with a median PFS of 18 months.

The Vancouver group have recently reported their results of ABMT with 4-HC purged marrow in 14 patients in initial response (<10% plasma cells) after two cycles of VAD.[62] Median age was 49 years and the oldest patient was 60 years. Conditioning was intensive, with BuCy (16 mg/kg /120 mg/kg) plus HDM 90 mg/m^2, and there were three deaths, two due to veno-occlusive disease and one to fungal infection. The remaining 11 patients achieved CR (6) or PR (5). Engraftment was not delayed (median 19 days to neutrophils $0.5 \times 10^9/1$ and median duration of platelet support 32 days). At a median follow-up of 20 months seven patients had relapsed and the projected median PFS was 18 months (Fig. 7).

It is difficult to compare these results directly with those of unpurged ABMT. However the results of the two series where patients were autografted in remission, which both showed a median PFS of 18 months, do not appear to be significantly different from those of unpurged ABMT, where median PFS in several studies is between 18 and 24 months. Given the difficulty in establishing whether or not purging is of value in acute leukaemia, its role in myeloma is unlikely to be clarified without a large randomized study. Meanwhile, the possible advantage of 'negative purging' by positive selection of normal CD34 positive stem cells, as has been performed in ABMT for breast cancer [63] is being explored in relation to myeloma.

Peripheral blood stem cell transplantation

During the past few years there has been increasing interest in the use of peripheral blood stem cells (PBSC) for restoration of haematopoiesis after myelo-

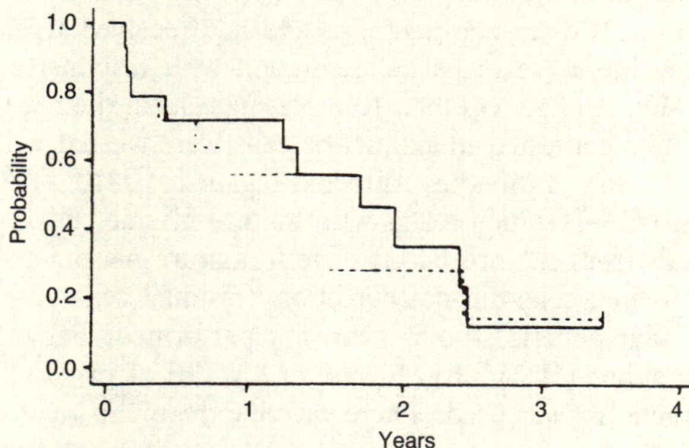

Fig. 7. Probability of survival and progression-free survival after BU CY MEL and autologous 4HC-purged BMT (from Reece et al 1993).[62]

ablative treatment (for review see Craig et al).[64] These cells can be mobilized by intensive chemotherapy and the yield can be increased enormously by the use of GM-CSF or G-CSF. The introduction of these growth factors into general use has made it logistically easy to harvest adequate numbers of PBSC with only one or two leucaphereses in the majority of patients. There is now a large experience of the use of PBSCT in a wide variety of haematological malignancies and solid tumours, and it is evident that PBSCT, especially using cells harvested with the use of growth factors, results in earlier engraftment than that observed after ABMT. The average period of neutropenia is shortened by about 7 days, and this is a major advantage in terms of hospital stay and patient turnover. Another advantage is that PBSC can be successfully harvested in patients who are unsuitable for marrow harvest because of prior local radiotherapy or heavy marrow infiltration.

An additional reason for the current interest in PBSCT in myeloma is the possibility that PBSC are less likely to be contaminated with malignant cells than is the marrow, based on the fact that circulating plasma cells are rarely observed in myeloma, even when the marrow is heavily infiltrated. However, there is considerable evidence from a variety of sources that the peripheral blood in myeloma patients contains mononuclear cells which belong to the malignant clone. Circulating B cells with tumour-specific Ig rearrangements can be detected by Southern blotting and more frequently by PCR-based techniques. [65–70] Circulating B lymphocytes in myeloma may express plasma cell antigens[71,72] and myeloma colonies can be grown from the peripheral blood.[73, 74]

Bell et al[75] used anti-idiotype antibodies and immunoglobulin gene analysis (Southern blotting) to look for myeloma cells in PBSC harvests in six patients and compared the results with those of bone marrow harvests obtained just before PBSC collection. The number of idiotype (Id)-positive cells in the marrows varied from 0.1% to 19%, while in the peripheral blood the number varied from 0% in two cases to 2%. Southern blotting detected Ig gene rearrangements in five of the six marrow samples but only two of the PBSC harvests. These data suggest that there are fewer myeloma cells in the blood than in the marrow, especially during remission, but given the limits of detection of the methods, which is of the order of 2% for Southern blotting, it is not possible to exclude contamination of the majority of PBSC harvests. It therefore remains probable that harvested circulating cells could be a cause of relapse after PBSCT.

There are a number of early reports indicating that PBSC can be successfully used to reconstitute bone marrow after myeloablative therapy in myeloma patients,[75–80] but these studies were small and follow-up was too short to evaluate long-term relapse risk. Fermand et al[81] have since reported longer-term results of PBSCT in a series of over 70 patients, all with stage III myeloma, of whom 48% had newly diagnosed disease. PBSC were harvested after primimg with combination chemotherapy (CHOP regimen), but growth factors were not used. An adequate number of stem cells was obtained after one course in 76% patients; if this was not successful there was only a 30% chance of obtaining sufficient cells after a second course. Previous chemotherapy had a significant effect on the ability to recruit PBSC; adequate harvests (minimum 2×10^4 CFU-GM/kg) were obtained in 31 of 33 previously untreated patients and in ten of 11 patients with minimal previous treatment, but only 15 of 26 patients with refractory disease. The number of GFU-GM collected was also lower in pretreated patients. While the use of growth factors will clearly improve the yield of PBSC, it is likely that there will continue to be a problem in heavily pretreated patients. In all, 58 patients in whom adequate PBSC had been obtained were considered for ABMT. Two progressed prior to transplant and six received other treatment. 50 patients underwent PBSCT; 43 of these were treated with a protocol including CCNU 120 mg m^2, etoposide 750 mg m^2, cyclophosphamide 60 mg/kg, HDM 140 mg/m^2 and TBI (dose not stated), and seven with busulphan and melphalan alone. The results in the 43 patients treated with chemotherapy and TBI are shown in Fig. 8. The eight deaths were related to postgraft aplasia or late infection. The median progression-free survival had not been reached at 40 months, but only eight were in CR. These patients represent a selected group of the 73 patients enrolled; 74% had responsive disease and 62% were newly diagnosed patients. They represent a similar group therefore to the Marsden series where ABMT was carried out after initial combination chemotherapy, in which median PFS was 24 months; while the results of the PBSCT series appear more promising, follow-up was shorter and only eight of the patients were in CR, so it is likely that more relapses will occur. As Fermand et al point out, differences in patient selection and in transplant protocols preclude any definitive comparison between ABMT and PBSCT at the present time. The current data from the French Autograft Registry[49] referred to above indicate that in a heterogenous group of patients there is no overall difference in relapse risk between PBSCT and ABMT. Whether it is possible to purge PBSC more effeciently than bone marrow remains to be determined.

Meanwhile the use of PBSC for haematological support is likely to increase for practical reasons. More work is needed to define, in the contest of the use of growth factors, whether or not intensive chemotherapy is still required to recruit adequate numbers of PBSC. It may be that standard combination chemotherapy alone is sufficient, particularly in patients who have received little previous treatment. A note of caution concerning the use of growth factors in myeloma is, however, warranted, in view of the evidence that both GM-CSF and G-CSF can stimulate myeloma growth in vitro and in vivo.[82,83]

Interferon maintenance after autologous transplant

Attal et al[26,27] have reported the results of a nonrandomized study of interferon maintenance in 29 patients who had received ABMT for poor-risk

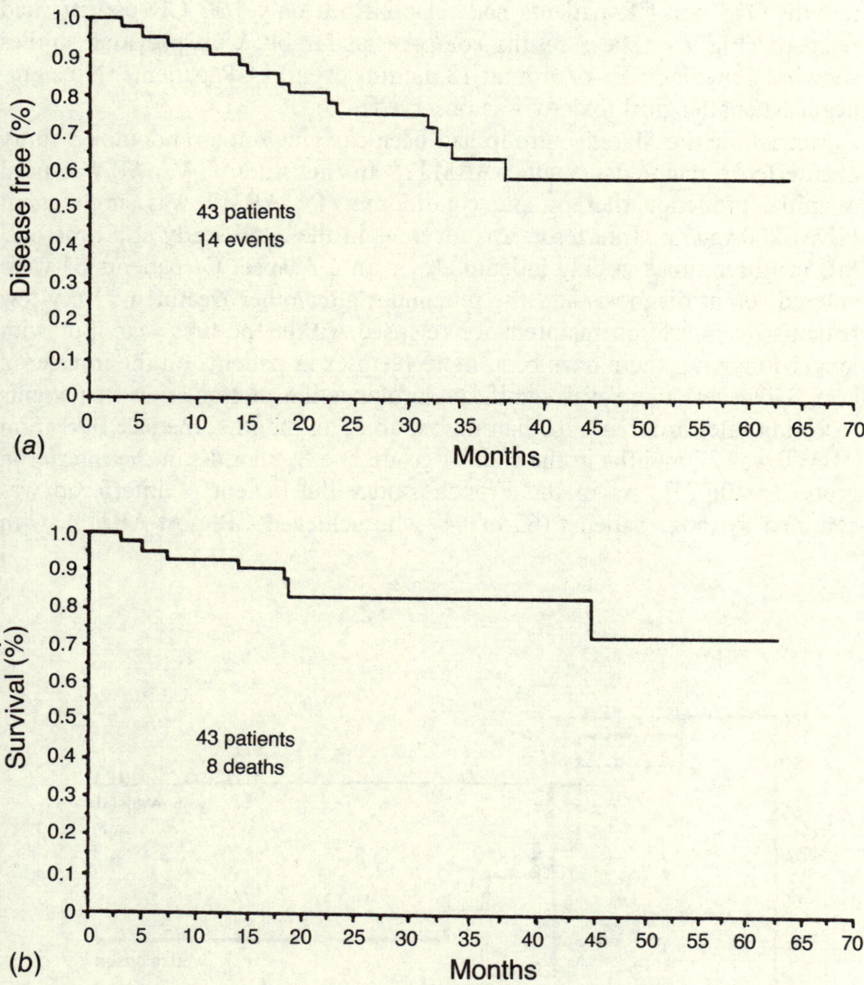

Fig. 8. Disease-free (*a*) and overall (*b*) survival of patients treated with high-dose chemotherapy and total body irradiation and autologous peripheral blood stem cell transplantation (from Fermand et al 1992).[81]

myeloma in first response. Initial induction therapy was with either VAD or VBMCP. Conditioning was with melphalan 140 mg/m² and TBI (8 Gy in four fractions); marrow was unpurged. Interferon alpha was started as soon after ABMT as granulocytes were >0.5 × 10⁹/1 and platelets >75 × 10⁹/1 which proved to be at a median time of 2.6 months (range 1 to 7.7). Interferon was given at a dose of 3 mU/m² three times weekly and continued indefinitely or until relapse. Of patients 15 reached CR after ABMT (14 of these after starting interferon) and 15 did not. At a median follow-up of 15.5

D Samson

months 7/15 non-CR patients had relapsed but only 1/15 CR patients had relapsed (Fig 9.). These results compare favourably with previous studies showing a median PFS of around 18 months even in CR patients. No significant haematological toxicity was observed.

Meanwhile the Marsden group had been carrying out a randomized study of interferon maintenance after ABMT.[14] In this study C-VAMP was used as initial induction therapy and conditioning for ABMT was single agent HDM 200 mg/m^2. Interferon was given as in the Attal study at a dose of 3 mU/m^2 three times weekly indefinitely or until relapse. Of patients 84 were entered, 66 at diagnosis and the remainder after other treatment. Very few patients on interferon maintenance relapsed within the first year, but with longer follow-up there have been more relapses in patients on the interferon arm. However, there was significant prolongation of remission in patients receiving interferon: at a median follow-up of 24 months, median PFS from ABMT was 27 months in the control group and 39 months in the interferon group (p<0.025). As in the French study, the benefit of interferon was confined to those patients (62 of 84) who achieved CR post-ABMT, with

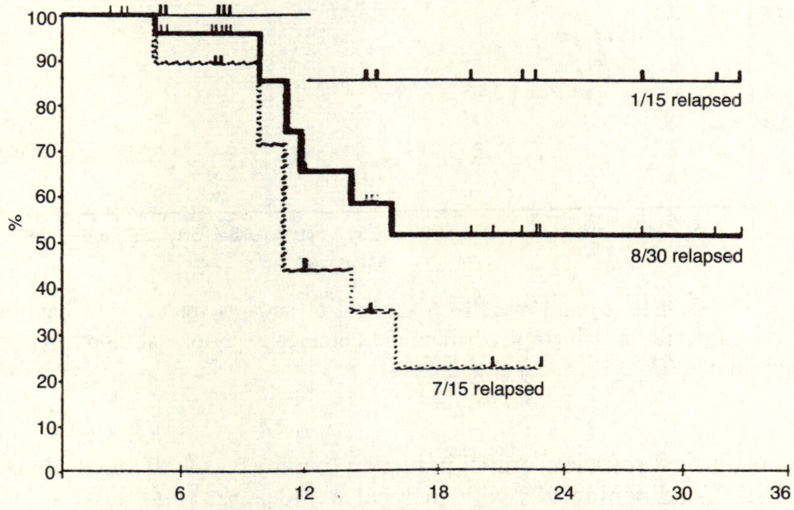

Fig. 9. Progression-free survival after ABMT with interferon maintenance (from Attal et al, 1992).[27]
solid line = all patients,
thin solid line = patients in CR after ABMT,
dotted line = patients not in CR.

138

53% remaining in remission at 4 years, while for nonresponders and PR patients there was no prolongation of PFS. The shapes of the PFS curves suggest that interferon is delaying relapse by approximately 2 years in the CR patients, but that ultimately all will relapse.

In the EBMT Registry study of autologous transplants, 22 of 86 responders received post-transplant interferon. There was no difference in PFS between these patients and those who did not receive interferon (PFS median 14 months in both groups) but this was not a randomized study and the interferon-treated group is small. In the French Autograft Registry Study, on the other hand, post-transplant interferon was correlated with improved survival (72% at 3 years v 46%, p = 0.0001).

Results of autologous versus allogeneic BMT

It is interesting that, whereas the attainment of CR post-BMT was the most significant factor affecting survival and PFS after allo-BMT, none of the studies of ABMT has observed this difference. The proportion of patients entering CR after ABMT is similar to that seen after allogeneic BMT (c. 50% overall and c 70% for those in first PR), but these remissions are not durable. Since the initial response is so similar, relapse from reinfused cells seems highly likely. Some authors have felt that the lack of correlation between bone marrow plasmacytosis at harvest and time to relapse made it more likely that relapse was from residual disease than from reinfused cells, but an alternative explanation is that the number of plasma cells is irrelevant if in all cases there are sufficient reinfused myeloma stem cells to regrow. The time to relapse might theoretically depend on other factors such as IL-6 levels during the post-transplant period. The question of the origin of relapse will only be answered definitively by genetic marking of the reinfused cells, as has recently been done in acute lymphoblastic leukaemia.[84]

Autologous transplant versus chemotherapy

There is no evidence from the current data that any form of autologous transplant is curative. However, prolongation of survival, especially progression-free survival is also a reasonable goal. What is the evidence that relapse-free survival after autologous transplant is better than after conventional chemotherapy plus interferon maintenance? More patients enter CR after myelo-ablative therapy than after conventional chemotherapy, and although patients not receiving maintenance interferon after autologous transplant relapse at the same rate whether or not CR has been achieved, it seems that interferon can prolong response duration in those patients who have achieved CR. The longest progression-free survivals have been observed in patients transplanted following response to first-line treatment, who achieve CR and who then receive maintenance interferon. The median PFS of such a patient group was 4 years in the Marsden series[14] and not reached at 3 years in the

D Samson

Toulouse study.[27] These represent the best currently reported results of ASCT. The best reported results of conventional chemotherapy and interferon are those observed in the current ECOG study, in which cyclical chemotherapy and interferon are given together for a 2-year period.[85] Median response duration is currently 46 months for the 30% of patients achieving CR and 35 months overall. It is thus not clear that ABMT improves outcome compared with conventional chemotherapy. This question can only be answered by randomized studies.

Future directions and current recommendations

Allogeneic BMT for myeloma carries a relatively high risk of procedure-related death, and relapse is also an important cause of failure. Nevertheless, it appears that some patients may be cured of their disease, and this justifies the use of allogeneic BMT earlier in the course of the disease, when mortality is less and the probability of CR and long-term survival is correspondingly greater. Given the existing regimen-related toxicity observed in myeloma patients, there would seem to be little room to increase the intensity of conditioning. The use of interferon maintenance after allogeneic BMT might be even more effective than in the autologous situation, since it could potentiate a graft-versus-myeloma effect. Whether it is possible to administer interferon early after allogeneic BMT, without unacceptable haematological toxicity and without exacerbating GVHD remains to be determined. The EBMT is currently carrying out a pilot study to evaluate this.

Autologous BMT is increasingly being used to treat patients with myeloma early in the course of their disease, and a number of randomized controlled trials are now in progress, comparing autologous transplant with conventional chemotherapy.

Meanwhile it is important to continue to explore new approaches to autologous transplant, including the use of positive stem cell selection. The clinical use of either purged marrow or positively selected normal progenitor cells needs to be combined with molecular techniques for assessment of residual contamination, or it will remain unclear whether relapse after purging is due to a failure of the purging method used or to residual myeloma. Such techniques may also elucidate whether PBSC can be more efficiently purged than bone marrow.

At present, the following would appear to be reasonable recommendations for patient management:

1. Patients under age 55 years with a matched sibling donor should be considered for allogeneic BMT after first-line treatment, especially if they have poor prognosis features and/or are refractory to initial therapy.
2. Patients under age 65 years and those without a sibling donor are suit-

able for autologous transplant after first-line treatment. This should preferably be carried out as part of a defined study.

3. At present, there is no evidence that the source of stem cells used for autologous transplant has a significant effect on the duration of response, and the choice betwen PBSC and marrow can therefore be made on practical grounds.
4. Recommended conditioning regimens for allogeneic BMT include Cy/TBI (12 Gy in 6 fractions), BuCy (Bu 14 mg/kg plus Cy 120–147 mg/kg) or HDM/TBI (HDM 120 mg/m^2/TBI 12 Gy in 6 fractions).
5. Recommended conditioning regimens for autologous BMT in patients up to 65 years include HDM 200 mg/m^2 or HDM 140 mg/m^2 plus TBI 8 Gy in 4 fractions. For patients below 55 years there may be an advantage in using one of the more intensive regimens proposed for allogeneic BMT.
6. Administration of interferon after ABMT appears to prolong response in CR patients but a survival benefit is not established, and interferon should therefore ideally be given in the context of a randomized study.

References

(1) MacLennan ICM, Chapman C, Dunn J, Kelly K, for the MRC Working Party for Leukaemia in Adults. Combined chemotherapy with ABCM versus melphalan for treatment of myelomatosis. *Lancet* 1992; 339: 200–5.
(2) Selby PJ, McElwain TJ, Nandi AC et al. Multiple myeloma treated with high-dose intravenous mephalan. *Br J Haematol* 1987; 66: 55–62.
(3) Samson D, Gaminara E, Newland AC et al. Infusion of vincristine and doxorubicin with oral dexamethasone as first-line therapy for multiple myeloma. *Lancet* 1989; ii: 882–5.
(4) Mandelli F, Avvisati G, Amadori S et al. Maintenance with recombinant interferon alfa-2b in patients with multiple myeloma responsive to conventional induction chemotherapy. *N Eng J Med* 1990; 322: 1430–4.
(5) Peest D, Deicher H, Colewey R et al. Melphalan and prednisone (MP) versus vincristine, BCNU, adriamycin, melphalan and dexamethasone (VBAMDex) induction chemotherapy and interferon maintenance treatment in multiple myeloma; current results of a multicenter trial. *Onkologie* 1990; 13: 458–60.
(6) Cooper MR, Dear K, McIntyre OR et al. A randomized clinical trial comparing melphalan/prednisone with or without interferon alfa 2b in newly diagnosed patients with multiple myeloma: a Cancer and Leukaemia Group B Study. *J Clin Oncol* 1993; 11: 155–60.
(7) Bird J, Samson D, Newland AC et al. VAD with concurrent IFN or VAD followed by maintenance IFN in newly-diagnosed myeloma: updated results of a randomised study. *Br J Haematol* 1993; 84 (suppl 1): 44.
(8) Mellstedt G. MP/alpha IFN in the induction treatment of multiple myeloma and as maintenance therapy: a randomised trial from MGCS. *Proc Workshop on Multiple Myeloma: from Biol to Therapy* 1991; 115–6 (abstr).

(9) Westin J, Rodjer S, Turesson I. Interferon-alpha 2b as maintenance therapy in multiple myeloma: effect on plateau phase duration and survival. *Abst 24th Congr Int Soc Haematol* 1992; 279.

(10) Barlogie B, Alexanian R, Smallwood L et al. Prognostic factors with high dose melphalan for refractory multiple myeloma. *Blood* 1988; 72: 2015–9.

(11) Barlogie B. Management of multiple myeloma. *Blut* 1990; 60: 1–7.

(12) Gore ME, Selby PJ, Viner C et al. Intensive treatment of multiple myeloma and criteria for complete remission. *Lancet* 1989; ii: 879–82.

(13) Montes A, Cunningham D, Paz-Ares L et al. High dose melphalan and autologous bone marrow transplant in multiple myeloma: long term follow up. Abstracts of 19th Annual Meeting of EBMT. Garmisch-Partenkirchen 1993; p. 68.

(14) Cunningham D, Powles R, Malpas JS et al. A randomised trial of Intron-A following high dose melphalan and ABMT in myeloma. Abstracts of 19th Annual Meeting of EBMT. Garmisch-Partenkirchen 1993; p. 68.

(15) Glenn L, Vesole D, Jagannath S, Barlogie B. Double autotransplant with melphalan for multiple myeloma. *Blood* 1992; 80 (suppl 1): 122a.

(16) Jagganath S, Vesole D, Glenn L, Barlogie B. Total therapy (TT) with intensive remission induction (IRI) and double autotransplants (Tx) for multiple myeloma. *Blood* 1992; 80 (suppl 1): 362a.

(17) Barlogie B, Alexanian R, Dicke KA et al High-dose chemoradiotherapy and autologous bone marrow transplantation for resistant multiple myeloma. *Blood* 1987; 70: 869–72.

(18) Barlogie B, Epstein J, Selvanayagam P, Alexanian R. Plasma cell myeloma – new biological insights and advances in therapy. *Blood* 1989; 73: 865–79.

(19) Jagannath S, Barlogie B, Dicke K et al. Autologous bone marrow transplantation in multiple myeloma: Identification of prognostic factors. *Blood* 1990; 76: 1860–6.

(20) Gahrton G, Tura S, Ljungman P et al. Allogeneic bone marrow transplantation in multiple myeloma. *N Eng J Med* 1991; 325: 1267–73.

(21) Helenglass G, Powles RL, McElwain TJ et al. Melphalan and total body irradiation (TBI) versus cyclophosphamide and TBI as conditioning for allogeneic matched sibling bone marrow transplants for acute myeloblastic leukaemia in first remission. *Bone Marrow Transpl* 1988; 3: 21–9.

(22) Phillips GL, Shepherd JD, Barnett MJ et al. Busulfan, cyclophosphamide, and melphalan conditioning for autologous bone marrow transplantation in hematologic malignancy. *J Clin Oncol* 1991; 9: 1880–8.

(23) Barlogie B, Gahrton G. Bone marrow transplantation in multiple myeloma. *Bone Marrow Transpl* 1991; 7: 71–9.

(24) Harrousseau JL, Milpied N, Jouet JP et al. High dose melphalan as 'in-vivo purging' before autologous transplantation in multiple myeloma. *Bone Marrow Transpl* 1990; 5 (suppl 2): 182 (abstr).

(25) Stoppa AM, Blaise D, Viens P, Baume D, Bataille R. Double bone marrow transplant with high dose alkylating agents for poor prognosis multiple myeloma. *Abst 18th Annual Meeting of EBMT*, Stockholm 1992; 188.

(26) Attal M, Huguet F, Schlaifer D et al. Maintenance treatment with recombinant

alpha interferon after autologous bone marrow transplantation for aggressive myeloma in first remission after conventional induction chemotherapy. *Bone Marrow Transpl* 1991; 8: 125–8.

(27) Attal M, Huguet F, Schlaifer D, et al. Intensive combined therapy for previously untreated aggressive myeloma. *Blood* 1992; 79: 1130–6.

(28) Gottlieb DJ, Prentice HG, Heslop HE et al. Effects of recombinant interleukin-2 administration on cytotoxic function following high dose chemo-radiotherapy for hematological malignancy. *Blood*, 1989; 74: 2335–42.

(29) Heslop HE, Gottlieb DJ, Bianchi ACM et al. In vivo induction of gamma interferon and tumor necrosis factor by interleukin-2 infusion following intensive chemotherapy or autologous bone marrow transplantation. *Blood* 1989; 74: 1374–80.

(30) Gahrton G, Tura S, Flesch A et al. Bone marrow transplantation for multiple myeloma: Report from the European Cooperative Group for Bone Marrow Transplantation. *Blood* 1987; 69: 1262–4.

(31) Tura S, Cavo M, Rosti G et al. Allogeneic BMT for multiple myeloma (MM). Prior responsiveness to chemotherapy predicts a favourable outcome of the procedure. Abstracts of 19th Annual Meeting of EBMT. Garmisch-Partenkirchen 1993; p. 69.

(32) Santos GW, Tutschka PJ, Brookmeyer R et al. Marrow transplantation for acute non-lymphocytic leukaemia after treatment with busulfan and cyclophosphamide. *N Eng J Med* 1983; 309: 1347–53.

(33) Tutschka PJ, Copelan EA, Klein JP. Bone marrow transplantation for leukaemia following a new busulfan and cyclophosphamide regime. *Blood* 1987; 70: 1382–8.

(34) Copelan EA, Tutschka PJ. Marrow transplantation following busulphan and cyclophosphamide for multiple myeloma. *Bone Marrow Transpl* 1988; 3: 363–5.

(35) Bensinger WI, Buckner CD, Clift RA et al. Phase I study of busulfan and cyclophosphamide in preparation for allogeneic marrow transplantation for patients with multiple myeloma. *J Clin Oncol* 1992; 10: 1492–7.

(36) Reece DE, Shepherd JD, Nantel SH et al. Intensive therapy (IT) and allogeneic bone marrow transplantation (alloBMT) for multiple myeloma patients: the Vancouver experience. *Blood* 1992; 80 (suppl 1): 362a.

(37) Fefer A, Greenberg PD, Cheever MA et al. Treatment of multiple myeloma with chemoradiotherapy and identical twin bone marrow transplantation. *Proc Am Soc Clin Oncol* 1982; 1: C731.

(38) Osserman EF, Di Re LB, Di Re J, Sherman WH, Hersman JA, Storb R. Identical twin transplantation in multiple myeloma. *Acta Haematol* (Basel) 1982; 68: 215–23.

(39) Buckner CD, Fefer A, Bensinger W1 et al. Marrow transplantation for malignant plasma cell disorders: summary of the Seattle experience. *Eur J Haematol* 1989; 43 (suppl 51): 186–90.

(40) McGlave PB, Beatty P, Ash R, Hows JM. Therapy for chronic myelogenous leukaemia with unrelated donor bone marrow transplantation. *Blood* 1990; 75: 1728–32.

(41) Bird JM, Samson D, Russell NH. Minimal residual disease after bone marrow transplantation for multiple myeloma: evidence for cure in long-term survivors. 1993; *Bone Marrow Transpl* 1993; 12: 651–4.

(42) Deane M, Norton JD. Immunoglobulin gene 'fingerprinting': an approach to analysis of B lymphoid clonality in lymphoproliferative disorders. *Br J Haematol* 1991; 77: 274–81.

(43) Deane M, Samson D. Detection of minimal residual myeloma after bone marrow transplantation. *Br J Haematol* 1991; 78: 134–135.

(44) Hughes TP, Morgan GJ, Martiat P, Goldman J. Detection of residual leukaemia after bone marrow transplantation: role of PCR in predicting relapse. *Blood* 1991; 77: 874–8.

(45) Bell JGB, Millar JA, Maitland JA, Nandi A, Gore M, McElwain TJ. Increased clonogenic tumour cells in bone marrow after VAMP therapy. *Lancet* 1988; ii: 931–3.

(46) Grogan TM, Durie BGM, Lomen C et al. Delineation of a novel pre-B cell component in multiple myeloma: immunochemical, immunophenotypic, genotypic, cytologic, cell culture and kinetic features. *Blood* 1987; 70: 932–42.

(47) Caligaris-Cappio F, Bergui L, Tesio L et al. Identification of malignant plasma cell precursors in the bone marrow of multiple myeloma. *J Clin Invest* 1985; 76: 1243–51.

(48) Harousseau JL, Milpied N, Laporte JP et al. Double-intensive therapy in high-risk multiple myeloma. *Blood* 1992; 79: 2827–33.

(49) Harousseau JL, Attal M, Divine M et al. Autologous hemopoietic stem cell transplantation (ASCT) in multiple myeloma. A report of the French Registry. Abstracts of 19th Annual Meeting of EBMT. Garmisch-Partenkirchen 1993; p. 68.

(50) Bjorkstrand B, Ljungman P, Brunet S et al. Autologous stem cell transplantation in multiple myeloma – a European Registry Study. *Blood* 1992; 80 (suppl 1): 362a.

(51) Gribben JG, Saporito L, Blake KW et al. Bone marrows of non-Hodgkin's lymphoma patients with a bcl-2 translocation can be purged of polymerase chain reaction-detectable lymphoma cells using monoclonal antibodies and immunomagnetic bead depletion. *Blood* 1992; 80: 1083–9.

(52) Foon KA, Todd RF. Immunological classification of leukaemia and lymphoma. *Blood* 1986; 68: 1–31.

(53) Anderson KC, Cochran M, Barut BA. Phenotypic and functional characterisation of normal and malignant terminal B (plasma) cells. *Eur J Haematol* 1989; 43 (suppl 51): 19–26.

(54) Grogan TM, Durie BGM, Spier C et al. Myelomonocytic antigen positive multiple myeloma. *Blood* 1989; 73: 763–9.

(55) Spier CM, Grogan TM, Durie BGM et al. T-cell antigen positive multiple myeloma. *Mod Pathol* 1990; 3: 302–7.

(56) Chan C, Stephenson R. Immunophenotyping and genotyping evaluation of efficiency in immunopurging of myeloma cells. *Blood* 1990; 76 (suppl 11): 344a.

(57) Rhodes EGH, Baker P, Rhodes JM, Davies JM, Cawley JC. Peanut agglutinnin in combination with CD19 monoantibody has potential as a purging agent in myeloma. *Exp Hematol* 1991; 19: 833–7.

(58) Rhodes EGH, Baker PK, Duguid JKM, Davies JM, Cawley JC. A method for clinical purging of myeloma bone marrow using peanut agglutinin as an anti-plasma cell agent, in combination with CD19 monoclonal antibody. *Bone Marrow Transpl* 1992; 10: 485–9

(59) Gobbi M, Tazzari PL, Cavo M et al. Autologous bone marrow transplantation with immunotoxin purged marrow in multiple myeloma. Long term results in 14 patients with advanced disease. *Bone Marrow Transpl* 1991; 8(suppl 2): 30.

(60) Dinota A, Tazzari PL, Bontadini A et al. Production and characterisation of monoclonal antibodies for the ex-vivo purging of the bone marrow in patients with multiple myeloma. *J Exp Pathol* 1987; 3: 363–7.

(61) Anderson KC, Barut BA, Ritz J et al. Monoclonal antibody-purged autologous bone marrow transplantation therapy for multiple myeloma. *Blood* 1991; 77: 712–20.

(62) Reece DE, Barnett MJ, Connors JM et al. Treatment of multiple myeloma with intensive chemotherapy followed by autologous BMT using marrow purged with 4-hydroperoxycyclophosphamide. *Bone Marrow Transpl* 1993; 11: 139–46.

(63) Berenson RJ, Bensinger WI, Hill RS et al. Engraftment after infusion of CD34$^+$ marrow cells in patients with breast cancer or neuroblastoma. *Blood* 1991; 77: 1717–22.

(64) Craig JIO, Turner ML, Parker AC. Peripheral blood stem cell transplantation. *Blood Rev* 1992; 6: 59–67.

(65) Berenson J, Wong R, Kim K, Brown N, Lichtenstein A. Evidence for peripheral blood B lymphocyte but not T lymphocyte involvement in multiple myeloma. *Blood* 1987; 70: 1550–3.

(66) Neri A, Murphy JP, Cro L et al. RAS oncogene mutation in multiple myeloma. *J Exp Med* 1989; 170: 1715–25.

(67) Chiu EKW, Ganeshaguru K, Hoffbrand AV, Mehta AB. Circulating monoclonal B lymphocytes in multiple myeloma. *Br J Haematol* 1989; 72: 28–31.

(68) Baldini L, Cro L, Delia D, Chiorboli O, Neri A, Maiolo AT. Analysis of tumor-specific immunoglobulin gene rearrangement in peripheral blood B-cells of multiple myeloma patients. *Am J Hematol* 1991; 37: 1–5.

(69) Billadeau D, Quam L, Thomas W et al. Detection and quantitation of malignant cells in the peripheral blood of multile myeloma patients. *Blood* 1992; 80: 1818–24.

(70) Bird JM, Samson D. Use of immunoglobulin gene fingerprinting for the detection of clonally rearranged cells in the peripheral blood of myeloma patients. *Br Haematol* 1993; 84 (suppl 2): 392.

(71) Omede P, Boccadoro M, Gallone G et al. Multiple myeloma: increased circulating lymphocytes carrying plasma cell-associated antigens as an indicator of poor survival. *Blood* 1990; 76: 1375–9.

(72) Shimizaki C, Fried J, Perez AG et al. Immunophenotypic analysis of lymphocytes and myeloma cells in patients with multiple myeloma. *Acta Haematol* 1990; 83: 123–9.

(73) Millar B, Bell J, Lakhani A et al. A simple method of culturing myeloma cells from human bone marrow aspirates and peripheral blood in vitro. *Br J Haematol* 1988; 69: 197–203.

(74) Caligaris-Cappio F, Bergui L, Gaidano GL et al. Circulating malignant

precursor cells in monoclonal gammopathies. *Eur J Haematol* 1989; 45 (suppl 51): 27–29.

(75) Bell AJ, North J, Stevenson EK, Hamblin TJ. Peripheral blood stem cell autografts in myeloma. *Bone Marrow Transpl* 1990; 5 (suppl 1): 52–54.

(76) Bell AJ, Williamson PJ, North J, Watts EJ, Stephens JR. Circulating stem cell autografts in high-risk myeloma. *Br J Haematol* 1989; 71: 162–163.

(77) Fermand JP, Levy Y, Gerota J et al. Treatment of aggressive multiple myeloma by high-dose chemotherapy and total body irradiation followed by blood stem cells autologous graft. *Blood* 1989; 73: 20–3.

(78) Reiffers J, Marit G, Boiron JM. Autologous blood stem cell transplantation in high-risk multiple myeloma. *Br J Haemat* 1989; 72: 296–297.

(79) Henon PR. for the France Autogreffe Group. Blood stem cell autograft in malignant blood disease: The French experience with a special focus on myeloma. *Haematologica* 1990; 75 (suppl 1): 53.

(80) Ventura GJ, Barlogie B, Hester JP et al. High dose cyclophosphamide, BCNU and VP-16 with autologous blood stem cell support for refractory multiple myeloma. *Bone Marrow Transpl* 1990; 5: 265–8.

(81) Fermand JP, Chevret S, Levy Y et al. The role of autologous blood stem cells in support of high-dose therapy for multiple myeloma. *Hematol Oncol Clin N Am* 1992; 6: 451–462.

(82) Zhang X–G, Bataille R, Jourdan M et al. Granulocyte-macrophage colony-stimulating factor synergizes with interleukin-6 in supporting the proliferation of human myeloma cells. *Blood* 1991; 76: 2599–605.

(83) Klein B, Bataille R. Cytokine network in human multiple myeloma. *Hematol Oncol Clin N Am* 1992; 6: 273–84.

(84) Brenner MK, Rill DR, Moen RC et al. Gene-marking to trace origin of relapse after autologous bone-marrow transplantation. *Lancet* 1993; 341: 85–6.

(85) Oken MM, Kyle RA, Greipp PR, Kay NE, Tsiatis A, O'Connell MJ. Possible survival benefit with chemotherapy plus interferon (r IFN α 2) in the treatment of multiple myeloma. *Proc ASCO* 1992 p.358 (abst).

Peripheral blood stem cells for therapeutic use

C A JUTTNER and L B TO

Introduction

High dose therapy is used increasingly in the management of cancer, even though its efficacy is far from proven. Reviews by Hryniuk and colleagues suggest that the intensity of *conventional dose* chemotherapy, ie delivered dose and time over which it is given, correlates with response rate in several cancers including breast, small cell lung, and ovarian cancer, Hodgkin's disease and non-Hodgkin's lymphoma.[1] Whether these increased response rates translate to more cures is uncertain. Less is known about *higher dose* therapy. Relapse is apparently decreased in some patients receiving high dose therapy and allogeneic bone marrow transplants. Examples include acute and chronic myeloid leukaemia (AML and CML) and acute lymphoblastic leukaemia (ALL). In CML, but less certainly in AML and ALL, these decreased relapse risks translate to increased leukaemia-free survival. It is uncertain whether the decreased relapse results from the high dose therapy or immune-mediated anticancer effects collectively termed graft-versus-leukaemia (GVL), or from a combination of the two. Studies from the International Bone Marrow Transplant Registry comparing twin transplants and allogeneic transplants, conventional and T-cell depleted, without graft-versus-host disease, support immunological antileukaemia effects.[2] Recent studies where donor blood cell infusions produced remission in patients with CML who relapse after high dose therapy and an allogeneic transplant lend further support to this notion.[3]

The contribution of high dose therapy and autotransplants to decreased relapse and increased survival is even more unclear. Some studies report cures in advanced Hodgkin's disease and non-Hodgkin's lymphoma, but it is uncertain that these results differ from those produced by chemotherapy

All correspondence to: Dr C A Juttner, Hanson Centre for Cancer Research, Institute of Medical and Veterinary Science, Frome Road, Adelaide, South Australia 5000.

Cambridge Medical Reviews: Haematological Oncology Volume 3
© Cambridge University Press 1994

alone. The most convincing data supporting a benefit for high dose therapy and autotransplants come from studies in advanced breast cancer, where up to 20% of patients with metastatic disease become long-term survivors. This is never achieved by conventional therapies.

Early studies in advanced non-Hodgkin's lymphoma (NHL) showed long-term benefit only in patients whose disease was responsive to conventional dose chemotherapy pretransplant. This may not be so in Hodgkin's disease (HD) where there may be long-term benefit even in resistant disease.[4] One study prospectively randomized patients with intermediate grade NHL still responsive to chemotherapy to conventional chemotherapy and total lymphoid radiation or to high dose therapy and an autotransplant. No benefit is yet reported for high dose therapy.[5] Another small unrandomized study of early high dose therapy and autotransplants in patients with intermediate grade NHL and poor prognostic features suggests a benefit for high dose therapy.[6] Preliminary data from another similar study also suggests a benefit for intensive treatment.[7]

Despite these uncertainties, autologous bone marrow transplantation (ABMT) has been in widespread use since the early 1980s. Large numbers of patients have received ABMT and long term clinical results are available. Peripheral blood stem cell transplantation (PBSCT) has been used widely only in the last 3–4 years, and clinical results are much less mature with fewer patients treated and briefer follow-up. This is despite the recognition of haemopoietic stem and progenitor cells in the circulation before 1970. Successful animal studies of PBSCT were carried out in the 1960's and 1970s. Initial human studies in syngeneic twins suggested inadequate engraftment although other early studies using peripheral blood stem cells (PBSC) from patients in the chronic phase of CML demonstrated engraftment, if not satisfactory long-term tumour control.[8]

Initial interest in PBSC was based on several potential advantages. It is theoretically possible that these stem cells might contain fewer clonogenic malignant cells than bone marrow, and PBSC could therefore be used in patients whose bone marrow was contaminated with cancer. PBSC could also be collected from patients with bone marrow impaired from fibrosis or previous radiation therapy. PBSC could be collected by apheresis in a conscious patient rather than by multiple bone marrow aspirations under general anaesthesia. PBSC collections might provide a richer source of stem cells for transplant, as suggested by the marked increase in PB progenitors seen during recovery after myelosuppressive chemotherapy, initially observed by Richman.[9]

The first reported transplants using recovery phase PBSC revealed the advantage of rapid haemopoietic reconstitution (HR).[10–12] Subsequent studies have identified some of the factors contributing to this advantage, including the need to collect an adequate dose of PBSC and the need to collect the

148

cells in a state of perturbed haemopoiesis ('mobilized' PBSC) in order to achieve rapid HR. The adequacy of lifelong HR after PBSCT is not yet confirmed in man, although animal studies demonstrate that PBSC can reconstitute haemopoiesis long-term up to 10 years after allogeneic transplant in the dog[13] and up to 13 months after sex mismatched transplant in the mouse.[14]

Although firm conclusions cannot yet be drawn about clinical outcomes in terms of tumour control and disease-free survival in comparison with either ABMT or conventional therapy, there has been an explosion in the use of PBSC autografting, largely because of the advantages of rapid HR.

This review sets out to consider a number of important questions basic to PBSC transplantation. In particular:

- Is HR after PBSCT significantly faster than after bone marrow transplant (BMT) and, most importantly after BMT with post graft administration of haemopoietic growth factors (HGF)? Is PBSC mobilization necessary?
- What determines an adequate number of PBSC for rapid early and sustained late HR, how is this 'adequate number' best measured and when is PBSC release maximal?
- What is the best method to mobilize?
- What is the molecular or biological mechanism of mobilization?
- What is the best technology for PBSC collection?
- Are there fewer cancer cells in PBSC than bone marrow?
- Do the initial clinical results allow valid comparison between PBSC and BM transplant?
- Do the particular characteristics of PBSC allow potential further development of haemopoietic support for high dose therapy?

These questions will be addressed and opinions or answers provided where possible. However, it must be emphasized that PBSC transplantation is relatively new and firm conclusions can often not yet be drawn.

Comparisons of haemopoietic reconstitution after PBSCT and BMT with and without post-transplant haemopoietic growth factors

Transplantation of PBSC collected during steady phase or unperturbed haemopoiesis produces HR which is not significantly different from ABMT.[15,16] In contrast, when PBSC mobilized by chemotherapy or HGF are used, granulocyte recovery is regularly and predictably faster than with BM. Fig. 1 shows that the mean time to achieve a granulocyte count of 0.5 $\times$ 10^9/l is usually between 7 and 10 days faster.[17,18] Platelet reconstitution is similarly rapid in some but not in all studies (see Fig. 2).[17–19] Both parameters are faster with large PBSC doses as measured by the number of CFU-GM infused but some patients receiving large numbers of CFU-GM may paradoxically have delayed and unsatisfactory platelet recovery, at least in AML.[20]

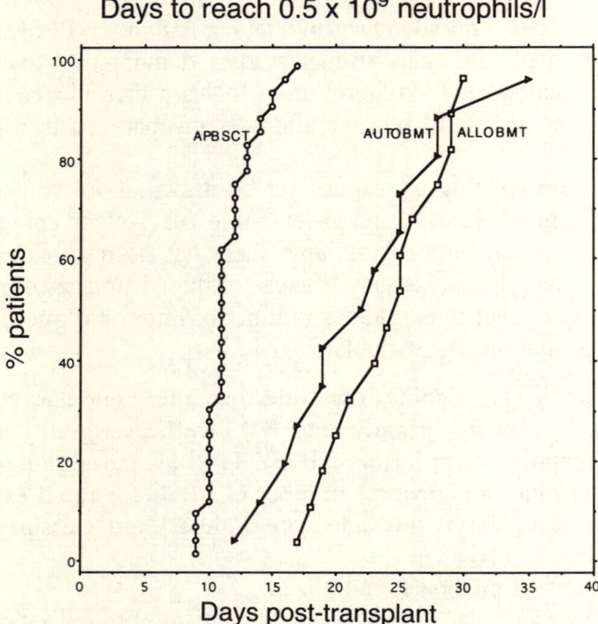

Fig. 1. Comparison of the time to recover a neutrophil count of 0.5×10^9/l in 38 patients receiving autologous peripheral blood stem cell transplant (APBSCT), 13 patients receiving autologous bone marrow transplant (AUTOBMT) and 14 patients receiving allogeneic bone marrow transplant (ALLOBMT). (Figure reproduced by permission of *Bone Marrow Transpl.*)

Several studies have suggested a minimum threshold dose for rapid, early reconstitution.[21,22] Red cell reconstitution is also faster, measured by the time to recover a specified absolute reticulocyte count in the peripheral blood. The rapid recovery is associated with reduced hospitalization, lower use of blood products, fewer febrile days and fewer days on parenteral antibiotics.[18]

Mobilized PBSC containing low numbers of CFU-GM produce HR which is not usually different from that after autologous bone marrow, although rapid granulocyte recovery may occur.[19] Similarly, combining relatively small doses of mobilized PBSC with autologous bone marrow often produces rapid HR.[23,24] This may result from the infusion of rapid repopulating cells not measured by the CFU-GM assay or from the high number of lymphocytes and monocytes infused, which may stimulate the bone marrow directly (cell–cell interactions) or may themselves release haemopoietic growth factors (endocrine effect). When steady phase PBSC are given with BM, early recovery is not enhanced.[25]

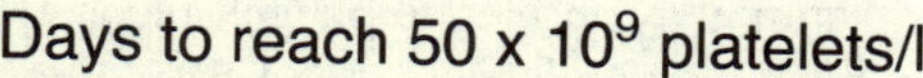

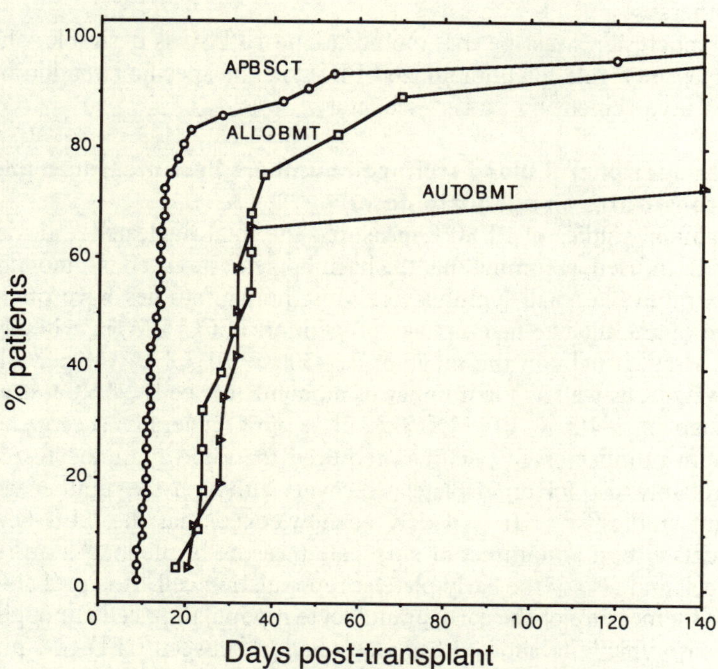

Fig. 2. A comparison of the time to recover a platelet count of 50×10^9l in 38 patients receiving autologous peripheral blood stem cell transplant (APBSCT), 13 patients receiving autologous bone marrow transplant (AUTOBMT) and 14 patients receiving allogeneic bone marrow transplant (ALLOBMT). (Figure reproduced by permission of *Bone Marrow Transpl.*)

Is the HR after mobilized PBSCT any better than that seen with ABMT and post graft haemopoietic growth factors? Granulocyte colony stimulating factor (G-CSF) and granulocyte-macrophage colony stimulating factor (GM-CSF) enhance granulocyte recovery after ABMT to a similar extent to mobilized PBSC. Importantly, however, there is no acceleration of platelet recovery.[26,27] Presumably, these HGF stimulate granulocytic progenitor cells in the graft but not megakaryocytic progenitors. Thus, PBSCT has an important clinical advantage because it produces rapid recovery of both platelets and granulocytes whereas HGF administration after ABMT only produces rapid granulocyte recovery. However, no studies have yet been reported using HGF such as IL-3, IL-6, IL-11 or leukaemia inhibitory factor (LIF) with known stimulatory effects on megakaryocyte progenitors after

ABMT. These factors may accelerate platelet reconstitution, and IL-3 has a demonstrable effect on platelet recovery after conventional dose chemotherapy.

The conclusion must be that mobilization of PBSC is desirable, although there may be a role for unmobilized PBSC in the specific situation of bone marrow involvement by cancer (see later).

How are peripheral blood stem cell numbers best measured and what constitutes an adequate dose?

Early animal studies of PBSCT measured the total nucleated and mononuclear cells infused, assuming that the haemopoietic stem cell is a mononuclear cell resembling a small lymphocyte. Most human studies have quoted the number of granulocyte-macrophage progenitors (CFU-GM) in a 14 day clonogenic assay, usually in the range of 0.5–500×10^4 CFU-GM per kilogram body weight, as well as the number of mononuclear cells (MNC), usually in the range of 2–10×10^8 MNC/kg. It is now generally accepted that a minimum number of CFU-GM is required for rapid granulocyte recovery and probably also for rapid platelet recovery although the number varies in different studies[21,22,28]. It is widely acknowledged that the CFU-GM dose represents at best an indirect or surrogate measure of the long-term repopulating cell and also of the early platelet repopulating cell. It is probably most useful as a measure of the early granulocyte repopulating cell although many studies are unable to show either a correlation between CFU-GM numbers and granulocyte recovery or a threshold effect with impaired granulocyte recovery below a minimum dose. The assay is highly dependent on technical factors, particularly the source of colony stimulating factor(s) used, the batch of fetal calf serum and the density at which cells are plated.[29] This explains some of the differences in minimum dose quoted by different institutions. In contrast, in PBSCT using steady phase PBSC, the mononuclear cell number is as useful as the CFU-GM number in quantitating the graft.[16]

Much current research is aimed at establishing laboratory measures of HR capacity which are more accurate, more convenient and more informative than the CFU-GM assay for both early and long-term reconstitution. Increasing use of recombinant growth factors may improve standardization of the assay, but serum deprived systems are not yet optimized and high levels of recombinant HGF almost certainly stimulate different progenitor cell populations from the various conditioned media previously used. If recombinant factors are used in combination, particularly if synergistic factors such as IL-1, IL-6 and stem cell factor (SCF) are included, more primitive progenitors are stimulated and the number of 'CFU-GM' will be higher.

There is increasing interest in using the $CD34^+$ cell as a measure of graft competency. The $CD34^+$ cell can probably be quantitated more reproducibly, and simple methods using whole blood lysis, directly conjugated antibody to the $CD34^+$ antigen and flow cytometry are being applied widely.[30] Initial studies in a non human primate model show that highly purified bone marrow $CD34^+$ cells produce haemopoietic reconstitution, while bone marrow deprived of $CD34^+$ cells does not.[31] Similar studies in humans have produced similar results.[32]

The most practical advantage of CD34 measurement is the fact that this assay can be performed rapidly to assess the adequacy of a stem cell collection. Clonogenic assays require between 7 and 14 days culture, and results are only available retrospectively and cannot help decide in 'real time' whether enough cells have been collected during apheresis. Siena has suggested that 7.8×10^6 $CD34^+$ cells/kg BW is adequate for rapid reconstitution based on a CFU-GM target of 50×10^4 CFU-GM/Kg BW.[30] Since rapid HR has been reported in PBSCT with half or even less than this CFU-GM number, $3–4 \times 10^6$ $CD34^+$ cells/kg BW seems a reasonable target. CD34 measurement also allows the recognition of high levels of PBSC on a daily basis and can thus help determine when apheresis should start.

Other rapid techniques under current investigation include measurement of tritiated thymidine incorporation on the assumption that high levels of PBSC will be associated with a large number of late progenitors which will be metabolically active and incorporating thymidine. Thymidine kinase levels in the serum may provide a similar assessment. Cytokine levels may also be increased during PBSC release, but initial studies have not demonstrated a consistent increase in levels. However, the PBSC release phenomenon may well be associated with significant changes in the levels of important cytokines, preceding the release by hours or days, and more study is clearly required. Techniques which initially allowed the identification of high PBSC levels during recovery after myelosuppressive chemotherapy were based on rapid increases in platelet and white cell counts.[33] Fig. 3 shows the close correlation in time between platelet and granulocyte recovery and high CFU-GM levels in a patient entering remission from AML. This is not totally predictable between individual patients, and high levels of PBSC, assessed by both CFU-GM content and HR after transplant, often occur when white cell and platelet counts are not rising rapidly. The move to more controlled and predictable PBSC mobilization using haemopoietic growth factors may make the need to assay PBSC on a 'real time' basis redundant.

Further work on the subsets of the $CD34^+$ cell suggests that it will be possible to delineate quantitatively, reproducibly and accurately which cells are responsible for initial rapid and short-term haemopoietic reconstitution and which cells are responsible for long-term reconstitution. Thus, the short-term repopulating cells are likely to have the phenotype $CD34^+/CD33^+/CD38^+$/lineage$^+$ and Rhodamine[BRIGHT], whereas the long-term repopulating cells are likely to be $CD34^+/CD33^-/CD38^-$/lineage$^-$ and Rhodamine[DULL]. These subpopulations of $CD34^+$ cells need to be measured

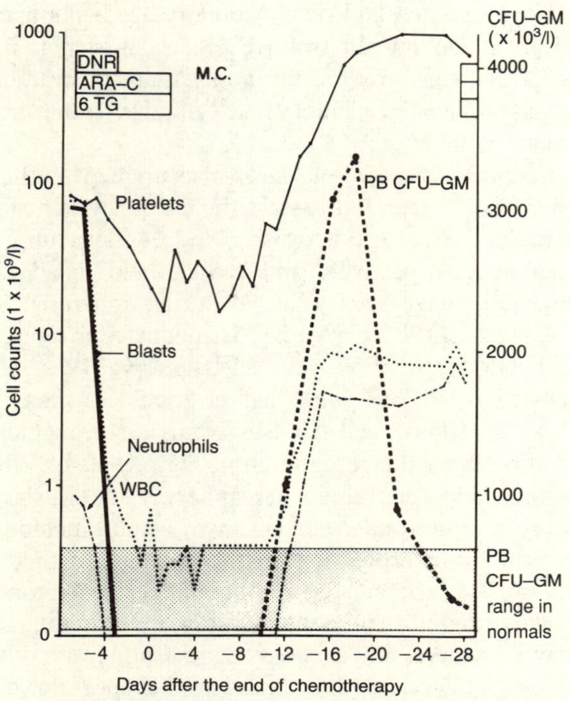

Fig. 3. Serial changes in platelets, leukaemic blasts, total white cells, neutrophils and peripheral blood CFU-GM following remission induction chemotherapy in a patient with AML. (Figure reproduced by permission of *B J of Haemat.*)

in PBSC transplants and correlated with short-term and long-term HR. Interestingly, initial studies in man suggest that CD34[+] cells in PBSC mobilized by cyclophosphamide alone, G-CSF alone, or the combination of cyclophosphamide and GM-CSF, have a Rhodamine[DULL] primitive phenotype with quite variable coexpression of CD33.[34] Early suggestions that circulating stem cells might be effete and incapable of long-term haemopoietic reconstitution[35] appear unlikely to be correct given more recent reports.[13,14] The finding that CD34[+] cells in mobilized PBSC are Rhodamine[DULL] certainly suggests otherwise.

Long-term reconstitution probably results from primitive stem cells not measured in the CFU-GM assay. Whether these come from endogenous recovery of cells in the recipient which survive high dose therapy, from the graft or both is uncertain. The animal data suggests origin from the graft in dogs and mice. Several new in vitro assays appear to correlate with the stem cells responsible for longer term reconstitution. The competitive repopulating unit (CRU) assay in mice is an example but the assay is not feasible in humans although gene marking studies may make such an approach possible in the future. The long-term culture initiating cell (LTCIC) assay, where haemopoietic cells are cultured over fibroblast or BM stromal layers for 5 to 8 weeks with a CFU-GM assay performed on the supernatant cells after that period correlates with the competitive repopulating unit assay and with long-term haematological recovery in mice. The LTCIC assay is used mostly to study normal haemopoiesis. There is a need to apply this approach to PBSC transplants.

An alternate approach is based on the pre-CFU-GM or 'delta' assay. The haemopoietic cell population of interest is cultured in medium with growth factors for 7 days and the cultured cells are then assayed for CFU-GM. The 'delta' or difference is the number of CFU-GM after 7 days compared with the number of CFU-GM present at the beginning. The assay is thought to identify more primitive cells than CFU-GM. This approach also needs to be used to quantitate PBSC and correlated with long-term HR.

Techniques for mobilization of stem cells into the circulation

Animal experimental data in the 1960s and 1970s showed that haemopoietic stem cells with bone marrow repopulating capacity were present in the peripheral circulation. This was seen in bone marrow reconstitution from a shielded limb in animals receiving supralethal irradiation to the rest of the bone marrow and in cross-circulation experiments between normal and irradiated primates. In addition, apheresis of dogs yielded a product capable of long-term haemopoietic reconstitution.

Initial human studies demonstrated a modest 2–3 fold increase in CFU-GM numbers in the peripheral blood following exercise[36], administration of dextran sulphate,[37] and administration of endotoxin.[38] Richman described a marked increase in CFU-GM levels during haemopoietic recovery after conventional dose myelosuppressive chemotherapy.[9] Lohrmann subsequently described the same phenomenon in lung cancer.[39] No transplants were performed, and it was 5 years before apheresis was performed during early remission from AML, demonstrating an average 27-fold increase above normal in PBSC levels when platelet and white cell counts were rising rapidly.[33] These cells were used for autologous transplantation in man and first demonstrated the rapid haemopoietic reconstitution now commonly associated with PBSCT.[10,12] Similar results were reported in Burkitt's lymphoma using cells collected after high dose cyclophosphamide chemotherapy mobilization.[11]

Many subsequent studies showed that PBSC levels were increased more or less with various single agent or combination chemotherapy regimens.

It appeared necessary to use cytotoxic regimens that produced a significant nadir in the white cell count below $0.5 \times 10^9/l$. It was less certain that a significant nadir in the platelet count was also important.[40] Conventional dose regimens like standard dose CHOP did not usually produce high levels of PBSC. Alkylating agents such as cyclophosphamide with major action on late progenitors were more effective than alkylating agents such as melphalan with major effect on early progenitors.

The next phase in PBSC mobilization involved the use of haemopoietic growth factors alone or in combination with cytotoxic chemotherapy. Phase I studies with G-CSF and GM-CSF demonstrated an increase in levels of progenitor cells in the peripheral blood.[41,42] The levels were even higher after the combination of cytotoxic chemotherapy followed by HGF.[42,43] The initial studies using G-CSF alone demonstrated an increase in levels of CFU-GM, BFU-E and CFU megakaryocyte, suggesting G-CSF had a capacity to act as a multilineage stimulant or else that G-CSF caused secondary release of other cytokines with the capacity to release lineages other than just granulocytic.

The first clinical studies of PBSC by mobilized chemotherapy and HGF with subsequent transplant were reported by Gianni.[43,44] GM-CSF was given after 7 g/m^2 of cyclophosphamide, PBSC were collected by three aphereses and autotransplantation was performed after high dose melphalan and total body irradiation. Bone marrow and PBSC were both reinfused and GM-CSF was given after transplant. The regimen produced rapid granulocyte and platelet recovery but whether the mobilized PBSC or the post-transplant GM-CSF contributed to the rapid HR was not readily assessable. Other studies have demonstrated rapid granulocyte and platelet reconstitution either using cyclophosphamide mobilized PBSC without bone marrow or cytokine administration either during mobilization or after the transplant.[18]

More recent human studies have examined the effect of PBSC collected following HGF alone. However, it is important to consider the animal studies which tend to be more advanced than those in the humans. Fibbe has demonstrated in the mouse that a single injection of IL-1 causes the release of high levels of PBSC into the peripheral blood, capable of both short- and long-term HR.[45] The exact mechanism is uncertain and IL-1 releases multiple other cytokines which may themselves be responsible for the phenomenon. Molineux has shown that high doses of G-CSF in a murine model release high levels of CFU-GM and CFU-S which can reconstitute haemopoiesis short and long term.[46] In a sex mismatched model, Testa has shown that haemopoiesis at 13 months post G-CSF mobilized PBSC transplant is entirely donor derived.[14] Preliminary studies with stem cell factor in primates suggest the capacity to release very high numbers of PBSC.[47]

The human studies are much less complete. Haas reported that GM-CSF mobilized PBSC produced granulocyte and platelet engraftment rates no faster than in ABMT but the CFU-GM dose given was less than 1×10^4/kg BW.[48] Sheridan reported transplants using a combination of G-CSF stimulated PBSC, bone marrow and post-transplant G-CSF which produced marked acceleration of platelet reconstitution compared with similar patients receiving ABMT and the same schedule of post-transplant G-CSF. Granulocyte recovery to $0.5 \times 10^9/1$ was one day faster.[49] Subsequent studies reported in abstract form show that G-CSF stimulated PBSC alone are capable of rapid granulocyte and platelet reconstitution without bone marrow although postgraft G-CSF was still given.[50]

Full and accurate assessment of the HR capacity of HGF mobilized PBSC requires collection after HGF alone and not after combined cytotoxic chemotherapy and HGF, that the transplant be performed using only the HGF collected PBSC without BM, and that no HGF be administered post-graft. Such studies are planned but no results are yet available.

Mechanism of mobilization

The reason why PBSC circulate in the peripheral blood is essentially unknown. It may represent an overflow of expanded numbers of haemopoietic stem cells present in the bone marrow. It may represent a residual mechanism from early embryonic life when haemopoietic stem cells circulate physiologically and sequentially between the yolk sac, the liver, the spleen and the bone marrow. It may represent a primary 'release' phenomenon without any stem cell expansion. It is uncertain why these cells are released in response to a variety of perturbations by exercise, dextran, chemotherapy or haemopoietic growth factors. It is probable that the mobilization phenomenon results from a perturbation of haemopoiesis which causes an endogenous release of haemopoietic growth factors. Which growth factors are released, in what order and at what level remains undefined. The mechanism may relate to changes in adhesion molecules on the stromal cells of the haemopoietic microenvironment or on the stem cells themselves. Preliminary data from our own laboratory suggest that there is down regulation of c-kit expression on $CD34^+$ cells, whether mobilization is induced by chemotherapy alone, G-CSF alone, or the combination of chemotherapy and GM-CSF.[34] In addition, the ligands which normally mediate adhesion between stem cells and stroma may be interfered with or abrogated by mobilization phenomena. The biology of the microenvironment/stem cell interaction is gradually being dissected, aided by the increasing availability of reagents such as cytokines, cytokine receptors, adhesion molecules and their ligands, and antibodies to each, which allow these mechanisms to be investigated.

PBSC collection

The basic practical requirements for collection, processing and cryopreservation include cell separators and experienced operators, an established cell culture facility, flow cytometry, a controlled rate freezer and liquid nitrogen storage vessels, although some reports suggest that haemopoietic stem cells can be stored satisfactorily for short periods of time in electric freezers at higher temperatures ($-70\ ^\circ C$ or $-130\ ^\circ C$). The techniques of PBSC harvesting, processing and storage used by several experienced centres have been published in manual form.[51]

The Haemonetics V30 and V50 operate in an intermittent flow mode which tends to produce greater cardiovascular fluctuations than continuous flow cell separators. The efficiency of PBSC collection with these machines has been improved by application of the 'lymphosurge' technique but they still require skilled operator input.

The Fenwal CS3000 and the Cobe Spectra are the two cell separators most commonly used for PBSC collection. They operate in a closed continuous flow mode and are easier to use. The Spectra requires that the operator position the buffy coat. The product has minimal red cell and platelet contamination. The CS3000 is fully automated with 2 inbuilt procedures (1 and 3) suitable for PBSC apheresis with minor modification. Its use in PBSC collection has been well described. Procedure 1 yields a product with minimal red cell contamination but high levels of platelets. The platelets may cause clumping on thawing, but their number can be reduced by a 'soft spin' before cryopreservation. Procedure 3 has less platelet but more red cell contamination. The combined use of procedure 1 and a new small volume collection chamber provides a cleaner product which minimizes prestorage processing.[52] Other continuous flow separators such as the Fresenius AS104 are under evaluation. Complications of PBSC apheresis include hypocalcaemia, clotting and bleeding around central venous access catheters and occasional postapheresis thrombocytopenia.

Sustained cytopenia after PBSC apheresis was seen in two 3-year-old children with cancer, suggesting that the PBSC may be a major physiological component of haemopoietic recovery in small children.[53] This has not been reported in adults after PBSC collections although transient leucopenia with leukocyte counts of 1.7 to 3.4 $\times$ 10^9/1 has been observed 2 weeks following G-CSF mobilization in three patients.[54]

Collection efficiency (CE) can be defined as the percentage of PBSC collected relative to the number of PBSC processed. The published mononuclear cell and CFU-GM CE of the Fenwal CS3000 has ranged from 55% – 73%.[55,56] A recent report has demonstrated a significant difference between the overall CFU-GM CE of 56% (based on the number of cells at the start of apheresis and the nominal blood volume processed) and the instantaneous CE of 95% (based on a comparison of the cells at the intake and output lines of the cell separator).[56] This discrepancy can be attributed to three factors which are not related to machine performance: 1) a fall of 20–30% in mononuclear cell and CFU-GM levels during apheresis, 2) an 8–10% dilution of blood by anticoagulant and 3) the operational dead space in the blood cell separator at the start of apheresis. This suggests that current PBSC collection technology based on mononuclear cell collection is already optimal, and little further improvement in collection efficiency is likely to be possible. The overall CE for the Spectra is similar to that of the CS3000,[57] although no data on instantaneous CE are available for this machine.

The next generation of PBSC harvesters will probably be further automated, closed, continuous flow systems with the additional capacity to capture stem and progenitor cells specifically. Positive selection of CD34$^+$ cells may offer the advantage of a smaller volume of cells, reducing storage costs and PBSC infusion side effects like circulatory overload and DMSO toxicity. Selection of CD34$^+$ cells may also allow depletion of cancer cells.

Contamination of PBSC with cancer cells

Current techniques for analysis of residual cancer include the study of cancer associated gene rearrangements by cytogenetics, polymerase chain reaction (PCR), fluorescence in situ hybridization (FISH), and long-term tumour cell cultures.[58–60] Most reported data are based on steady-state collections, not now commonly applied to PBSC transplantation. Malignant contamination of the PBSC collection might be increased by the perturbations of haemopoiesis which increase CFU-GM, but might also be decreased during early recovery from bone marrow aplasia as suggested by Carella for CML[61] and To for AML.[33] Reports of long-term disease-free survival following high dose therapy and autotransplantation with unmobilized PBSC from patients with bone marrow involvement in Hodgkin's disease and non-Hodgkin's lymphoma suggest that these PBSC may have low malignant contamination.[62] Similar data are not yet available for mobilized PBSC in lymphoma. In AML the results are less encouraging, although the relapse rate for PBSC transplants appears similar to ABMT. The major cause of relapse in AML autotransplants of either type is probably the failure to eradicate tumour within the recipient and the lack of a graft versus leukaemia effect. Better techniques to quantify small numbers of residual cancer cells may permit malignant contamination to be assessed with greater accuracy. However, randomized clinical studies remain vitally important and are yet to be done. It is desirable that all groups involved in PBSC transplantation have access to the newest techniques for assessing malignant contamination. Gene marking of the infused cells can potentially detect whether relapse occurs from cells in the graft or from residual cancer in the patient.

Clinical studies of autologous peripheral blood stem cell transplantation versus autologous bone marrow transplantation

There are no prospective randomized trials evaluating the kinetics of HR, tumour response and disease-free survival after APBSCT compared with ABMT in any disease. However, some preliminary data can be presented for AML. Reiffers retrospectively analysed data from the European Bone Marrow Transplant Group for AML patients transplanted in first complete remission (CR).[63] Patients receiving PBSCT were compared with ABMT patients or patients who received purged autologous marrow grafts (pABMT) and were matched for age, FAB subclassification and the interval from CR to transplantation. The actuarial risk of relapse was not significantly different for PBSCT, ABMT and pABMT patient cohorts, whereas the median number of days after transplant to reach 0.5×10^9 granulocytes/litre in the peripheral blood after transplant was significantly less in the APBSCT patient group. Platelet reconstitution was not different.

In a single institution study, the kinetics of haemopoietic reconstitution and DFS after PBSCT in 20 patients were compared with pABMT in 23 patients using mafosfamide purged bone marrow.[64] All transplants were performed in first CR of AML. White cell and granulocyte reconstitution occurred significantly earlier after PBSCT, but there was only borderline significance in favour of PBSCT for platelet HR. The hospital stay was significantly shorter following PBSCT.

The probability of DFS 2 years after transplantation was higher in the pABMT group (51%) compared with the APBSCT group (35%) but the difference was not statistically significant. In Korbling's study, the PBSCT group lacked a stable DFS plateau with relapses occurring more than 1 year post-transplant, unusual in pABMT. A phase II study of PBSCT in AML reported by Szer was associated with rapid haemopoietic reconstitution and an actuarial DFS of 38% at 26 months, equivalent to the 2 studies mentioned above.[65] The period of hospitalization was shorter than that reported by Korbling. HR was not completely predictable with a wide range in the time to initial platelet recovery.[63] This may reflect differences in the quality of mobilized PBSC in AML compared with nonmyeloid malignancies, and may result from AML remission sometimes being a differentiation of the underlying malignant clone rather than true clonal deletion. Table 1 summarizes relapse data and disease-free survival for these 3 studies.

Most studies in CML have used Ph^1+ve chronic phase PBSC. Surprisingly, some of these patients develop partial or complete Ph^1 negativity post-transplant, suggesting the chronic phase PBSC contain some Ph^1−ve 'normal' long-term reconstituting cells.[66] Recent immunophenotyping and sorting techniques allow selection of putative normal cells in the chronic phase of CML which may be used for autotransplants.

Most published results in lymphoma have used nonmobilized PBSC from patients with bone marrow involvement with lymphoma or irradiated bone marrow sites.[62] The preliminary results suggest an advantage for PBSC from marrow involved cases compared with bone marrow from cases without bone marrow involvement, with disease-free survival better for the PBSCT group than the ABMT group. The results are similar in Hodgkin's disease.[67] In breast cancer and solid tumours, PBSC have been used as an adjunct to ABMT to reduce cytopenia and hospitalization, although PBSC have been used alone in breast cancer with bone marrow involvement.[15] Small patient

Table 1. *Disease-free survival and relapse of AML after first remission autotransplant with peripheral blood stem cell or bone marrow*

	Korbling[64]		Reiffers[63]		Szer[65]
	PBSC	pABMT	PBSC	ABMT	PBSC
Number of patients	20	23	28	683	36
Median time to relapse (months)	8.1	NR	NS	NS	13.5
Actuarial risk of relapse	NS	NS	57 ± 10%	48 ± 6%	NS
DFS	35 ± 21% (2 years)	51 ± 21% (2 years)	39 ± 10% (time not stated)	42 ± 5% (time not stated)	38 ± 8% (26 months)

NR = not reached.
NS = not stated.
Acturial risk of relapse and DFS are shown as percentages ± standard errors.

numbers and short follow-up do not allow analysis of disease control. In multiple myeloma, PBSC autografting has been used alone to purge myeloma cells[28] and in combination with BM to expedite HR. A prospectively randomized collaborative international study is currently examining the effect of GM-CSF on PBSC mobilization after chemotherapy with cyclophosphamide 7 gm/m^2 in patients with multiple myeloma (see Fig. 4). Transplants use only the PBSC without bone marrow or post-transplant GM-CSF. This will clearly elucidate the effect of GM-CSF on PBSC mobilization after cyclophosphamide and will also provide response data.

**PBSC transplant in myeloma:
CSF 39–300**

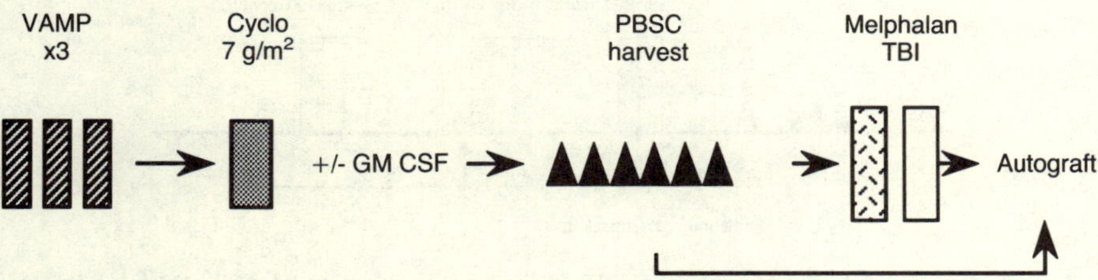

Fig. 4. Randomized study of the effect of GM-CSF after high dose cyclophosphamide immobilization of PBSC in multiple myeloma. Note: No administration of bone marrow or GM-CSF post-transplant.

Future prospects and conclusions

The shortening of total aplasia is the most striking advantage of PBSCT over ABMT. Reduction of the period of aplasia may allow the design of new approaches to the treatment of cancer such as repeated myeloablative treatment cycles, an attractive option for the further study of dose intensification. Fig. 5 shows the schema for one such study using G-CSF mobilized PBSC and repeated courses of high dose epirubicin and cyclophosphamide. Three Australian centres (Royal Melbourne Hospital, Alfred Hospital Melbourne and Royal Adelaide Hospital) are collaborating in this study based on previous dose escalation of high dose epirubicin and high dose cyclophosphamide using G-CSF alone developed by Dr Michael Green, Royal Melbourne Hospital. The principal investigators are Dr WP Sheridan, Dr J Szer and Dr LB To. Ten patients have already been treated on this protocol which appears both feasible and tolerable.

Significant expansion of PBSC is demonstrably feasible using the combination of IL-1, IL-3, IL-6, G-CSF, GM-CSF and SCF.[68] This is directed towards the complete abrogation of cytopenia after HDT and is an important further step towards increasing the safety of these procedures, potentially allowing safe outpatient transplants and fully exploring dose intensification in older and sicker patients. The same general approach may eventually allow true expansion of long-term repopulating cells, so that autotransplants can be performed with very small cell collections.

Currently, PBSCT is the preferred option when the pelvis has been irradiated, or where bone marrow is infiltrated with cancer. The latter situation

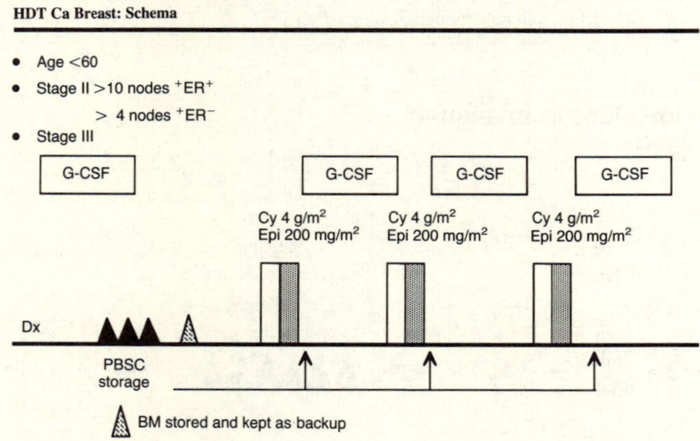

Fig. 5. Repeated high dose therapy for poor prognosis stage II and stage III breast cancer using cellular support with G-CSF mobilized PBSC and postinfusion G-CSF following each course of high dose therapy.

might also coincide with high contamination of PBSC with cancer cells, although available evidence suggests otherwise.[58,60]

Preliminary studies of cost analysis have been reported. Three studies report significantly briefer hospitalization with PBSC autotransplants compared with ABMT, less days of fever, less antibiotic use and fewer transfusions.[69,18,70] These factors contribute to substantial saving even if the cost of the mobilization including cytokines, aphereses and multiple cryopreservation procedures is considered. In each case, the overall cost of PBSC transplants including multiple collection and cryopreservation procedures was approximately one-half that of a bone marrow transplant. Many centres performing PBSC transplants still collect bone marrow, a substantial additional expense which is probably unnecessary since few of these series report the need to infuse backup bone marrow.

More effective cytokine-induced mobilization of stem cells using sequential IL-3 and GM-CSF or combinations of SCF, IL-1, IL-3 and GM-CSF might further expand the circulating stem cell pool. This makes the more uniform blood stem cell population the ideal target for selection of $CD34^+$ cells or $CD34^+$ subpopulations for further genetic and cellular modifications. Currently, however, G-CSF appears the most effective single HGF for PBSC mobilization, and the combination of G-CSF with conventional dose chemotherapy may allow the collection of enough PBSC for transplant with just a single apheresis.

References

(1) Hryniuk WM. The importance of dose intensity in the outcome of chemotherapy. In: Hellman S, De Vita V, Rosenberg S, eds. *Important advances in oncology*. Philadelphia: Lippincott, 1988: 121–41.

(2) Horowitz MM, Gale RP, Sondel PM et al. Graft-versus leukaemia reactions after bone marrow transplantation. *Blood* 1990; 75; 3: 555–62.

(3) Kolb HJ, Mittermuller J, Clemm CH et al. Donor leukocyte transfusions for treatment of recurrent chronic myelogenous leukemia in marrow transplant patients. *Blood* 1990; 76; 12: 2462–5.

(4) Jagannath S, Dicke KA, Armitage JO et al. High-dose cyclophosphamide, carmustine, and etoposide and autologous bone marrow transplantation for relapsed Hodgkin's disease. *Ann Intern Med* 1986; 104; 163–8.

(5) Bron D, Philip T, Guglielmi C et al. The Parma international randomized study in relapsed non-Hodgkin lymphoma analysis on the first 153 pre-included patients. *Exp Hematol* 1991; 19; 546. Abst 339.

(6) Gulati SC, Shank B, Black P et al. Autologous bone marrow transplantation for patients with poor-prognosis lymphoma. *Journal of Clin Oncol* 1988; 6; 8; 1303–13.

(7) Gianni AM, Bregni M, Siena S et al. Prospective randomized comparison of MACOP-B vs rhGM-CSF-supported high-dose sequential myeloablative

chemo-radiotherapy in diffuse large cell lymphomas. *Proc ASCO* 1991; 10; 274. Abst 951.

(8) Goldman JM, Johnson SA, Islam A et al. Haematological reconstitution after autografting for chronic granulocytic leukaemia in transformation: the influence of previous splenectomy. *Br J Haemat* 1980; 45: 223–31.

(9) Richman CM, Weiner RS, Yankee RA. Increase in circulating stem cells following chemotherapy in man. *Blood* 1976; 47: 1031–9.

(10) Juttner CA, To LB, Haylock DN, Branford A, Kimber RJ. Circulating autologous stem cells collected from acute non-lymphoblastic leukaemia produce prompt but incomplete haemopoietic reconstitution after high dose melphalan or supralethal chemoradiotherapy. *Br J Haemat* 1985; 61: 739–46.

(11) Korbling M, Dorken B, Ho AD, Pezzuto A, Hunstein W, Fliedner TM. Autologous transplantation of blood-derived haemopoietic stem cells after myeloablative therapy in a patient with Burkitt's lymphoma. *Blood* 1986; 67: 529–32.

(12) Reiffers J, Bernard P, David B et al. Successful autologous transplantation with peripheral blood haemopoietic cells in a patient with acute leukaemia. *Exp Hematol* 1986; 14: 312–5.

(13) Carbonnell F, Calvo W, Fliedner TM et al. Cytogenetic studies in dogs after total body irradiation and allogeneic transfusion with cryopreserved blood mononuclear cells: Observations in long-term chimeras. *Int J Cell Cloning* 1984; 2: 81–8.

(14) Testa NG, Molineux G, Hampson IN, Lord BI, Dexter TM. Comparative assessment and analysis of peripheral blood and bone marrow stem cells. *Int J Cell Cloning* 1992; 10; (suppl 1): 30–2.

(15) Kessinger A, Armitage JO, Landmark JD & Weissenberger DD. Reconstitution of hematopoietic function with autologous cryopreserved circulating stem cells. *Exp Hematol* 1986; 14: 192–6.

(16) Kessinger A, Armitage JO, Lanadmark JD, Smith DM, Weisenburger DD. Autologous peripheral hematopoietic stem cell transplantation restores hematopoietic function following marrow ablative therapy. *Blood* 1988; 71: 723–7.

(17) Juttner CA, To LB, Ho JQK et al. Early lympho-hemopoietic recovery after autografting using peripheral blood stem cells in acute non-lymphoblastic leukemia. *Transpl Proc* 1988; 20: 40–3.

(18) To LB, Roberts M, Haylock DN et al. Comparison of haematological recovery times and supportive care requirements of autologous recovery phase peripheral blood stem cell transplants, autologous bone marrow transplants and allogeneic bone marrow transplants. *Bone Marrow Transpl* 1992; 9 (4): 277–84.

(19) Castaigne S, Calvo F, Douay L et al. Successful haematopoietic reconstitution using autologous peripheral blood mononucleated cells in a patient with acute promyelocytic leukaemia. *Br J Haemat* 1986; 63: 209–11 (letter).

(20) To LB, Haylock DN, Dyson PG, Thorp D, Roberts M, Juttner CA. An unusual pattern of haemopoietic reconstitution in patients with acute myeloid leukaemia transplanted with autologous recovery phase peripheral blood. *Bone Marrow Transpl* 1990; 6: 109–14.

(21) To LB, Dyson PG, Juttner CA. Cell-dose effect in circulating stem cell autografting. *Lancet* 1986; ii: 404–5 (letter).

(22) Reiffers J, Leverger G, Marit G et al. Hematopoietic reconstitution after autologous blood stem cell transplantation. Bone marrow transplantation: current controversies. In: R.P. Gale & R.E. Champlin, eds. *Proceedings of Sandoz-UCLA symposium*, Colorado, 1988; 313.

(23) Bell AJ, Oscar DG, Figes A, Hamblin TJ. Use of circulating stem cells to accelerate myeloid recovery after autologous bone marrow transplantation. *Br J Haematol* 1987; 67: 252–3.

(24) Lopez M, Mortel O, Pouillart P et al. Acceleration of hemopoietic recovery after autologous bone marrow transplantation by low doses of peripheral blood stem cells. *Bone Marrow Transpl* 1991; 7: 173–81.

(25) Lobo F, Kessinger A, Landmark JD et al. Addition of peripheral blood stem cells collected without mobilization techniques to transplanted autologous bone marrow did not hasten marrow recovery following myeloablative therapy. *Bone Marrow Transpl* 1991; 8: 389–92.

(26) Sheridan WP, Morstyn G, Wolf M et al. Granulocyte colony-stimulating factor (G-CSF) and neutrophil recovery after high-dose chemotherapy and autologous bone-marrow transplantation. *Lancet* 1989: 891–5.

(27) Brandt SJ, Peters WP, Atwater SK et al. Effect of recombinant human granulocyte-macrophate colony-stimulating factor on hematopoietic reconstitution after high-dose chemotherapy and autologous bone marrow transplantation. *N Eng J Med* 1988; 318; 14: 869–76.

(28) Fermand JP, Levy Y, Gerota J et al. Treatment of aggressive multiple myeloma by high-dose chemotherapy and total body irradiation followed by blood stem cell autologous graft. *Blood* 1989; 73; 1: 20–3.

(29) To LB, Haylock DN, Juttner CA & Kimber RJ. The effect of monocytes on the peripheral blood CFU-c assay system. *Blood* 1983; 62: 112–7.

(30) Siena S, Bregni M, Brando B et al. Flow cytometry for clinical estimation of circulating hematopoietic progenitors for autologous transplantation in cancer patients. *Blood* 1991; 77: 400–9.

(31) Berenson RM, Andrews RG, Bensinger WI et al. Antigen CD34+ marrow cells engraft lethally irradiated baboons. *J Clin Invest* 1988; 81: 951–5.

(32) Berenson RJ, Bensinger WI, Hill RS et al. Engraftment after infusion of CD34+ marrow cells in patients with breast cancer or neuroblastoma. *Blood* 1991; 77: 1717–22.

(33) To LB, Haylock DN, Kimber RJ, Juttner CA. High levels of circulating haemopoietic stem cells in very early remission from acute non-lymphoblastic leukaemia and their collection and cryopreservation. *Br J Haematol* 1984; 58: 399–410.

(34) Simmons PJ, Haylock DN, Niutta S, To LB, Juttner CA. *Unpublished observations* 1992.

(35) Micklem HS, Anderson N, Ross E. Limited potential of circulating haemopoietic stem cells of CBA mice. *Nature* 1975; 256: 41–3.

(36) Barrett AJ, Longhurst P, Sneath P, Watson JM. Mobilization of CFU-C by exercise and ACTH induced stress in man. *Exp Hematol* 1978; 6: 590–4.

(37) Ma EP, Guo SH, Wei HD et al. Experimental study and normal individual trial of hemopoietic stem cell mobilizer DS. *Int J Cell Cloning* 1992; 10: 41–4.

(38) Cline MJ, Golde DW. Mobilization of hematopoietic stem cells (CFU-C) into the peripheral blood of man by endotoxin. *Exp Hematol* 1977; 5: 186–90.

(39) Lohrmann HP, Schreml W, Fliedner TM, Heimpel H. Reaction of human granulopoiesis to high-dose cyclophosphamide therapy. *Blut* 1979; 38: 9–16.

(40) To LB, Sheppard KM, Haylock DN et al. Single high doses of cyclophosphamide enable the collection of high numbers of haemopoietic stem cells from the peripheral blood. *Exp Hematol* 1990; 18: 442–7.

(41) Duhresen U, Villeval JL, Boyd J, Kannourakis G, Morstyn G, Metcalf D. Effects of recombinant human granulocyte-colony stimulating factor on haemopoietic progenitor cells in cancer patients. *Blood* 1988; 72: 2074–81.

(42) Socinski MA, Cannistra SA, Elias A, Antman KH, Schnipper L & Griffin JD. Granuloctye macrophage colony stimulating factor expands the circulating haemopoietic progenitor cell compartment in man. *Lancet* 1988; i: 1194–8.

(43) Gianni AM, Siena S, Bregni M, et al. Granulocyte-macrophage colony-stimulating factor to harvest circulating haemopoietic stem cells for autotransplantation. *Lancet* 1989; 2: 580–5.

(44) Gianni AM, Bregni M, Siena S et al. Recombinant human granulocyte-macrophage colony-stimulating factor reduces hematologic toxicity and widens clinical applicability of high-dose cyclophosphamide treatment in breast cancer and non-Hodgkin's lymphoma. *J Clin Oncol* 1990; 8: 768–8.

(45) Fibbe WE, Hamilton MS, Laterveer LL et al. Sustained engraftment of mice transplanted with IL-1-primed blood-derived stem cells. *J Immunol* 1992; 148: 417–21.

(46) Molineux G, Pojda Z, Hampson IN, Lord BI, Dexter TM. Transplantation potential of peripheral blood stem cells induced by granulocyte colony stimulating factor. *Blood* 1990; 76: 2153–8.

(47) Andrews RG, Knitter GH, Bartelmez SH et al. Recombinant human stem cell factor, a c-kit ligand, stimutates hematopoiesis in primate. *Blood* 1991; 78: 1975–80.

(48) Haas R, Ho AD, Bredthauer U et al. Successful autologous transplantation of blood stem cells mobilized with recombinant human granulocyte-macrophage colony-stimulating factors. *Exp Hematol* 1989; 18: 94–8.

(49) Sheridan WP, Begley CG, Juttner CA et al. Effect of peripheral-blood progenitor cells mobilized by filgrastim (G-CSF) on platelet recovery after high-dose chemotherapy. *Lancet* 1992; 339: 640–4.

(50) Sheridan WP, Begley G, Juttner C et al. Effect of different doses and schedules of R-METHUG-CSF (Filgrastim) on mononuclear cell and PBPC collections and haematopoietic recovery after high dose chemotherapy (HDC) and infusion of R-METHUG-CSF mobilized peripheral blood progenitor cells (PBPC) without bone marrow. *Blood* 1992; 80; 10: 331a.

(51) Juttner CA, To LB. Collection, processing, storage and quantitation of peripheral blood stem cells. In: EM Areman, HJ Deeg, RA Sacher, eds. *Bone marrow and stem cell processing: a manual of current techniques*. 1992: 68–73.

(52) Bender JG. Harvesting of peripheral blood stem cells with the Fenwal CS3000 plus cell separator and and a small volume collection chamber. *Int J Cell Cloning* 1992; 10 (suppl 1): 79–82.

(53) Takaue Y, Watanabe T, Kawano Y et al. Sustained cytopenia after

leukapheresis for collection of peripheral blood stem cells in small children. *Vox Sang* 1989; 57: 168–71.

(54) To LB, Dyson PG, Bayly JL, Rawling CM, Juttner CA. *Unpublished observations* 1992.

(55) Lasky LC, Smith JA, McCullough J, Zanjani ED. Three-hour collection of committed and multipotent hematopoietic progenitor cells by apheresis. *Transfusion* 1987; 27: 276–8.

(56) Haylock DN, Canty A, Thorp D, Dyson PG, Juttner CA, To LB. A discrepancy between the instantaneous and the overall collection efficiency of the Fenwal CS3000 for peripheral blood stem cell apheresis. *J Clin Apheresis* 1992; 7: 6–11.

(57) Craig JIO, Anthony RS, Smith SM et al. Comparison of the Cobe Spectra and Baxter CS3000 cell separators for the collection of peripheral blood stem cells from patients with hematological malignancies. *Int J Cell Cloning* 1992; 10; (suppl 1): 82–5.

(58) To LB, Russell J, Moore S, Juttner CA. Residual leukaemia cannot be detected in very early remission peripheral blood stem cell collections in acute non-lymphoblastic leukaemia. *Leuk Res* 1987; 11: 327–9.

(59) Hutchins C, White D, Suttle J, Haylock D, To LB, Juttner C. Fluorescence in situ hybridization (FISH) can detect residual disease in acute myeloid leukaemia. *Blood* 1992; 80 (10): 438a (abst).

(60) Sharp JG, Kessinger A, Vaughan WP et al. Detection and clinical signficance of tumour cell contamination of peripheral stem cell harvests. *Int J Cell Cloning* 1992; 10 (suppl 1): 92–4.

(61) Carella AM, Podesta M, Carlier P, Raffo MR, Pollicardo N, Gualandi F. Conventional intensive therapy can lead to overshoot of Ph-negative blood cells in chronic myelogenous leukaemia. *Int J Cell Cloning* 1992; 10 (suppl 1): 1117–213.

(62) Kessinger A, Armitage JO, Smith DM, Landmark JD, Bierman PJ, Weisenburger DD. High-dose therapy and autologous peripheral blood stem cell transplantation for patients with lymphoma. *Blood* 1989; 74: 1260–5.

(63) Reiffers J, Korbling M, Labopin M, Henon Ph, Gorin NC on behalf of the EBMT Group Working Party for Autologous Bone Marrow Transplantation. Autologous blood stem cell transplantation versus autologous bone marrow transplantation for acute myeloid leukaemia in first complete remission. *Int J Cell Cloning*; 10 (suppl 1): 111–3.

(64) Korbling M, Fliedner TM, Holle R et al. Autologous blood stem cells (ABSCT) versus purged bone marrow transplantation (pABMT) in standard risk AML: influence of source and cell composition of the autograft on haemopoietic reconstitution and disease-free survival. *Bone Marrow Transpl* 1991; 7: 343–9.

(65) Szer J, Juttner CA, To LB et al. Post remission therapy for acute myeloid leukaemia with blood-derived stem cell transplantation. Results of a collaborative Phase II trial. *Int J Cell Cloning* 1992; 10 (suppl 1): 114–6.

(66) Butturini A, Keating A, Goldman J, Gale RP. Autotransplants in chronic myelogenous leukaemia: strategies and results. *Lancet* 1990; 335: 1255–8.

(67) Kessinger A, Bierman PJ, Vose JM, Armitage JO. High-dose cyclophosphamide, carmustine and etoposide followed by autologous

peripheral stem cell transplantation for patients with relapsed Hodgkin's disease. *Blood* 1991; 77: 2322–5.

(68) Haylock DN To LB, Dowse TL, Juttner CA, Simmons PJ. Ex vivo expansion and maturation of peripheral blood CD34$^+$ cells into the myeloid lineage. *Blood* 1992; 80: 1405–12.

(69) Elias A, Mazanet R, Anderson K et al. GM-CSF mobilized peripheral blood stem cell autografts: the DFCI/BIH experience. *Int J Cell Cloning* 1992; 10 (suppl 1): 149–51.

(70) Henon PR, Liang H, Beck-Wirth G et al. Comparison of hematopoietic and immune recovery after autologous bone marrow or blood stem cell transplants. *Bone Marrow Transpl* 1992; 9: 285–91.

The laboratory aspects of myelodysplasia

D J CULLIGAN and A K BURNETT

Introduction

The myelodysplastic syndromes (MDS) were clearly defined in morphological terms by the French – American – British group (FAB) in 1982.[1] As such they were presented as five conditions each with their own diagnostic criteria, but with the shared characteristic features of ineffective blood cell production in one or more cell line, dysplasia, and a propensity to evolve into acute myeloid leukaemia. There has followed much interest in the biological processes involved in these conditions as they represent a transitory though variable phase in the multistep leukaemogenic process.[2,3] Whilst the mainstay of clinical practice is based on the morphological classification of MDS based on the FAB criteria, this can be fraught with difficulty. Patients often have different characteristics at different times suggesting an evolving process and making it difficult to allocate them to a specific disease entity. There is overlap between the five groups and in some cases with myeloproliferative disease and aplasia, and whilst typical cases are easily diagnosed there is considerable difficulty and disagreement regarding the minimal diagnostic criteria required in early or equivocal cases. This was recently emphasized by several attempts to provide minimal diagnostic criteria.[4] The availability of more advanced laboratory techniques has led them to be applied to MDS in an attempt to supplement the fundamental morphological approach in improving diagnostic and prognostic accuracy and helping characterize the pathological basis of these acquired preleukaemic conditions. These include cytogenetics, immunohistochemistry and immunophenotyping, progenitor growth studies and molecular biological analysis of mutated genes and tissue clonality. This article will attempt to review these techniques as applied to the diagnosis, prognosis and briefly the pathogenesis of MDS.

All correspondence to: Dr D J Culligan, Department of Haematology, University Hospital of Wales, Heath Park, Cardiff, UK.

Cambridge Medical Reviews: Haematological Oncology Volume 3

D J Culligan and A K Burnett

Classification and morphological criteria of MDS

The defining features for the FAB groups of refractory anaemia (RA), acquired idiopathic sideroblastic anaemia (AISA), refractory anaemia with excess blasts (RAEB), refractory anaemia with excess blasts in transformation (RAEB-t) and chronic myelomonocytic leukaemia (CMML) are shown in Table 1. The key to confirming the diagnosis of MDS and assigning a given case to one of these subgroups is a careful morphological examination of blood and bone marrow. The peripheral blood often provides evidence of dysplastic haemopoiesis with cytopenias, macrocytosis and monocytosis. There are variable degrees of aniso-poikylocytosis and fragmented red cells, basophilic stippling, and Howell–Jolley bodies are seen. Marked dysgranulo-poiesis in the peripheral blood involves hypogranulation of neutrophils which can lead to a negative peroxidase reaction and a false automated neutrophil count.[5] The nuclei are usually hyposegmented or dumbbell shape (pseudo-Pelger–Huët abnormality). The nuclear chromatin appears clumped and can appear fragmented giving a ring structure. Less commonly, granulo-cytes are hypersegmented and hypergranular or contain abnormally large granules. Myeloblasts may be seen especially in the more advanced forms of MDS with the presence of Auer rods making the diagnosis at least RAEB-t. The most conspicuous platelet abnormality in the blood is thrombocytopenia, though patients with the so-called 5q-syndrome can have increased platelet numbers[6] as can patients with CMML especially early in the disease when they tend towards a myeloproliferative state rather than cytopenia. Variation

Table 1. *The FAB classification of the myelodysplastic syndromes*

Category	Blood and marrow characteristics
Refractory anaemia (RA)	Refractory cytopenias, with peripheral monocytes $<1 \times 10^9/1$, peripheral blasts $<1\%$, bone marrow blasts $<5\%$, and ring sideroblasts $<15\%\star$
Acquired idiopathic sideroblastic anaemia (AISA)	As for RA but with ring sideroblasts $>15\%\star$
Chronic myelomoncytic leukaemia (CMML).	Monocytes $>1 \times 10^9/1$, peripheral blasts $<5\%$, bone marrow blasts $<20\%$
Refractory anaemia with excess blasts (RAEB)	As for RA but with peripheral blasts $<5\%$ and bone marrow blasts 5–20%
Refractory anaemia with excess blasts in transformation (RAEB-t)	As for RA but with peripheral blasts $>5\%$, or bone marrow blasts 20–30%, or Auer rods in the blasts

Adapted from Culligan et al. in *Rec Adv Haematol* 7. 1993.
$\star$ As a percentage of total numbers of erythroblasts.

in platelet size with prominent giant platelets are seen and again these can have abnormal granulation.

These dysplastic features of the peripheral blood are in typical cases magnified in the marrow upon which the diagnosis is made. In general, the marrow is normo-hypercellular and caution is needed when making a diagnosis of MDS in the presence of a hypocellular marrow as this may reflect a different process such as aplasia or myelofibrosis, though hypoplastic MDS and MDS with fibrosis are described. The characteristic features of dyserythropoiesis, dysgranulopoiesis, and dysmegakaryopoiesis are well reviewed[7,8] with the most notable red cell changes including megaloblastoid change, binucleate erythroblasts and erythroblasts showing nuclear budding, bridging and fragmentation. Micromegakaryocytes and large forms containing single nuclei or multiple separate nuclei are common, megakaryocyte abnormalities and granulocytic dysplasia similar to that seen in the blood is found in the marrow especially hypogranularity and Pelgerization. It is essential for the classification of MDS to perform an iron stain of the marrow. Sideroblastic anaemia is based on a minimum of 15% of erythroblasts being ring sideroblasts where the iron granules form a ring applied to at least one-third of the nuclear rim, and these are often associated with so called pathological sideroblasts which have more than five iron granules per cell though not in a ring structure. The cut of point of 15% ring sideroblasts in the division of RA from AISA is useful for classification of MDS but as with other morphological classifications of MDS is of necessity arbitary, and must be viewed in the light of a range of 1–86% in all groups of MDS.[9,10] According to Juneja's study of 43 patients with AISA, the average number of ring sideroblasts per case was 40%. As such, the percentage sideroblast count probably bears little relevance to the biological differences between cases, and what seems more important in respect to prognosis in AISA is the involvement of other lineages. A study by Gattermann et al[11] has defined two distinct subtypes of AISA. On morphological and clinical grounds one group has trilineage myelodysplasia with ring sideroblasts and the other group has apparent erythroid restricted disease with ring sideroblasts. The 5-year cumulative chance of survival is reported as 69% in the pure red cell form and only 19% in the trilineage form. However, the detectable stage of evolution of individual cases at the time of study may explain some of these differences and Bowen and Jacobs[12] have shown that AISA can be diagnosed at a stage when the only peripheral blood abnormality is macrocytosis though undoubtedly some of these cases would go on to demonstrate trilineage involvement if studied over a long period of time.

The above morphological features help diagnose and classify MDS, however, the most important laboratory and morphological feature at diagnosis is the percentage of blasts in the marrow. As shown in Table 1 the accurate assessment of the percentage marrow blast count is vital to the subclassification of MDS, and in our institution we count at least 400 nucleated cells. The progressive worsening of prognosis from RA through RAEB to RAEB-t is well documented[13–15] and reflects the deterioration in prognosis with increasing blast count and leukaemic phenotype. Sanz et al[16] have studied the effect of blast count over a smaller range than used by the FAB group for classification purposes and showed that, in patients with 5–10% blasts, the mean survival is considerably better (16 months) than in those cases with 11–20% blasts (5 months). Recently, there has been much debate regarding the precise definition of blast cells in MDS with the dysplastic process making their separation from more mature granulocytic precursors difficult. The FAB group defined type one blasts as having no primary azurophilic granules and no Auer rods, and type two blasts as having some granules but no Golgi apparatus. Goasguen et al[17] have studied 18 cases of MDS and defined a further type three blast as having more than 20 primary azurophilic granules. By counting the three blast types in these 18 cases, seven cases were reassigned to RAEB-t from RAEB, and RAEB was redefined as RAEB I (blast type 1+2+3 >5% <10%) or RAEB II (blast type 1+2+3 >10% <20%). This approach to classification is more in keeping with the prognostic groups of Sanz et al.

Most morphological description of the dysplastic process is based on the bone marrow aspirate, though this can be misleading, given the patchy distribution of haemopoietic tissue. There have been attempts to use specific features of bone marrow trephine biopsies to improve on the morphological diagnosis. In this way MDS with myelofibrosis has been defined as a distinct entity[18] and, in difficult cases, MDS can be distinguished from aplasia. However, most studies have been interested in the distribution of immature cells in the trephine biopsy and more recently their immunophenotypic characteristics. Tricot et al[19] were the first to describe the so called abnormal localization of immature precursors (ALIPs) in plastic embedded thin bone marrow biopsy specimens. ALIPs were defined as myeloblasts and promyelocytes clustered (3–5 cells) or aggregated (>5 cells) within the marrow away from the paratrebeculae area. Several studies have shown that, if you divide MDS into ALIP positive and ALIP negative cases, then this has prognostic significance but this varies from study to study and may reflect the interobserver variation in detecting ALIPs. Mangi et al[20a,b] have used immunohistochemical techniques to define three types of immature cell aggregates which can be difficult to distinguish morphologically: these are two types of pseudo-ALIP consisting of erythroid or megakaryocytic precursors and true ALIPs consisting of aggregates of myeloblasts and monoblasts.

Cytogenetics

Whilst morphological techniques provide the mainstay of diagnosis and subclassification of MDS and have allowed the development of prognostic scoring systems such as the Bournemouth score[13] based simply on the blood count and conventional morphology, more sophisticated laboratory techniques have, over the last few years, attempted to supplement these in improving diagnostic and prognostic subclassification of MDS whilst adding insight into the pathogenesis of these conditions which morphology is unable to do. The most important of these techniques, to date, has been bone marrow cytogenetics. Clonal chromosomal abnormalities have been described in 23–85% of MDS, with the incidence in different studies depending on the number of each subtype of MDS included, whether cases of secondary MDS are included and the use of conventional or higher resolution banding.[21-25] A non-random clonal cytogenetic abnormality is defined as two or more cells with the same structural abnormality or the same chromosome gained, or three or more cells with the same chromosome lost. The most common abnormalities are shown in Table 2. Except for the so-called 5q-syndrome[6,26] described as typically affecting elderly females who present with macrocytosis, thrombocytosis or normal platelet counts, dyserythropoiesis and micromegakaryocytes or megakaryocytes with hypolobulated nuclei, specific cytogenetic abnormalities are not associated with specific clinical syndromes or FAB type. However, patients with RA and AISA have a lower incidence of karyotypic abnormalities than those with RAEB/RAEB-t which is prognostically consistent with the observations that chromosomal abnormalities appear to be associated with leukaemic change and more rapid

Table 2. *Cytogenetic abnormalities in MDS*

del (5q)/ monosomy 5	trisomy 8
del (7q)/ monosomy 7	trisomy 21
del (13q)	trisomy 19
del (17p or 17q)	trisomy 11
del/rearrangement (3q)	
del (12)(p11p13)	t(1;7)(p11;p11)
del (20)(q11q13)	t(1;15)(p12;p11)
del/trans(21q)	t(2;11)(p11;q23)
del/trans(19p or q)	t(3;12)(p22;q15)
del/trans(6p)	t(5;20)(q15;q13)
	t(5;7)(q11–2;p11–2)
abscent Y	
	t(6;9)(p22–3;q34)
	t(11;21)(q22;q21)
	trans/dup(X)(q13)
	trans(X)(p11)
	inv(5)(q14;q32)
	i(17q)

progression of disease. White et al[27] have presented an extended cytogenetic follow-up of 177 patients with MDS over a 5-year period. They defined three prognostic subgroups according to the presence of normal karyotype, single abnormalities or multiple abnormalities at presentation. In poor prognosis MDS (RAEB/RAEB-t) karyotype status had independent prognostic significance. Those cases with a normal karyotype did not differ significantly in terms of survival from cases of RA and, as such, survived significantly longer than those with an abnormal karyotype. Abnormal versus normal cytogenetics had similar prognostic significance in CMML. As has been noted before, survival and risk of leukaemic change were significantly worse in those who subsequently developed an abnormality from normality at presentation compared with those who remained normal on sequential follow-up.

As well as complex changes having a worse prognosis than single abnormalities, distinct abnormalities also carry different prognostic significance. It has been shown that average survival was longer than 2 years in patients with the lone abnormality of 5q-, between 1 and 2 years for those with the sole abnormality of trisomy 8 and less than 1 year for the lone abnormality of monosomy 7.[28]

An important distinct disease group which cytogenetics has helped to define is that of secondary or treatment-related MDS (t-MDS). Bloomfield[29] described an overall incidence of cytogenetic abnormalities in cases secondary to treatment with chemotherapy or radiotherapy of 66% and other studies have indicated it to be as high as 80–97%.[30,31] In Bloomfield's study the most common single abnormalities were monosomy 7 in 35%, 5q- in 18% and monosomy 5 in 14% and abnormalities of chromosome 5 and 7 including total monosomy. Deletions of the long arms of these chromosomes and unbalanced translocations involving these chromosomes, eg t(3; 5), t(5; 7), and t(1; 7) are now recognized as common abnormalities in therapy related MDS.[32–35] Another characteristic feature of secondary MDS is multiple complex cytogenetic abnormalities sometimes with a number of different clones, but with the same stem abnormality, suggesting a very unstable and progressive clonal disorder. All cases of secondary MDS tend towards rapid transformation to AML and a poor prognosis and this is particularly true of this latter group with the complex cytogenetic abnormalities. The cytogenetic abnormalities described in treatment related MDS are also described more commonly in MDS and de novo AML following exposure to myelotoxic chemicals such as benzene.[36,37] Fenaux et al[38] have described the clinical and laboratory features of 37 young persons (age less than 50 years) with primary MDS, which accounted for 6.7% of their total adult cases. There was a preponderance of RAEB, RAEB-t and CMML and five had a family history of MDS. When this group were compared with the over-50 age group there was a higher incidence of karyotypic abnormalities (62.5% vs 29%) and especially involving chromosome 7 (44% vs 4.5%). In these respects, this group of young patients behave like secondary MDS and suggest MDS in this age group may commonly be related to some environmental mutagen, though in only three cases was there a history of potential chemical exposure. A recent description of 33 cases of childhood MDS[39] again emphasizes the high incidence of poor risk MDS, RAEB, RAEB-t and CMML associated with poor prognosis Bournemouth score (3 or 4 points) high leukaemic transformation rate and short overall survival. Again, MDS in this very young age group behaves like secondary MDS and at least some cases may represent environmental exposure at an early stage in life though in this study cytogenetic data was only available for five patients with one showing monosomy 7 and one trisomy 19.

Recently, an additional use of cytogenetic analysis in MDS has been in the attempt to help resolve the conflicting data regarding which cell lines are part of the neoplastic clone. Using conventional karyotyping Lawrence et al[40] demonstrated the cytogenetic abnormality 13q- to be present in granulocytes and B- cells but not T- cells from two cases of AISA. Kere et al[41] showed that, in four cases of MDS with monosomy 7, none of the lymphocytes had the abnormality. The eloquent technique of fluorescent in situ hybridization (FISH) of chromosomes has been applied to a few cases of MDS whereby the visual presence or absence of a numerical chromosomal abnormality can be correlated with conventional cell morphology. Gerritsen et al[42] have studied 8 patients with monosomy 7 using this technique to enumerate the number of chromosome sevens in interphase cells with a specific chromosome 7 probe. They persistently showed two chromosome sevens in T and B cells and concluded that, in these cases of MDS, monosomy seven is restricted to the myeloid line hence suggesting the lymphocytes are not part of the clonal process. Kibbelaar et al[43] similarly studied two patients with trisomy 8 and one with t(1; 7) using fluorescent probes for the three chromosomes. Again, the analysis showed that the cytogenetic abnormalities were confined to non-lymphoid cells. The abnormality t(1; 7) was recognized as three chromosome 1 spots, one of which colocalized with the chromosome 7 spot. This exciting new technique has strengthened the argument recently suggested by several molecular genetic studies of clonality in MDS that in many cases lymphocytes are not part of the abnormal clone, and as such the idea of MDS being a disorder of the pluripotential stem cell in the same fashion as chronic myeloid leukaemia (CML) is probably not always true. These studies will be returned to later in this review.

Studies of haemopoietic progenitors

In a similar fashion to cytogenetic studies in vitro culture of haemopoietic progenitors has contributed to the diagnosis and prognosis of MDS, and has added to the understanding of the pathophysiology of these conditions. When confirming the diagnosis of MDS proves difficult because of minimal marrow dysplasia, abnormal progenitor growth provides biological evidence of the dysplastic process, in the same way that cytogenetics or X-linked clonality studies can provide evidence of clonal haemopoiesis. In Cardiff 79% of patients had abnormal growth of BFU-E (burst forming unit erythroid) and 45% abnormal growth of CFU-GM (colony forming unit granulocyte and monocyte) at diagnosis.[4]

Although comparison of data between different groups working in this field is difficult because of variation in techniques, interpretation of results and whether peripheral blood or marrow is studied, some general consensus opinion has emerged. Erythroid colony growth is decreased or absent in most marrow or peripheral blood cultures from patients with MDS.[44-47] However, most studies have concentrated on patterns of myeloid colony growth especially in the context of being a predictor of risk of leukaemic transformation. Milner et al[48] showed that cultures of CFU-GM from bone marrow show a reduction of both colony (>40 cells) and cluster (<40 cells) growth in patients with RA and RAEB, and this general tendency to poor progenitor growth has been identified in all types of MDS.[49-51] Attempts have been made to describe leukaemic and nonleukaemic patterns of growth, and five categories have been described which could be related to prognosis and propensity to evolve into acute leukaemia.[50,52] In general, leukaemic patterns tend to be characterized by reduced numbers of colonies and increased numbers of microclusters. Tennant et al[53,54] have used a peripheral blood CFU-GM assay and defined patterns of prognostic significance. In keeping with studies of marrow cultures, undetectable myeloid colony growth or a low colony/cluster ratio is associated with poor prognosis and shorter survival. In patients with low risk MDS, defined in these studies as less than 5% myeloblasts, median survival is reduced in those patients with >15 clusters per ml. In patients with AISA, survival is related to colony numbers whereas in RAEB survival is independent of the absolute colony number but clearly related to the colony/cluster ratio. A combination of high colony/cluster ratio (>0.3) and <15 clusters per ml defines the group of MDS with the best prognosis of all. As might be predicted from this data, increased expression of the myeloblast surface marker CD34 is associated with a low colony/cluster ratio in myeloid growth studies and a poor prognosis.[55]

Perhaps of more therapeutic significance will be the newer in vitro growth studies which can now rely on the use of highly purified growth factors in an attempt to strictly regulate the growth environment for different progenitors. Such studies may help define deficiencies or abnormalities in the cytokine network in MDS or in the ability of the progenitors to respond to individual or combinations of growth factors. This may, in turn, predict which factors are likely to have clinical benefit and stimulate clinical trials. Some such studies have already attempted to define the in vitro kinetics of myeloid colony growth in response to purified growth factors. The delayed colony growth of MDS seems to result from the increased time dysplatic myeloid progenitors spend in GO compared to normal progenitors. Schipperus et al[56, 57] have shown that optimum proliferation can only be returned by a combination of an early acting factor IL-3 and a later acting factor G-CSF suggesting that the MDS progenitors require both a pluripotential colony stimulating factor and a lineage specific factor. However, Baines et al[58] have found combinations of factors largely unhelpful in improving the indolent growth of MDS myeloid progenitors.

A separate approach to defining potential growth factor deficiency in MDS is to measure the level of the factor in the peripheral blood and compare it to the normal. Of course, this approach suffers from the fact that serum or plasma levels may not reflect what is happening in the microenvironment of the marrow. Serum levels of erythropoietin are generally related to the degree of anaemia in MDS, though there is a wide range of values between different patients with the same haemoglobin concentrations and some patients have relatively low levels[59–61] suggesting that, at least in some instances, deficiency in the EPO response mechanism may compound the anaemia of MDS. This may help explain why several studies have now shown that some patients with MDS have anaemia which responds to exogenous EPO therapy.[63–65] Levels of serum macrophage colony stimulating factor (M-CSF) have been shown to be raised in MDS, but there is no relationship to white cell count, monocyte count or the percentage of marrow blast cells and no difference between FAB types.[66] We have measured serum stem cell factor (SCF) concentrations in 85 patients with MDS and shown that the mean concentration in MDS is significantly lower than that in 234 normal subjects.[67] What these laboratory measurements mean in terms of the pathophysiology of aberrant myeloid growth patterns in MDS and whether they will indeed predict therapeutic response to the likes of M-CSF and SCF have yet to be determined.

Immunological abnormalities in MDS

Immunological abnormalities are well documented in MDS. Lymphopenia is a common feature, most commonly the result of low numbers of T-cells.[68–70] Low natural killer (NK) cell activity is also described in the small numbers of patients studied.[71–73] However, most interest has been in the humoral immune system in MDS. Polyclonal hypergammaglobulinaemia is well described. Solal-Celigny et al[74] described 23/35 patients with CMML and such a polyclonal rise in IgG above 14 g/l. Similarly, Economopoulos et al[75] showed 17 of 52 patients with all types of MDS had a polyclonal rise in immunoglobulin (Ig) as did Mufti et al[76] in 27/84 cases (32%). Autoimmune disease is described in MDS[74,76] including hypothyroidism, pernicious anaemia and autoimmune haemolytic anaemia. More commonly occurring associations with MDS which probably have an immune basis are cutaneous and systemic vasculitis[77,78] (with a single case recently being described in which the vasculitis was associated with antineutrophil cytoplasmic antibodies (ANCA)[79] and Sweet's syndrome)[80,81] the appearance of which may herald acceleration of the MDS and imminent transformation to acute leukaemia.

The association of MDS and neoplasms of the lymphoid system is now well recognized and is perhaps more important in attempting to unravel the role of lymphoid involvement in the dysplastic process than the other immunological abnormalities described above which may represent epiphenomena. The earliest association was between MDS and myeloma[82] and this has now been well described.[83–85] In Copplestone's study, 20 cases out of 190 (10.5%) with MDS had coexistent lymphoid or plasma cell neoplasms distributed as follows: eight cases of myeloma, three cases of benign monoclonal gammopathy, one case of monoclonal gammopathy of uncertain significance, three cases of CLL, three cases of B-NHL and two cases of T- cell lymphoma. In 14 of the B-cell malignancies, a paraprotein was present. The association of MDS with these B-cell malignancies has been reviewed by Hamblin[86] and begs the question do they occur by chance in an aged population or is the MDS and the B-cell proliferation part of the same process? Hamblin et al[87] showed that the prevalence for both conditions in 1300 volunteers over the age of 55 was one in 500 and hence the combined frequency of approximately 10% observed by Copplestone et al was highly unlikely to have occurred by chance alone. However, transformation to acute lymphoblastic leukaemia (ALL) is a very rare event in the evolution of MDS with only 16 cases reported[87] unlike the other typical pluripotential disorder chronic myeloid leukaemia (CML) where it is relatively frequent.

Molecular studies of gene defects and clonality

The most recent laboratory technology to be applied to the study of MDS has been the molecular study of potential oncogenes involved in the pathogenesis of these preleukaemic conditions and the study of X-chromosome inactivation in order to confirm the clonal nature of these disorders and demarcate as closely as possible which cell lineages within the marrow are part of the abnormal clone. These molecular genetic studies have been reviewed in depth[2,3] and the salient points will be briefly summarized. Though many oncogenes have been studied in MDS, to date, the RAS family of genes and the FMS gene have proven the most important. The three RAS genes H-RAS, K-RAS and N-RAS encode for an inner membrane guanine nucleotide-binding protein p21 which has a pivotal role in signal transduction. These genes can be activated by point mutations at codons 12, 13 and 61 and such mutations leave p21 constitutively locked in the active GTP bound form and able to transform NIH3T3 fibroblasts. Of all the haematological malignancies studied, the highest incidence of such mutations are found in MDS. Bartram[2] has summarized the data from 282 published cases compiled from several studies. The incidence of RAS mutations varies between laboratories from 9% to 40%, however, there is consensus of opinion that the most common mutations are found in N-RAS and the most frequently affected subgroup of MDS is CMML. In general, RAS mutations in MDS are associated with poor prognosis in tems of survival and progression to AML, though they have now been described in both early and late stages of the disease including haematologically normal people who are known to be at risk of secondary MDS and AML because of previous chemotherapy for malignant disease and rarely in normals who are not apparently at increased risk.[88,89]

The FMS gene encodes the functional receptor for the monocyte growth factor M-CSF. Mutations at codon 301 of FMS mimic the ligand induced conformational change produced by M-CSF binding which produces constitutional protein tyrosine kinase activity and transformation in NIH3T3 cells. Additional mutations at codon 969 enhance this transforming ability. Such mutations have been demonstrated in up to 18% of cases of MDS[90,91] and again these mutations are more common in CMML.

In females heterozygous for polymorphic X-linked genes in which the maternal and paternal alleles can be distinguished by restriction fragment length polymorphisms (RFLPs) the active from the inactive allele can be further defined by differences in the methylation patterns of the two genes.[92] According to Lyon's hypothesis[93] such X-gene inactivation occurs randomly in each female cell at an early stage in embryogenesis so that normal polyclonal female tissues demonstate mosaicism for the paternal and maternal X-chromosome. By contrast, in a monoclonally derived tissue, all the cells will have the same X-chromosome in the active and inactive state as the cell of origin. The genes phosphoglycerate kinase (PGK) and hypoxanthine phosphorybosyl transferase (HPRT) and more recently the variable number tandem repeat sequence at DXS255 recognized by the probe M27B have been used to perform this clonal analysis of blood and bone marrow cells from patients with MDS. The combined heterozygosity frequency for PGK and HPRT is at best 50% but that for M27B is about 80%,[94,95] therefore using all three X-linked probes allows this form of clonal assessment in practically all females. The initial results of Janssen et al[96] and Tefferi et al[97] using this RFLP approach confirmed the pioneering work of Prchal et al[98] and Raskind et al[99] who, using the same principle of X-inactivation but detected via analysis of G6PD isoenzymes, demonstrated the clonal nature of haemopoiesis in MDS. In 2 patients with sideroblastic anaemia erythrocytes, granulocyte, platelets and lymphocytes expressed the same isoenzyme only and hence were of a common clonal origin. In Janssen's study, as well as showing monoclonality of total blood or bone marrow DNA, they showed the same RAS mutation to be present in myeloid and lymphoid fractions in 2 patients with CMML. Tefferi's study demonstrated monoclonality of granulocytes and T-cells in 4 of 6 cases and of monocytes in one of these cases. Taken together, these studies suggest that MDS is a disease of the pluripotential stem cell. However, three recent studies have allowed analysis of many more patients according to X-inactivation and these have cast doubt on the universal pluripotential stem cell origin of MDS. Abrahamson et al,[100] Culligan et al[101] and Van kamp et al[102a] have all shown that the majority of cases demonstrate polyclonal lymphocytes including mixed lymphocyte populations, and separated B, T, and NK cells. This is in keeping with the newly described FISH data outlined previously. In our study,[101] a few cases had monoclonal lymphocytes in keeping with the earlier reports and some of the cytogenetic studies, and as this review was going to press a further study using PGK and HPRT but not M27B has been published showing only monoclonal T-cells.[102a] Interestingly, this study describes 3 cases, 1 RA, 1 AISA and 1 RAEB in which unseparated nucleated cells were polyclonal. We, to date, have found 5 cases of MDS diagnosed according to the FAB classification which demonstrate polyclonal granulocytes and separated lymphocytes (unpublished data). Such cases may represent mosaicism of the dysplastic and normal clones, some may represent erythroid restricted disease, or some may not be MDS in the true sense of a clonal preleukaemic condition. Further long-term follow-up and analysis of pure red cell precursors may help resolve this. It is worth mentioning that a word of caution is needed in assessing those recent studies which rely heavily on data from M27B analysis in that there are discrepancies in the way some of these results are interpreted. We have shown how some X-inactivation patterns commonly obtained with M27B cannot be interpreted in terms of Lyon's hypothesis and may represent methylation patterns not related to gene activation status.[95] It must also be emphasized that, wherever possible, normal nonhaemopoietic tissue should be analysed to exclude constitutional extremes of Lyonization as a cause for the monoclonal pattern. This is not an issue in the recent studies as they have demonstrated polyclonal results in MDS, but may account for some of the monoclonal results where normal tissue was not available. One further important practical advance has been the successful application of the polymerase chain reaction (PCR) to X-inactivation analysis of the PGK locus.[103,104] This allows the added advantage of being able to analyse small populations of cells, eg those separated by fluorescent activated cell sorting (FACS). In conclusion, this fascinating area of clonal analysis in MDS has, on the one hand, allowed confirmation of the clonal nature of these disorders, however, it has failed to allow agreement as to which lineages are part of this clone, and hence what is the level of commitment of the cell of origin. It is likely and sensible to assume that the clinical heterogeneity of these diseases is a reflection of the heterogeneity of the initiated progenitor giving rise to them. In some cases, this is a true myeloid/lymphoid pluripotential progenitor and, in others, it is a committed myeloid/ erythroid progenitor. Obviously, this is important in insuring that the correct cell populations are used

180

in future genetic studies into the pathogenesis of MDS, and further efforts using pure cell populations and genetic markers of disease will allow a better understanding of lineage involvement and evolution in the different subtypes of MDS.

References

(1) Bennett JM, Catovsky D Daniel MT. Proposals for the classification of the myelodysplastic syndromes. *Br J Haematol* 1982; 51: 189–99.

(2) Bartram CR. Molecular genetic aspects of myelodysplastic syndromes. In: Koeffler HP, guest eds. *Haematol/oncol Clin of N Am: myelodysplastic syndromes*, 1992; 6: 557–70.

(3) Culligan D, Jacobs A, Padua RA. The genetic basis of myelodysplasia. In: Hoffbrand AV and Brenner MK, eds. *Rec Adv Haematol* 7: 1993.

(4) Hamblin T, Culligan DJ, Jacobs A et al. Minimal diagnostic criteria for the myelodysplastic syndrome in clinical practice. *Leuk Res* 1992; 16: 3–11.

(5) Davey ER, Erber WN, Gatter KC et al. Abnormal neutrophils in acute myeloid leukaemia and myelodysplastic syndromes. *Hum Pathol* 1988; 19: 454.

(6) Van den Berghe H, Cassiman J, David G. Distinct haematological disorder with deletion of the long arm of no 5 chromosome. *Nature* 1974; 251: 437–8.

(7) Bain BJ. *Leukaemia diagnosis a guide to the FAB classification*. Gower Medical Publishing 1990.

(8) Kouides PA, Bennett JM. Morphology and classification of myelodysplastic syndromes. In: Koeffler HP, guest ed. *Haematol/oncol Clin N Am: Myelodysplastic Syndromes* 1992; 6: 485–99.

(9) Juneja SK, Imbert M, Sigaux S et al. Prevalence and distribution of ringed sideroblasts in primary myelodysplastic syndromes. *J Clin Pathol* 1983; 36: 566–7.

(10) May A, De Souza P, Barnes K et al. Erythroblast iron metabolism in sideroblastic marrows. *Br J Haematol* 1982; 52: 611–21.

(11) Gattermann N, Aul C, Schneider W. Two types of acquired idiopathic sideroblastic anaemia (AISA). *Br J Haematol* 1990; 74: 45–52.

(12) Bowen D, Jacobs A. Primary acquired sideroblastic erythropoiesis in non-anaemic and minimally anaemic subjects. *J Clin Pathol* 1989; 42: 56–8.

(13) Mufti GJ, Stevens JR, Oscier DG et al. Myelodysplastic syndromes: a scoring system with prognostic significance. *Br J Haematol* 1985; 59: 425.

(14) Goasguen JE, Garand R, Bizet M et al. Prognostic factors of myelodysplastic syndromes – a simplified 3-D scoring system. *Leuk Res* 1990; 14: 255.

(15) Third MIC Cooperative Study Group. Recommendations for a morphologic, immunologic and cytogenetic (MIC) working clasification of the primary and therapy related myelodysplastic disorders. *Cancer Genet Cytogenet* 1988; 32: 1.

(16) Sanz GF, Sanz MA, Vallepspi T et al. Two regression models and a scoring system for predicting survival and planning treatment in myelodysplastic syndromes: a multivariate analysis of prognostic factors in 370 patients. *Blood* 1989; 74: 395.

(17) Goasguen JE, Bennet JM, Cox et al. Prognostic implication and

characterization of the blast cell population in the myelodysplastic syndrome. *Leuk Res* 1991, 15: 159–65.

(18) Pagliuca A, Layton DM, Manoharan A et al. Myelofibrosis in primary myelodysplastic syndromes: a clinico-morphological study of 10 cases. *Br J Haematol* 1989; 71: 499–504.

(19) Tricot G, De Wolf-Peeters C, Vlientinck R et al. Bone marrow histology in myelodysplastic syndromes II. Prognostic value of abnormal localization of immature precursors in MDS. *Br J Haematol* 1984; 58: 217–25.

(20a) Mangi MH, Mufti GJ. Primary myelodysplastic syndromes: diagnostic and prognostic significance of immunohistochemical assessment of bone marrow biopsies. *Blood* 1992; 79: 198–205.

(20b) Mangi MH, Salisbury JR, Mufti GJ. Abnormal localisation of immature precursors (ALIP) in the bone marrow of myelodysplastic syndromes: Current state of knowledge and future directions. *Leuk Res* 1991; 15: 627–39.

(21) Second International Workshop on Chromosomes in Leukaemia. Chromosomes in preleukaemia. *Cancer Genet Cytogenet* 1979; 2: 108–13.

(22) Nowell PC. Cytogenetics of preleukaemia. *Cancer Genet Cytogenet* 1982; 5: 265–78.

(23) Nowell PC, Besca EC. Prognostic significance of single chromosome abnormalities in preleukaemic states. *Cancer Genet Cytogenet* 1989; 42: 1–7.

(24) Yunis JJ, Rydell RE, Oken MM et al. Refined chromosome analysis as an independent prognostic indicator in de novo myelodysplastic syndromes. *Blood* 1986; 67: 1721–30.

(25) Geddes AD, Bowen DT, Jacobs A. Clonal karyotipic abnormalities and clinical progress in the myelodysplastic syndromes. *Br J Haematol* 1990; 76: 194–202.

(26) Van den Berghe H, Vermaden K, Mecucci C et al. The 5q- anomaly. *Cancer Genet Cytogene* 1985; 17: 189–255.

(27) White AD, Culligan DJ, Hoy TG, Jacobs A. Extended cytogenetic follow-up of patients with myelodysplastic syndrome (MDS). *Br J Haem* 1992, 81: 499–502.

(28) Yunis JJ, Lobell M, Arnesen MA et al. Refined chromosome study helps define prognostic subgroups in most patients with primary myelodysplastic syndrome and acute myelodysplastic syndrome and acute myelogenous leukaemia. *Br J Haematol* 1988; 68: 189–194.

(29) Bloomfield CD. Chromosomal abnormalities in secondary myelodysplastic syndromes. *Scand J Haematol* 1986; 45: suppl 82.

(30) Pedersen-Bjergaard J, Philip P, Larsen SD et al. Chromosome aberrations and prognostic factors in therapy related MDS and acute non-lymphocytic leukaemia. *Blood* 1990; 76: 1087–91.

(31) Le Beau MM, Albain KS, Larson RA et al. Clinical and cytogenetic correlation in 63 patients with therapy related myelodysplastic syndromes and acute non-lymphocytic leukaemia: further evidence for characteristic abnormalities of chromosome 5 and 7. *J Clin Oncol* 1986; 4: 325–45.

(32) Thangaveleu M, Bitter MA, Larson RA et al. der (5) t (5;7) (q11.2;p11.2): a new recurring abnormality in malignant myeloid disorders. *Cancer Genet Cytogenet* 1989; 32: 1–10.

(33) Van den Berghe H, Mecucci C, Delannoy A et al. Deletion of 5q by t(5;17)

in therapy related myelodysplastic syndrome. *Cancer Genet Cytogenet* 1990; 48: 49–52.

(34) Scheres JMJC, Hustinx TWS, Geraedts JPM et al. Translocation 1;7 in haematological disorders. A brief review of 22 cases. *Cancer Genet Cytogenet* 1985; 18: 207–13.

(35) Iurlo A, Mecucci C, Van Orshoven A et al. Cytogenetic and clinical investigations in 76 cases with therapy related leukaemia and myelodysplastic syndrome. *Cancer Genet Cytogenet* 1989; 43: 227–41.

(36) Mitelman F, Brandt L, Nilsson PG. Relation among occupational exposure to potential mutagenic/carcinogenic agents, clinical findings and bone marrow chromosomes in acute non-lymphocytic leukaemia. *Blood* 1978; 52: 1229–37.

(37) Van den Berghe H, Louwagie A, Broeckaert-Van Orshoven A et al. Chromosome analysis in two unusual malignant blood disorders presumably induced by benzene. *Blood* 1979; 53: 558–66.

(38) Fenaux P, Preeudhomme C, Estienne MH. De novo myelodysplastic syndromes in adults aged 50 or less. A report on 37 cases. *Leuk Res* 1990; 14: 1053–9.

(39) Tuncer MA, Pagliuca A, Hicsonmez S et al. Primary myelodysplastic syndrome in children: the clinical experience in 33 cases. *Br J Haematol* 1992; 82: 347–53.

(40) Lawrence HJ, Broudy VC, Magenis RE et al. Cytogenetic evidence for involvement of B lymphocytes in acquired idiopathic sideroblastic anaemias. *Blood* 1987; 70 1003–5.

(41) Kere J, Ruutu T, Chapelle A. Monosomy 7 in granulocytes and monocytes in myelodysplastic syndromes. *N Engl J Med* 1987; 316: 499–503.

(42) Gerritsen WR, Bourhis JH, Donohue J et al. Frequency of monosomy 7 in different cell lineages in myelodysplastic syndromes. *Blood* 1991; 78 Suppl 1, 136.

(43) Kibbelaar RE, van Kamp H, Dreef EJ et al. Cytogenetically restricted lineage involvement in myelodysplasia as demonstrated by combined in situ hybridization and immunocytochemistry. *Blood* 1991; 78 Suppl 1 134.

(44) Chui DHK, Clarke BJ. Abnormal erythroid progenitor cells in human preleukaemia. *Blood* 1982; 60: 362–7.

(45) Amato D, Khan NR. Erythroid burst formation in cultures of bone marrow and peripheral blood from patients with refractory anaemia. *Acta Haematol* 1983; 70: 1–10.

(46) Ruutu T, Partanen S, Lintula R et al. Erythroid and granulocyte-macrophage colony formation in myelodysplastic syndromes. *Scand J Haematol* 1984; 32: 395–402.

(47) May SJ, Smith SA, Jacobs A et al. The myelodysplastic syndromes: analysis of laboratory characteristics in relation to the FAB classification. *Br J Haematol* 1985; 59: 311–9.

(48) Milner GR, Testa NG, Geary CJ et al. Bone marrow culture studies in refractory cytopenia and 'smouldering leukaemia'. *Br J Haematol* 1977; 32: 251.

(49) Greenberg PL. In vitro culture techniques defining biological abnormalities in the myelodysplastic and myeloproliferative disorders. *Clin Haematol* 1986; 15: 973–93.

(50) Spitzer G, Verma DS, Dicke KA et al. Sub-groups of oligoleukaemia as identified by in vitro agar culture. *Leuk Res* 1979; 3: 29–39.

(51) Yoshida Y, Yoshida C, Tohyamma K et al. Prognostic implication of sequential bone marrow cultures in the myelodysplastic syndromes. *Leuk Res* 1989; 13: 967–72.

(52) Verma DS, Spitzer G, Dicke KA et al. In vitro agar culture patterns in preleukaemia and their clinical significance. *Leuk Res* 1979; 3: 41.

(53) Tennant GB, Jacobs A. Undetectable peripheral blood CFU-GM as a prognostic indicator in myelodysplastic syndrome. *Leuk Res* 1988; 12: 961.

(54) Tennant GB, Bowen DT, Jacobs A. Colony-cluster ratio and cluster number in cultures of circulating myeloid progenitors as indicators of high risk myelodysplasia. *Br J Haematol* 1991; 77: 296.

(55) Guyotat D, Campos L, Thomas et al. Myelodysplastic syndromes. A study of surface markers and in vitro growth patterns. *Am J Haematol* 1990; 34: 26–31.

(56) Schipperus M, Sonneveld P, Lindemans J et al. The effects of interleukin-3, GM-CSF and G-CSF on the growth kinetics of colony forming cells in myelodysplastic syndromes. *Leukemia* 1990; 4: 267–72.

(57) Schipperus M, Sonneveld P, Lindemans J. The combined effects of IL-3, GM-CSF and G-CSF on the in vitro growth of myelodysplastic myeloid progenitor cells. *Leuk Res* 1990; 14: 1019–25.

(58) Baines P, Bowen D, Jacobs A. Clonal growth of haemopoietic progenitor cells from myelodysplastic marrow in response to recombinant haemopoietins. *Leuk Res* 1990; 14: 247–53.

(59) Jacobs A, Culligan D, Bowen D. Erythropoietin and the myelodysplastic syndrome. In Gurland HJ et al (eds) *Erythropoietin in renal and non-renal anaemias* 1990.

(60) Jacobs A, Janowska-Wieczorek A et al. Circulating erythropoietin in patients with myelodys plastic syndromes. *Br J Haematol* 1989; 73: 36–9.

(61) Bowen DT, Jacobs A, Cotes M et al. Serum erythropoietin and erythropoiesis in patients with myelodysplastic syndromes. *Eur J Haematol* 1989; 44: 30–2.

(63) Bowen DT, Culligan D, Jacobs A. The treatment of anaemia in the myelodysplastic syndromes with human recombinant erythropoietin. *Br J Haematol* 1991; 77: 419–23.

(64) Hirashima K, Besho M, Susaki L, et al. Improvement of anaemia by IV injections of recombinant erythropoietin in patients with MDS and aplastic anaemia. *Exp Haemat* 1989; 17: 385.

(65) Van Kamp H, Prinsze- Postema TC, Kluin PM et al. Effects of subcutaneously administered human recombinant erythropoietin on erythropoiesis in patients with myelodysplasia. *Br J Haematol* 1991; 78: 488–93.

(66) Janowska-Wieczorek A, Belch AR, Jacobs A et al. Increased circulating colony stimulating factor 1 in patients with preleukaemia, leukaemia and lymphoid malignancies. *Blood* 1991; 77: 1796–803.

(67) Bowen D, Yancik S, Bennett L, Culligan D, Resser K. Serum stem cell factor concentration in patients with myelodysplastic syndromes. *Br J Haematol* 1993: in press.

(68) Bynoe AG, Scott CS, Ford P, Roberts BE. Decreased T helper cells in myelodysplastic syndromes. *Br J Haematol* 1983; 54: 97–102.

(69) Baumann MA, Milson TJ, Patrick CW et al. Immunoregulatory abnormalities in myelodys-plastic disorders. *Am J Haematol* 1986; 22: 17–26.

(70) Hockland P, Kerndrup G, Griffin JD, Ellegaard J. Analysis of leukocyte differentiation antigens in blood and bone marrow from preleukaemia (refractory anaemia) patients using monoclonal antibodies. *Blood* 1986; 67: 898–902.

(71) Janowska-Wieczorek A, Jakobisiak M, Dobaczewska H. Decreased antibody-dependent cellular cytotoxicity in preleukaemia syndromes. *Acta Haematol* 1983; 69: 132–5.

(72) Kerndrup G, Meyer K, Ellegaard J, Hockland P. Natural killer (NK) cell activity and antibody-dependent cellular cytotoxicity (ADCC) in primary preleukaemic syndrome. *Leuk Res* 1984; 8: 239–47.

(73) Takagi S, Kitagawa S, Takeda A et al. Natural killer-interferon system in patients with pre-leukaemic states. *Br J Haematol* 1984; 58: 71–81.

(74) Solal-Celigny P, Desaint B, Herrera A et al. Chronic myelomonocytic leukaemia according to the FAB classification. Analysis of 35 cases. *Blood* 1984; 63: 634–8.

(75) Economopoulos T, Economidou J, Giannopoulos G et al. Immune abnormalities in myelodysplastic syndromes. *J Clin Pathol* 1985; 38: 908–11.

(76) Mufti GJ, Figes A, Hamblin TJ et al. Immunological abnormalities in myelodysplastic syndromes 1. Serum immunoglobulins and autoantibodies. *Br J Haematol* 1986; 63: 143–7.

(77) Green AR, Shuttleworth D, Bowen DT, Bentley DP. Cutaneous vasculitis in patients with myelodysplasia. *Br J Haematol* 1990; 74: 364–5.

(78) Pagliuca A, Higgins E, Samson D et al. Prodromal cutaneous vasculitis in myelodysplastic syndromes. *Br J Haematol* 1990; 75: 444–6.

(79) Savige JA, Smith C, Chang L, Duggan JC. Anti-neutrophil cytoplastic antibodies (ANCA) in a patient with the vasculitis of myelodysplasia. *Br J Haematol* 1991; 78: 583–4.

(80) Cooper PH, Innes DJ Jr, Greer KE. Acute febrile neutrophilic dermatosis (Sweet's syndrome) and myeloproliferative disorders. *Cancer* 1983; 51: 1518–26.

(81) Soppi E, Nousiainen A, Seppa A, Lahtinen R. Acute febrile neutrophilic dermatosis (Sweet's syndrome) in association with myelodysplastic syndromes: a report of three cases and a review of the literature. *Br J Haematol* 1989; 73: 43–7.

(82) Dacie JV, Mollins DL. Siderocytes, sideroblasts, and sideroblastic anaemia. *Acta Med Scand* 1966; 445: 237–42.

(83) Catovsky D, Shaw MT, Hoffbrand AV, Dacie JV. Sideroblastic anaemia and its association with leukaemia and myelomatosis: a report of five cases. *Br J Haematol* 1971; 20: 385–93.

(84) Mufti GJ, Hamblin TJ, Clein GP, Race C. Coexistent myelodysplasia and plasma cell neoplasia. *Br J Haematol* 1983; 54: 91–6.

(85) Copplestone JA, Mufti GJ, Hamblin TJ, Oscier DG. Immunological abnormalities in myelodysplastic syndromes II. Coexistent lymphoid or plasma cell neoplasms. *Br J Haematol* 1986; 63: 149–59.

(86) Hamblin TJ. Immunological abnormalities in myelodysplastic syndromes. In: Koeffler HP, guest ed. *Haematol/Oncol Clin N Am* 1992; 6: 571–86.

(87) Hamblin TJ, Copplestone JA, Mufti GJ, Oscier DG. Coexisting lymphoid or plasma cell neoplasms. *Br J Haemat* 1987; 65: 376.

(88) Carter G, Hughes DC, Clark RE et al. RAS mutations in patients following cytotoxic therapy for lymphoma. *Oncogene* 1990; 5: 411–6.

(89) Jacobs A. Genetic lesions in preleukaemia. *Leukaemia* 1991; 5: 277–82.

(90) Ridge SA, Worwood M, Oscier D et al. FMS mutations in myelodysplastic, leukaemic and normal subjects. *Proc Natl Acad Sci USA* 1990; 87: 1377–80.

(91) Tobal K, Pagliuca A, Bhatt B et al. Mutation of the human FMS gene (M-CSF receptor) in myelodysplastic syndromes and acute myeloid leukaemia. *Leukaemia* 1990; 4: 486–9.

(92) Vogelstein B, Fearon ER, Hamilton SR et al. Use of restriction fragment length polymorphisms to determine the clonal origin of human tumours. *Science* 1987; 227: 642–5.

(93) Lyon M. X-chromosome inactivation and developmental patterns in mammals. *Biol Rev* 1972; 47: 1–35.

(94) Fraser NJ, Boyd Y, Brownley GG, Craig IW. Multi-allelic RFLP for M27B, an anonymous single copy genomic clone at Xp11.3-Xcen (HGM9 provisional No DXS255). *Nucl Acids Res* 1987; 15: 9616.

(95) Cachia PG, Culligan DJ, Thomas ED et al. Methylation of the DXS255 hypervariable locus 5' CCGG site may be affected by factors other than X-chromosome activation status. *Genomics* 1992; 14: 70–4.

(96) Janssen JWG, Buschle M, Layton M et al. Clonal analysis of myelodysplastic syndromes: evidence of multipotent stem cell origin. *Blood* 1989; 73: 248–54.

(97) Tefferi A, Thibodeau SN, Soldberg LA. Clonal studies in the myelodysplastic syndrome using X-linked restriction fragment length polymorphisms. *Blood* 1990; 75: 1770–3.

(98) Prchal JT, Throckmorton DW, Carol AJ et al. A common progenitor for human myeloid and lymphoid cells. *Nature* 1978; 274: 590–1.

(99) Raskind WH, Tirumali N, Jacobsen R et al. Evidence for a multistep pathogenesis of a myelodysplastic syndrome. *Blood* 1984; 63: 1318–23.

(100) Abrahamson G, Boultwood J, Madden J et al. Clonality of cell populations in refractory anaemia using combined approach of gene loss and X-linked restriction fragment length polymorphism-methylation analysis. *Br J Haematol* 1991; 79: 550–5.

(101) Culligan DJ, Cachia P, Whittaker J et al. Clonal lymphocytes are detectable in only some cases of MDS. *Br J Haematol* 1992; 81: 346–51.

(102a) Van Kamp H, Fibbe WE, Rumo PM et al. Clonal involvement of granulocytes and monocytes, but not T and B lymphocytes and natural killer cells in patients with myelodysplasia: Analysis by X-linked restriction fragment length polymorphisms and polymerase chain reaction of the phosphoglycerate kinase gene. *Blood* 1992; 80: 1774–80.

(102b) Tsukamoto N, Morita K, Maehara T et al. Clonality in myelodysplastic syndromes: demonstration of pluripotent stem cell origin using X-linked restriction fragment length polymorphisms. *Br J Haematol* 1993; 83: 589–94.

(103) Gilliland DG, Blanchard KL, Levy J et al. Clonality in myeloproliferative disorders: analysis by means of the polymerase chain reaction. *Proc Natl Sci USA* 1991; 88: 6848–52.

(104) Van Kamp H, Jansen R, Willemze R et al. Studies on clonality by PCR analysis of the PGK-1 gene. *Nucl Acids Res* 1991; 19: 2794.

Retinoids in acute promyelocytic leukaemia

C CHOMIENNE, S CASTAIGNE, M CORNIC,
P LEFEBVRE, N BALITRAND, S BARBEY,
H DE THE, P FENAUX, L DEGOS

All-*trans*-retinoic acid, one of the active metabolites of vitamin A, is known to specifically induce fresh human promyelocytic leukaemic cells (AML3) to differentiate in vitro to mature functional granulocytes which lose their selfrenewal potency and spontaneously die. These results were confirmed in vivo: AML3 patients treated with oral all-*trans*-RA alone achieved complete remission. Two distinct classes of proteins directly interact with RA: nuclear receptors (RARs and RXRs) and specific cytoplasmic proteins (CRABP). The retinoic receptor alpha (RARα) gene located on chromosome 17, is rearranged through the t(15; A17) translocation observed in these cells and fused to a newly identified gene, PLM, localized on chromosome 15. The specificity of the PML/RAR fusion protein and RA sensitivity of the APL leukaemia points to a close relationship between the leukaemogenesis and the therapeutic efficacy. We show that multiple parameters, among which feature the normal RA binding proteins (RARα and CRABP) and the effective retinoid concentration, play a crucial role in the efficacy of RA therapy in these patients.

Effect of retinoids on AML3 leukaemic cells in vitro

Though retinoids have been shown to alter leukaemic cell growth,[1-7] only AML3 cells[8] are successfully induced to differentiate in vitro.[6,7,9-11] Morphologically, the modifications of the promyelocytic leukaemic cells during the differentiation induced by all-*trans*-RA are variable from one sample to another as are often the promyelocytic leukaemic cells before treatment. After 5 days' incubation with RA, however, all leukaemic cells have a smaller cell volume, a low nucleus cytoplasm ratio, and disappearance of nucleoli if initially present. The cells are granulocytic at the stage of metamyelocytes and

All correspondence to: C Chomienne, Laboratoire de Biologie Cellulaire Hématopoïétique, Institut d'Hématologie, Hôpital Saint Louis, 1 Av Claude Vellefaux 75010, Paris, France.

Cambridge Medical Reviews: Haematological Oncology Volume 3
© Cambridge University Press 1994

band cells, but with sometimes a true asynchrony of maturation between nucleus and cytoplasm, and persistence of Auer rods which confirms the differentiation of AML3 cells. These cells express the CD15 antigen but no mature surface antigen of polymorphonuclear cells or monocytes. The respiratory burst function is acquired rapidly (50% of the cell population is NBT positive after 3 days in culture with RA and 100% by day 7). The number of cells recovered after 5 days in culture with or without RA is little different from the initial cell concentration. These differentiated leukaemic cells can no longer produce leukaemic clones in soft agar and significant decrease of the BCL2 protein in these cells strongly suggest that, at least in vitro, the elimination of the leukaemic clone may be in part due to programmed cell death.[12]

Structure–function relationship for different existing retinoid molecules have been studied in myeloid leukaemic cell lines. All-*trans*-and 13-*cis*-forms are equally effective in the HL-60 cells.[13–17]. Other compounds are either more or, like the ethyl ester (Tigazon®), less effective[16] than the naturally occurring isomers. We observed that, of the three identified isomers, the all-*trans*- and 9-*cis*-retinoids are equally effective on AML3 cell differentiation and viable cell count. The 13-*cis*-isomer, however, induces an equivalent effect at only high concentration (10–6M).[10] We have also studied the effects of the major metabolites of RA: 4-oxo-13 *cis*- and 4-oxo-all *trans*-RA which both induce differentiation of AML3 cells.[10]

Treatment of APL with retinoids

The first available retinoid for in vivo use of RA treatment in acute leukaemias was the 13-*cis*-isomer. In AML3 patients, refractory to conventional chemotherapy, at a 45 to 100 mg/m^2 daily dose, little to no efficacy was observed.[11,17–23] The original experience of Huang and colleagues[24] with all-*trans*-RA in 24 AML3 patients treated with a daily dose of 45 mg/m^2 was striking: 23 patients obtained complete remission and coagulation disorders were rapidly corrected. Our own experience corroborates their data. In first relapse AML3 patients, 26 out 28 patients achieved complete remission (CR).[25,26] These data were rapidly corroborated by different groups.[27–29] In de novo patients, in the first 19 patients that were treated (17 of whom had major contraindication to chemotherapy, mainly old age or poor clinication condition) only 5 CR were obtained, death occurring in the 14 other patients.[30] In a recent European Multicentre Trial, 80 de novo patients with no initial increase in the WBC were treated with retinoic acid alone or conventional chemotherapy followed by chemotherapy consolidation. CR rate was of 91% in the RA group versus 80% in the chemotherapy group. Though the number of early deaths was identical in both groups, the percentage of event-free survival at 12 months was significantly greater with RA (75% versus 47%).[31]

190

The complete remission is obtained via a differentiation mechanism. An intermediate population expressing both mature (CD16) and immature (CD33) markers is detected during the 3rd and 4th week of treatment by cell surface immunophenotyping.[27] In situ hybridization with a chromosome 17 probe[27] and DNA polymorphism studies,[32, 33] confirmed the relationship between the clinical response and the maturation of the leukaemic clone. After 30 to 45 days of treatment, normal myeloid cells have replaced the leukaemic differentiated cells, and the remission is polyclonal.[33]

Coagulation disorders, when present, were rapidly controlled. The bleeding diathesis was recently attributed to a more general activation of fibrinolysis, with a minor DIC. Four patients investigated 8 days after treatment with ATRA had a normalization of the fibrinolytic disorder but persistence of DIC.[34]

The complete remission is achieved without any signs of aplasia. Most patients were treated on an outpatient basis and few (25%) patients needed antibiotics and transfusions.[17–23, 35] ATRA therapy is well tolerated and minor inconveniences (namely dryness of skin and mucosae, transient bone pain, increases of triglycerides and transaminases) are easily overcome by cream, eyedrops or analgesics. The major side effect is the occurrence of a hyperleucocytosis (WBC >10 to 100 10^9/ml) and the 'RA syndrome' (fever, respiratory distress, pulmonary infiltrates, pleural effusions and impaired myocardial function).[36] Hyperleucocytosis is frequent in de novo patients (60%) and less so in relapse (20%).[17–23] Early deaths are often concomitant to an increase in WBC and, though the WBC which mainly consist of AML3 cells are not resistant to ATRA in vitro, rapid decrease of the cell count to prevent fetal outcome is only achieved with the addition of chemotherapy. The frequency of the 'RA syndrome' is not yet known as it is often associated with hyperleucocytosis.[36] Short course, high dose corticosteroid treatment promptly reversed these symptoms in four out five patients treated in the Memorial Sloan Kettering Institute.[36] Little dose escalations studies have been performed. In an attempt to reduce the side effect of ATRA in vivo, Dr Castaigne launched a pilot study with 25 mg/m^2/d in 30 patients. CR rate and frequency of hyperleucocytosis was the same as with 45 mg dose. Median time to achieve CR was equally identical.[37] The similar AUC levels observed, suggest that doses may stil be lowered in vivo.

Length of complete remission was noted to be short if all-*trans*-RA alone or low dose chemotherapy were given as maintenance therapy (4–47 months).[7–10] Recent results suggest that consolidation therapy with conventional (daunorubicin and cytosine arabinoside) chemotherapy not only provides long disease-free complete remissions[30,31] but that these remissions may be longer than when induction chemotherapy consisted of only chemotherapy.

Resistance to ATRA therapy is currently observed in non-AML3 cases[18] though some AML2 or AML1 cases have been found to respond in vitro and in vivo to ATRA.[6,7,9,10] In 'virgin' AML3 cases (not previously treated by RA), sensitivity seems to be related to the history of the disease. Among four patients in second relapse, three had a partial response and one patient in third relapse had a resistance to the ATRA (in vitro and in vivo).[25] When AML3 cases relapse after ATRA-induced complete remission, failure to achieve a second remission with ATRA is the rule when these relapses occur soon after the withdrawal of ATRA.[17–23]

Hypotheses for the basis of RA's efficacy in APL cells

The mechanism(s) through which RA induces leukaemic cell differentiation have not been elucidated though many effects consecutive to RA action have been observed at different levels of the cell. Monitoring RA's efficacy and side effects during prolonged RA therapy has suggested that RA's outcome and biological consequences in tissues other than haematopoietic must be considered.

Structure and function of the PML/RAR fusion protein

Through the t(15;17) translocation[38], these AML3 leukaemic cells present with PML/RARα fusion transcripts and to a lesser frequency with the recip-rocal RARα/PML transcripts.[39–43] The transcripts are variable in sizes depending on the breakpoint localization on the PML gene, each AML3 patient being characterized by a specific fusion transcript. These transcripts are not easily detectable on Northern blots (poor cellular samples and weak expression of the messenger RNA)[44–47] but can now be observed in all AML3 cases by reverse transcriptase polymerase chain reaction.[48–53] So far, these different types of fusion transcripts do not allow to discriminate between different AML3 subtypes, or for a specific outcome or response to RA.

PML-RARa alters the *trans*activation of RARE reporter genes (either spon-taneously or in the presence of RA), depending on the type of the transfected cell, the promoter gene used and the quantity of plasmid transfected, sug-gesting cell type specific gene activation or inactivation.[54–56] In haematopoietic cells (HL-60) PML/RAR inhibits RA-mediate *trans*activation.[57] No data are yet available concerning the functional effect of the other abnormal PML proteins. However, it already appears that PML/RAR blocks the RA-mediated granulocytic differentiation of HL-60 cells[57] and that, on its own, the truncated RARa protein, has no repressor effect in *trans*activation assays.[54–57]

Putative roles of the PML/RARα and normal RAR proteins in the RA-induced differentiation

In the presence of high concentrations of ATRA, PML/RARα can activate RA-inducible reporter genes.[55–57] This is in agreement with the structural conservation of the ligand binding domain in the PM/RARα protein and its

192

identical binding affinity for all-*trans*-RA compared to RARα,[58] though it is not yet known how the tri-dimensional structure of the abnormal protein affects the stability of the RA binding in the cell. This may imply that the PML/RARα protein could be responsible both for the oncogenic effect and RA responsiveness of AML3 cells.

Another explanation which need not be exclusive is that RA-efficacy may be linked to the normal remaining RARα gene. Various data implicate RARα in normal granulocytic differentiation: RARα is highly expressed in normal differentiated granulocytes[44] and in the myeloid tissue by in situ hybridization (F Guidez personal communication). On normal myeloid progenitor cells, all-*trans*-RA increases granulocytic differentiation.[59] This has led us to postulate that RA and its receptor α may play a role in normal granulocytic differentiation. In AML3 cells, we noted a significant increase of the normal RARα gene expression after treatment with all-*trans*-RA. This appears as an early event of RA and forwards an explanation for the paradoxical effect of all-*trans*-RA in this disease. The level of expression of RARα gene was correlated to the concentration of all-trans-RA used.[60] RARα is known to form heterodimers both RXRα and PML, PML/RARα.[61] It is not yet known how the equilibrium between these different proteins affect *trans*activation and differentiation in AML3 cells.

Levels of all-trans-RA concentrations: a prerequisite for RA sensitivity of AML3 cells

Pharmacological studies of all-*trans*-RA in AML3 patients have brought forward interesting data. The plasma concentration of all-*trans*-RA achieved in AML3 patients was within the in vitro differentiating concentrations; time to peak concentration of all-*trans*-RA was between 60 and 120 minutes (median: 90 minutes) after ingestion, with maximum concentrations between 0.03 µg/ml and 2.5 µg/ml (median 0.4 µg/ml), median AUC 630 ng h/ml. These concentrations were within the in vitro differentiating concentration range of all-*trans*-RA for these patients' cells. Interpatient variations were linked to an increased clearance rate and to the leukaemic cell burden.[62,63] The great interpatient variability observed suggests that intracellular concentration determinations may prove essential in the pharmacological studies of all-*trans*-RA in AML3 patients undergoing RA therapy. A significant decrease of the area under the curve is found very early after onset of ATRA treatment.[63] Little is known about the exact physiological outcome of all-*trans*-RA in normal or AML3 patients. Different enzymes are implicated in the conversion of the exogenous Vitamin A to retinoic acid and its various metabolites. These enzymes depend on the presence of cytochrome P450, NAD and certain cellular binding proteins such as CRABP which have been recently shown to act as substrate for retinoic acid metabolism.[64] RA induces P450 metabolism and AML3 cells of patients after RA therapy have a hypercatabolytic state to RA. The quantity of CRABP detected is related to the length of ATRA therapy and decreases very slowly (months) after withdrawal of ATRA. These data strongly suggest a metabolism cause for the resistance of ATRA in relapse patients and the failure of continuous ATRA therapy as maintenance therapy. Drugs that reduce P450 activity or binding to CRABP may circumvent resistance to ATRA. Revision of the schedule, dose and length of ATRA therapy in the induction treatment of AML3 may prevent the induction of this 'salvage' cascade and therefore the induction of resistance.

Discussion

Terminal differentiation of acute myeloid leukaemic cells has opened both new perspectives on the understanding of leukaemogenesis, and new possibilities of therapies in malignancy. To date, in vitro and in vivo differentiation of acute promyelocytic leukaemic cells with all-*trans*-RA is the first model of differentiation therapy. Patients achieve complete remission with an oral therapy without the inconvenience of an aplastic phase. A true correlation is observed between the in vitro and in vivo differentiating characteristics (structure and dose) of the retinoids used. The plasma levels reached during ATRA therapy are within the in vitro differentiating concentrations, but intracellular determinations are required to correlate all-*trans*-RA concentrations and clinical outcome.

This novel approach to cancer therapy has stimulated a major interest in the study of RA's differentiating efficacy in AML3 cells as in normal haematopoietic cells. The concomitant cloning of the nuclear receptors of RA brought the awaited elements for this study. This resulted in the discovery that one allele of the RAR alpha gene was rearranged in AML3 cells through the chromosomal translocation specifically observed in these cells. The abnormal transcripts are under the regulation of a newly identified gene *PML* from chromosome 15. Altered expression of nuclear receptors has been proposed as one of the multiple steps leading to carcinogenesis:[65] in a human hepatoma, for example, the RAR beta gene is truncated by the insertion of a hepatitis B viral genome,[66] while the cellular homologue of the retroviral oncogene, v-*erb*A is a thyroid hormone receptor.[67,68] The PML/RARα gene may lead to the production of an altered, functionnally impaired RA binding protein which could interfere with the normal programme of granulocytic differentiation.

This discovery which implicates the PML/RAR gene product in the leukaemogenesis of APL has not side-tracked the original study of RA efficacy in AML3 patients. The coexpression of normal and abnormal RARα transcripts in AML3 cells proposes the normal RARα as a possible candidate receptor for mediating RA-induced granulocytic differentiation. Our results suggest that in vitro, the RARα expressed in AML3 cells may be induced by RA, the RARα gene appearing thus as a primary target for RA in M3 cells. Autoregulation of other members of the thyroid/steroid hormone receptor family have been shown in response to their ligand.[69–71] The data of CRABP induction during ATRA therapy in AML3 patients, place high levels of CRABP not as a tool but most probably as an impediment to RA efficacy: the capture of free cytoplasmic RA by CRABP might reduce the effective RA concentration reaching the nucleus and forwards thus as possible explanation for the secondary resistance observed in AML3 patients after RA therapy.

The monitoring of ATRA efficacy in AML3 patients requires a thorough knowledge of the biodisposability, cellular uptake and metabolism of all-*trans*-RA in AML3 cells along with the determination of the presence, quantity and affinity of the different RA binding proteins. The parallel studies on the role of the PML/RARα product on the blockage of myeloid differentiation and of the normal RARα in normal and leukaemic differentiation will provide the necessary elements.

References

(1) Douer D, Koeffler HP: Retinoic acid: Inhibition of the clonal growth of human myeloid leukemia cells. *J Clin Invest* 1982; 69: 277.

(2) Champelovier P, Seigneurin D. Proliferation and maturation of human leukemic cells in liquid culture: activity of human placenta conditioned medium and retinoic acid. *Exp Hematol* 1985; 13: 1094.

(3) Lawrence J, Conner K, Kelly MA, Hanslerr MR, Wallace P, Bagby GC Jr. *cis*-retinoic acid stimulates the clonal growth of some myeloid leukemia cells in vitro. *Blood* 1987; 69: 302.

(4) Gallagher RE, Lurie KJ, Leavitt RD, Wiernik PH. Effects of interferon and retinoic acid on the growth and differentiation of leukemic cells from acute myelogenous leukemia patients treated with recombinant leucocyte-alpha A interferon. *Leuk Res*, 1987; 11: 609.

(5) Findley HW, Steuber CP, Ruyman FB, Culbert S, Ragab AH. Effect of retinoic acid on the clonal growth of childhood myeloid and lymphoid leukemias: a pediatric oncology group study. *Exp Hematol* 1984; 12: 768.

(6) Breitman TR, Collins SJ, Keene BP. Terminal differentiation of human promyelocytic leukemic cells in primary culture in response to retinoic acid. *Blood* 1981; 57: 1000.

(7) Honma Y, Fujita Y, Kasukabe T et al. Induction of differentiation of human acute non-lymphocytic leukemia cells in primary culture by inducers of differentiation of human myeloid leukemia cell line HL-60. *Eur J Cancer Clin Oncol* 1983; 19: 251.

(8) Bennett JM, Catovsky D, Daniel MT et al. Proposals for the classification of the acute leukemia. *Br J Haematol* 1976; 33: 451.

(9) Imaizumi M, Breitman TR. Retinoic acid induced differentiation of the human

promyelocytic leukemia cell line, HL-60, and fresh human, leukemia cells in primary culture: a model for differentiation inducing therapy. *Eur J Haematol* 1987; 38: 19.

(10) Chomienne C, Ballerini P, Balitrand N et al. All-*trans* retinoic acid in acute promyelocytic leukemias: II In vitro studies: structure–function relationship. *Blood* 1990; 76: 1710.

(11) Chomienne C, Ballerini P, Balitrand N et al. Retinoic acid therapy for promyelocytic leukemia. *Lancet* 1989; i: 746.

(12) Chomienne C, Barbey S, Balitrand N, Degos L, Sachs L. Regulation of BCL-2 and cell death by all-*trans* retinoic acid in acute promyelocytic leukemic cells. *Biomed Pharmacother* 1992; 46 abstr 260.

(13) Yen A, Powers V, Fisbaugh J. Retinoic acid induced HL-60 myeloid differentiation: dependence of early and late events on isomeric structure. *Leuk Res* 1986; 10: 619.

(14) Tobler A, Dawson MI, Koeffler HP. Retinoids: structure–function relationship in normal and leukemic hematopoiesis in vitro. *J Clin Invest* 1986; 78: 303.

(15) Chomienne C, Balitrand N, Cost H, Degos L, Abita JP. Structure–activity relationships of the aromatic retinoids on the differentiation of the human histiocytic lymphoma cell line U-937. *Leuk Res* 1986; 10: 1301.

(16) Chomienne C, Balitrand N, Abita JP. Inefficacy of the synthetic aromatic retinoid etretinate and of its free acid on the in vitro differentiation of leukemic cells. *Leuk Res* 1986; 10: 1079.

(17) Sampi K, Honma Y, Hozumi M, Sakura M. Discrepancy between in vitro and in vivo inductions of differentiation by retinoids of human acute promyelocytic cells in relapse. *Leuk Res* 1985; 9: 1475.

(18) Hoffman SJ, Robinson WA. Use of differentiation-inducing agents in the myelodysplastic syndrome and the acute non-lymphocytic leukemia. *Am J Hematol* 1988; 28:124.

(19) Flynn PJ, Miller WJ, Weisdorf DJ, Arthur DC, Brunning R, Branda RF. Retinoic acid treatment of acute promyelocytic leukemia: In vitro and in vivo observations: *Blood* 1983; 62: 1211.

(20) Nilsson B. Probable in vivo induction of differentiation by retinoic acid of promyelocytes in acute promyelocytic leukemia. *Br J Haematol* 1984; 57:365

(21) Fontana JA, Rogers JS, Durham JP. The role of 13-*cis* -retinoic acid in the remission induction of a patient with acute promyelocytic leukemia. *Cancer* 1986; 57: 209.

(22) Daenen S, Vellenga E, van Dobbenburgh OA, Halie MR. Retinoic acid as antileukemic therapy in a patient with acute promyelocytic leukemia and A*spergillus* pneumonia. *Blood* 1986; 67: 559.

(23) Kramer ZB, Boros L, Wiernik PH et al. *Cis*-retinoic acid in the treatment of elderly patients with acute myeloid leukemia *Cancer* 1991; 67:1484.

(24) Huang ME, Ye YI, Chen SR et al. Use of all-*trans*-retinoic acid in the treatment of acute promyelocytic leukemia. *Blood* 1988; 72: 567.

(25) Castaigne S, Chomienne C, Daniel MT, Berger R, Fenaux P, Degos L. All *trans*-retinoic acid as a differentiation therapy for acute promyelocytic leukemia: I Clinical Results. *Blood* 1990; 336:1440.

(26) Degos L, Chomienne C, Daniel MT et al. Treatment of first relapse in acute promyelocytic leukemia with all-*trans*-RA. *Lancet*, 1990; 336:1440.

(27) Warrel RP, Frankel SR Miller WH et al. Differentiation therapy of acute promyelocytic leukemia with tretinoin (all-*trans*-retinoic acid). *N Engl J Med* 1991; 324: 1385.

(28) Chen ZX, Xue YQ, Zhang R et al. A clinical and experimental study on all-*trans*-retinoic acid treated acute promyelocytic leukemia patients. *Blood* 1991; 78: 1413.

(29) Warrel RP, Frankel SR, Miller WH, Eardley A, Dmitrovsky E. All-*trans*-retinoic acid for remission induction of acute promyelocytic leukemia: results of the New York study. *Blood* 1992; 80: 360a.

(30) Fenaux P, Castaigne S, Dombret H et al. All-*trans*-retinoic acid in newly diagnosed acute promyelocytic leukemia; a pilot study. *Blood* 1992; 80: 2176.

(31) Fenaux P, Castaigne S, Dombret H et al. All-*trans*-retinoic acid in newly diagnosed acute promyelocytic leukemia; a pilot study. ASCO meeting 1993 (in press)

(32) Fearon ER, Burke PJ, Schiffer CA, Zehnbauer BA, Vogelstein B: Differentiation of leukemia cells to polymorphonuclear leukcytes in patients with acute nonlymphocytic leukemia. *N Engl J Med* 1986; 315: 15.

(33) Elliott S, Taylor K, White S et al. Proof of differentiative mode of action of all-*trans*-retinoic acid in acute promyelocytic leukemia using X-linked clonal analysis. *Blood* 1992; 8: 1916.

(34) Scrobohacci ML, Dombret H, Ghorra P, Baurmann H, Castaigne S, Daniel MT. Disseminated intravascular coagulation and/or primary fibrinolysis in acute promyelocytic leukemia: effect of all-*trans*-RA acid treatment. *Blood* 1991; 78 Abst. 183 48a.

(35) Eardley A, Franlel SR, Heller G, Warrell RP. Cost benefit analysis of all-*trans*-retinoic acid compared to standard chemotherapy for remission induction of newly diagnosed patients with acute promyelocytic leukemia. *Blood* 1992; 80: 109a.

(36) Frankel S, Eardly A; Lauwers G, Weiss M, Warrel RP. The 'retinoic acid syndrome' in acute promyelocytic leukemia: reversal by corticosteroids. *Ann Intern Med*. 1992; 117:292.

(37) Castaigne S, Lefèbvre P, Rigal Huguet F et al. Lower all-trans retinoic acid (ATRA 2 mg/m^2/day) are effective in acute promyelocytic leukemia (APL). *Blood* 1992; 80:360a.

(38) Larson RA, Kondo K, Vardiman JW, Butler AE, Golomb HM, Rowley JD. Evidence for a 15;17 translocation in every patient with acute promyelocytic leukemia. *Am J Med* 1984; 76: 827.

(39) Chomienne C, Ballerini P, Balitrand et al. Normal RARa gene transcripts are modulated during RA induced granulocytic differentiation in APL cells. *Leukemia* 1990; 4802.

(40) de Thé H, Chomienne C, Lanotte M, Dejean A. The t(15;17) translocation of acute promyelocytic leukaemia fuses the retinoic acid receptor alpha gene to a novel transcribed locus. *Nature* 1990; 347: 558.

(41) Borrows J, Goddard AD, Sheer D, Solomon E. Molecular analysis of APL breakpoint cluster region on chromosome 17. *Science* 1990; 249: 15770.

(42) Longo L, Dionti E, Mencarelli A et al. Mapping of chromosome 17 breakpoints in acute myeloid leukemia. *Oncogene* 1990; 5: 1557.

(43) Chen Z, Chen SJ, Tong JH et al. The retinoic acid alpha receptor gene is frequently disrupted in its 5′ part in Chinese patients with acute promyelocytic leukemia. *Leukemia* 1991; 5: 288.

(44) Alcalay M, Zangrilli D, Padolfi PP et al. Translocation breakpoint of acute promyelocytic leukemia lies within retinoic acid receptor alpha locus. *Proc Natl Inst Acad Sci USA* 1991; 8: 1977.

(45) Chang KS, Trujillo JM. Rearrangement of the retinoic acid receptor gene in acute promyelocytic leukemia. *Leukemia* 1991; 5: 200.

(46) Miller WH, Warrell RP, Frankell SR et al. Novel retinoic acid receptor alpha transcripts in acute promyelocytic leukemia responsive to all-*trans*-retinoic acid *J Natl Cancer Inst* 1990; 82: 1932.

(47) Longo L, Pandolfi PP, Biondi A, Rambaldi A et al. Rearrangements and aberrant expression in the RAR alpha gene in acute promyelocytic cells. *J Exp Med* 1990; 172: 1571.

(48) Castaigne S, Balitrand N, de The H, Dejean A, Degos L, Chomienne C. A PML/RARa fusion transcript is constantly detected by RNA-based polymerase chain reaction in acute promyelocytic leukemia. *Blood* 1992; 79: 3110.

(49) Miller WH, Kakizuka A, Frankel SR et al. Reverse transcriptase polymerase chain reaction (RT-PCR) for the rearranged retinoic acid receptor alpha of acute promyelocytic leukemia clarifies diagnosis and detects minimal residual disease in clinical remission. *Proc Natl Acad Sci USA* 1992; 89: 2694.

(50) Chang KS, Lu JF, Wang G et al. The t(15.17) translocation breakpoint in acute promyelocytic leukemia cluster within two different sites of the myl gene: targets for detection of minimal residual disease by the polymerase chain reaction. *Blood* 1992; 79: 554.

(51) Chen SJ, Chen Z, Chen A et al. Occurrence of distinct PML-RARa fusion gene isoforms in patients with acute promyelocytic leukemia detected by reverse transcriptase polymerase chain reaction. *Oncogene* 1992; 7: 1223.

(52) Lo Coco F, Diverio D, Pandolfi PP. Molecular evaluation of residual disease as a predictor of relapse in acute promyelocytic leukemia. *Lancet* 1992; 340: 1437.

(53) de The H, Lavau C, Marchio A, Chomienne C, Degos L, Dejean A. The PML/RARa fusion mRNA generated by the t(15;17) translocation in acute promyelocytic leukemia encodes a functionally altered RAR. *Cell* 1991; 66: 675.

(54) Kakizuka A, Miller WH, Umesono K et al. Chromosomal translocation t(15;17) in human acute promyelocytic leukemia fuses RARa with a novel putative transcriptional factor PML. *Cell* 1991; 66: 663.

(56) Kastner P, Perez A, Lutz Y et al. Stucture localization and transcriptional properties of two classes of retinoic acid receptor alpha fusion proteins in acute promyelocytic leukemia: structural similarities with a new family of oncoprotein. *EMBO J* 1992; 11: 629.

(57) Rousselot P, Hardas B, Castaigne S et al. The PML-RARa gene product of the t(15;17) translocation inhibits retinoic acid induced granulocytic differentiation. *Blood* 1992; 80: 255a

(58) Nervi C, Poindexter C, Grignani F et al. Characterization of the PML/RAR

chimeric product of the acute promyelocytic specific t(15;17) translocation. *Cancer Res.* 1992; 52: 3687.

(59) Gratas C, Menot ML, Dresch C, Chomienne C. Retinoids support granulocytic but not erythroid differentiation of myeloid progenitor in normal bone marrow cells. *Leukemia* 1993; 7: 1156–62.

(60) Chomienne C, Ballerini P, Balitrand N et al. The retinoic acid receptor alpha gene is rearranged in retinoic acid-sensitive promyelocytic leukemias. *Leukemia,* 1992; 4: 802.

(61) Kliewer SA, Umesono K, Mangelsdorf DJ, Evans RM. Retinoic X receptor interacts with nuclear receptors in retinoic acid, thyroid hormone and vitamin D3 signalling. *Nature* 1992; 355: 446.

(62) Lefebvre P, G Thomas, Gourmel B, Dreux C, Castaigne S, C Chomienne. Pharmacokinetics of all-*trans* -RA in patients with acute promyelocytic. *J Clin Invest* 1991; 88: 2150.

(63) Muindi JRF, Frankel SR, Huselton C et al. Clinical pharmacology of oral all-*trans*-retinoic acid in patients acute promyelocytic leukemia. *Cancer Res* 1992; 52: 2138.

(64) Cornic M, Delva L, Balitrand N, Guidez F, Chomienne C. Characterization of cytoplasmic retinoic acid binding protein during therapy of RA in promyelocytic acute leukemia. *Cancer Res* 1992; 52: 3329.

(65) Greene S, Chambon P. A superfamily of potentially oncogenic hormone receptors. *Nature,* 1986; 615.

(66) Dejean A, Bougueleret L, Grzeschik KH, Tiollais P. Hepatitis B virus DNA integration a sequence homologous to v-erbA and steroid receptor genes in a hepatocellular carcinoma. *Nature* 1986; 322: 70.

(67) Sap J, Munoz A, Damm K et al. The c-erb A protein is a high-affinity receptor hormone for thyroid hormone. *Nature* 1986; 324: 635.

(68) Damm K, Thompson CC, Evans RM. Protein encoded by V-erbA functions as a thyroid hormone receptor antagonist. *Nature* 1989; 339: 593.

(69) de Thé H, Vivanvo-Ruiz MdM, Tiollais P, Stunnenberg H, Dejean A,: Identification of a retinoic acid responsive element in the retinoic acid receptor beta gene. *Nature* 1990; 343: 177.

(70) Okret S, Poellinger L, Dong Y, Gustafsson JA. Down-regulation of glucocorticoid receptor mRNA by glucocorticoid hormones and recognition by the receptor of a specific binding sequence within a receptor cDNA clone. *Proc Natl Acad Sci USA* 1986; 83: 5899.

(71) Saceda M, Lippman ME, Chambon P et al. Regulation of the estrogen receptor in MCF-7 cells by estradiol. *Mol Endocrinol* 1988; 2: 1157.

The cytogenetics of acute lymphoblastic leukaemia

L M SECKER-WALKER

Chromosomal abnormalities acquired by the bone marrow cells in patients with leukaemia are the microscopically visible signs of submicroscopic genetic change associated with the conversion of normal into malignant cells. Recognition of the clinical importance of cytogenetic changes in acute lymphoblastic leukaemia (ALL) dates from 1978 and the first demonstration of their prognostic significance.[1] The impact of chromosomal change on the biology of the leukaemias is seen in the chromosomal subgroups each identified by a particular chromosomal configuration and associated with remarkably similar clinical features and a predictable response to treatment.[2-4] Evidence for the central role of cytogenetic change in the aetiology of the disease is compelling. Chromosomal breakpoints are frequently located at the sites of cellular oncogenes;[5] chromosomal translocations bring about the unnatural juxtaposition of an oncogene with a cell-type specific gene which results in the aberrant expression of the oncogene.[6,7] Molecular probes to a number of chromosomally induced genetic abnormalities are now available. Using the techniques of Southern blotting, polymerase chain reaction (PCR), and fluorescence in situ hybridization (FISH) chromosomal abnormalities can now be detected in whole cell populations at different levels of sensitivity. The combination of cytogenetics and molecular techniques now provide powerful tools with which to detect and monitor these specific markers of the disease.

Clinical and biological features of acute lymphoblastic leukaemia

This kind of leukaemia is primarily a disease of childhood, with 3 cases per 100 000 per annum and a peak at ages 3 to 5 years. Approximately 25% of patients are adults aged >15 years at presentation. The best prognosis is

All correspondence: Professor Secker-Walker, Cytogenetics Laboratory Department of Haematology, The Royal Free Hospital, Pond Street, London NW3 2QG, UK.

Cambridge Medical Reviews : Haematological Oncology Volume 3 associated with leucocyte counts below $10 \times 10^9/l$ age 3–5 years, common (C-) ALL immunophenotype and female sex. An increasingly poor prognosis is seen with increasingly elevated leucocyte counts; age below 2 and above 9 years; T cell, pre-B, null or mature B immunophenotype.[8]

Cytogenetic abnormalities acquired by the leukaemic cells at diagnosis are another of the variable diagnostic features which define the biology of the disease and have an impact on prognosis. Chromosomal abnormalities include both structural and numerical change.

Detecting the abnormal clone

A chromosomally abnormal clone in the bone marrow at diagnosis has been reported in between 44% and >90% of patients analysed.[2-4, 9-18] The incidence of chromosomally normal cases is higher in T-ALL (30%) than in B-lineage ALL 10%–20%[19, 20] Confidence limits for the exclusion of a clone depend on the number of cells analysed. The finding of 20/20 normal cells excludes the presence of an 11% actively cycling clone with 90% confidence.[21]

Cases in which metaphases are absent, insufficient or of inadequate morphology are found in all surveys. Failure rates range from 7% in single centres to 45% in multicentre studies.[3, 14, 15, 18, 22-24] The success of a cytogenetic investigation and the detection of a clone are dependent on optimal sample and culture conditions.[3, 25-27]

Established chromosomal abnormalities and chromosomal classification

Recognized established or recurring primary abnormalities are those which have been detected as the only change in at least 2 individual cases of ALL from at least 2 different laboratories worldwide.[28] There are now at least 36 structural and 8 numerical established abnormalities. Numerical abnormalities include different monosomies, namely loss of 20, 21, X or Y and 5 different trisomies, gain of a single homologue namely 8,13,16,18 or 21.[28] The established chromosomal changes are of three kinds: (i) translocations associated with specific clinical features, blasts which express a particular immunophenotype and have a known impact on prognosis; (ii) abnormalities which are found in a large number of cases but have diverse clinical or blast cell features and have no apparent prognostic impact; (iii) translocations in mature B-cell and T-ALL which involve the chromosomal locations of one or more of the immunoglobulin or T-cell receptor genes, respectively. These last are particularly important for their contribution to our understanding of the mechanisms of leukaemogenesis.

Chromosomal classification of ALL has undergone several changes since classification by ploidy was first proposed in 1978.[1] Classification may now be (i) a hierarchical system first identifying patients with established chromosomal change and then entering the remainder to one of the ploidy groups.

Established changes present in small numbers are included in the appropriate ploidy groups. (ii) Patients are ascribed to a ploidy group but those with established chromosomal change are also described separately.[2–4, 29] In this chapter I shall describe chromosomal subgroups, those with other established structural change and then ploidy groups. The immunophenotype, clinical features, and incidence are shown for the most important structural abnormalities in Table 1 and for the ploidy groups in Table 5. The genes involved in structural change are shown for B-precursor and mature B-ALL in Table 2 and for T-ALL in Table 3.

Table 1. *Structural abnormalities in acute lymphoblastic leukaemia*

Chromosome abonormality	Immuno-phenotype	Associated features (means)	Incidence	
t(1;19)(q23;p13)[1]fder (19)[1]	Pre-B Cμ>80% (C-ALL)	WBC: 20 × 10⁹/l AGE: C[3] 5 y A[4] 25 y	ALL[2] Pre-B	3%–7% 25%
t(4;11)(q21;q23)[1]	early B/ pre-B Cμ/ Null	WBC: >100 × 10⁹/l AGE: C[3] 1 y A[4] >40 y	C[3] A[4]	2% 5%
t(9;22)(q34;q11)[1]	C-ALL/ Pre-B Cμ	WBC: >30 × 10⁹/l AGE: C[3] >10 y A[4] >40 y	C[3] A[4]	2%–5% 15%– 44%
t(2;8)(p12;q24)[1]	B-ALL	FAB: L3		
t(8;14)(q24;q32)[1]		WBC: 10 × 10⁹/l		5%
t(8;22)(q24;q11)[1]		M>F		
t(8;14)(q24;q11)	T-ALL	WBC: 95 × 10⁹/l AGE: 5 y		1%
del(6q)	C-ALL/ T-ALL		C-ALL[5] T-ALL[6]	4% 16%
del(9p)	C-ALL/ T-ALL	WBC: high lymphomatous	C-ALL[5] T-ALL[6]	5% 9%
t/del(12p)	C-ALL/ T-ALL	WBC: 30 × 10⁹/l		8–10%

[1] = chromosomal subgroup.
[2] = C-ALL & T-ALL; [3] = childhood; [4] = adult; [5] = CD10+; [6] = T-ALL.

t(1;19) and der(19)t(1;19)

This translocation is found in two forms: a balanced translocation t(1;19) (q23;p13) and an unbalanced form der(19)t(1;19) in which the reciprocal product der(1) is lost. The unbalanced form results in trisomy of the long arm of chromosome 1 distal to the q23 breakpoint and monosomy of chromosome 19 distal to the break at 19p13.[30–33]

Chromosomal abnormalities additional to the translocation are found in 55–70% of cases at diagnosis. These include additional copies of 1q, deletion of 6q, i(7)(q10), deletion and translocation of 9p, i(9) (q10), involvement of 13q and translocation of 14q.[34,35]

The translocation is found in between 3% and 6% of cases of ALL. It is strongly associated with a pre-B immunophenotype with >70% blasts expressing cytoplasmic immunoglobulin (CIg)[32] and probably accounts for 25% of pre-B cases.[31–33] It occurs in patients aged <1–45 years with a median age in children of 5 years and in adults of 25 years. Leucocyte counts range from 0.5–459 × 10^9/l (median 20.9 × 10^9/l). Studies in the United States have noted a high incidence (up to 38%) of black race among children in this subgroup.[35,36]

The molecular consequence of t(1;19) is to juxtapose a gene on chromosome 19 *E2A* with a gene on chromosome 1 *PBX1*. Rearrangement of the *E2A* gene can be detected by Southern blotting.[37–39] The more sensitive technique of PCR can be used to identify chimeric *E2A/PBX1* transcripts. Initial results comparing the two techniques indicate that these may not be fully concordant. PCR may fail to identify the translocation detected cytogenetically or may suggest an unusually high incidence in cytogenetically 'normal' samples. Equally, the relationship between PCR positivity in remission and disease status is at present unclear since this may be followed by early relapse or by prolonged remission.[40]

The prognostic implications of this abnormality were initially unclear. An association with poor risk features was noted by some[41] but not others.[31,32] In pre-B ALL t(1;19) has been identified as the major adverse feature.[16,35] More intensive treatment appears to improve survival of patients with this translocation.[35] Recently the variant form der(19)t(1;19) of the translocation was shown to be associated with a better prognosis than the balanced form. The 30 cases with t(1;19) had a median survival of 24 months while median survival had not been reached for the 36 cases with der(19) which had a projected median survival >120 months (p=0.002). The impact of karyotype was in marked contrast to that of age, white blood count and additional chromosomal change none of which was prognostically important in this group of patients.[34]

t(17;19) (q22;p13)

This translocation, a variant of t(1;19) involves fusion of the same *E2A* gene on 19 with a gene *HLF* for a novel basic leucine zipper (bZIP) protein on chromosome 17 which brings about leukaemogenic conversion of a bZIP transcription factor.[42] It has been described in at least five patients aged 2 to

17 (median 15.5) years with leucocyte counts 4.3–71.9 (median 16.1) $\times$ $10^9/l$ and with C-ALL (four cases) or null (one case) immunophenotype. Two of these patients presented with disseminated intravascular coagulation (DIC), a rare complication in ALL, that improved with antileukaemic therapy.[43,44]

t(4;11) (q21;q23)

In childhood t(4;11) has an incidence of 2%[3,45] and a median age of less than 1 year. In the infant age group but not at other ages it is associated with an excess of females to males. It appears to be twice as frequent in adults at 5%.[2,10] The translocation occurs as the only change in 70% of cases at diagnosis but in relapse 70% of cases show additional change with +6, +8, +13 and i(7)(q10).[46] This subgroup is remarkable for its association with very high white blood counts (>155 $\times$ $10^9/l$) and blasts of null immunophenotype (CD19+ve, CD10−ve, CIg+/−) which may have myelomonocytic characteristics indicative of a B precursor leukaemia originating in a pluripotent stem cell.[2,3,10,45–49] The majority of cases investigated have shown rearrangement of immunoglobulin genes (*IGH*) confirming B-cell clonality.[48,49]

The gene located at 11q23 which is rearranged in acute leukaemias involving this region has been named *MLL* or *ALL-1*. In t(4;11) *ALL-1* is cleaved within the coding region and results in fusion of the open reading frames of *ALL-1* and a gene on chromosome 4 in phase.[50–52]

Prognosis for the subgroup as a whole is poor with 75% of childhood cases achieving remission compared with 98% of other cases. Relapse occurs early and maximum survival in many surveys has been <6 months.[2–4] Adults fare exceptionally badly compared with those in other chromosomal groups.[2,10] There are reports of some long-term survivors (32+ to 84+ months) among children and it has been shown that, whereas prognosis is particularly poor for infants, older children in this subgroup and particularly those aged 1 to 9 years have a much better prognosis. Among children investigated by age group, neither sex nor leucocyte count less or greater than 100 $\times$ $10^9/l$ were prognostically important.[49,53]

t(4;11) in secondary leukaemia This translocation has been identified in at least 9 patients who developed ALL following chemotherapy and radiotherapy for a prior malignancy. Treatment had included a combination of topoisomerase II inhibitors (anthacyclines mitoxantione, or the epopodophillotoxin derivatives VP16 or VM26) and cyclophosphamide.[54–56] This kind of observation may provide clues to the etiology of the t(4;11) ALL de novo.

t(11;19)(q23;p13)

This translocation is also a feature of infant ALL and together with t(4;11) accounts for nearly 50% of patients <1 year at diagnosis.[57,58]

L M Secker-Walker

t(8;14)(q11;q32)

A translocation involving chromosomes 8 and 14 involving 14q32 and a second breakpoint at 8q11 has been described in at least 5 children and 1 young adult with early B-lineage ALL. The particular interest of this acquired translocation is an apparent association with congenital genetic disorders; among the first six cases described one patient was mentally retarded and of unusual appearance and two patients have had Down syndrome with trisomy 21.[59,60]

t(9;22)(q34;q11)

The truncated chromosome 22, the Philadelphia chromosome, was identified by Nowell & Hungerford in 1960 as the first leukaemia-related chromosomal abnormality.[61] This was later shown to be a reciprocal translocation between chromosomes 9 and 22.[62] Chiefly remarkable for its occurrence in >90% of cases of chronic myeloid leukaemia (CML)[63,64] it also identifies a major subgroup in adult ALL[2,10] and a small but important subgroup in acute myeloid leukaemia and ALL in childhood.[65-67] Ph+ acute and chronic leukaemias are distinct diseases, with different clinical presentations, but Ph+ CML inevitably converts to an acute phase from which Ph+ acute leukaemia is indistinguishable cytogenetically and morphologically. ALL de novo is distinguished from CML acute phase by its response to ALL therapy which may result in both haematological and cytogenetic remission. Patients with acute phase CML respond to treatment by reverting to chronic phase but, in CML, elimination of the Ph clone is achieved only by more innovative treatment such as the use of alpha interferon.[68]

Clonal evolution, change additional to the Ph is found at diagnosis in approximately 60% of children[67] and adults (own data); slightly lower than the 80% seen in CML at blast crisis.[64] Possibly unique to ALL is evolution of the derived chromosomes 9q+[69,70] and 22q−.[10]

The incidence of Ph+ cases in ALL shows a remarkable increase with increasing age. The incidence in childhood ranges from 2.3% to 5%.[3,65-67,71] The median age in one childhood survey was 9.6 years, compared with 4.8 years for other childhood cases.[67] Santana et al reported a lower incidence among 1–9 year olds (3.7%) than among 10–20 year olds (7.0%).[72] The mean age of Ph+ adults is also significantly older than that of Ph− patients. A mean age of 39.7 years for Ph+ and of 28.3 years for Ph− cases (p<0.0001) has been reported with a progressive increase in incidence from 10% at ages 15–20 years to 44% over the age of 50 years.[10] Ph+ cases have higher median leucocyte counts than other childhood cases (33×10^9/l vs 12×10^9/l p= 0.002)[67] but this is not necessarily so in adults.[10] With few exceptions the blast cell immunophenotype is B-precursor with blasts expressing the common ALL antigen CD10; pre-B immunophenotype has been found in 16–25% of those tested for CIg.[10,67] A minority of cases are of T-ALL.[67]

The genetics of t(9;22) (q34;q11) The translocation juxtaposes the oncogene *ABL* normally located at 9q34 with the *BCR* gene at 22q11 to produce a chimeric *BCR/ABL* gene. The breakpoint on 9q34 is between the first and second exons (a1 and a2) of the *ABL* oncogene but the site of the breakpoint in the *BCR* gene at 22q11 differs. In 50–70% of Ph+ acute leukaemias the *BCR* gene breaks between exons 1 and 2 (e1 and e2) (also known as the minor breakpoint cluster region or m-bcr) to form an e1/a2 chimeric gene with a p190 *ABL* related product. In the remaining acute leukaemias and in all cases of CML breakage is between exons 2 (b2) and 3 (b3) or exons 3 and 4(b4) of the major breakpoint cluster region (M-bcr) forming b2/a2 or b3/a2 junctions which both give rise to a p210 *ABL* related product. These mRNAs are both larger than the normal *ABL* product (p145 mRNA) and have markedly enhanced tyrosine kinase activity.[73,74]

The use of molecular techniques to detect Ph+ patients extends cytogenetic analysis to patients in whom metaphase cytogenetics has failed and provides a useful tool with which to monitor the clone in remission. One study using PCR to identify Ph+ in adults with ALL identified 55% Ph+ cases in B-lineage ALL, a higher incidence than has been recorded cytogenetically.[75] Among patients investigated by both techniques, PCR has indicated the presence of the Ph chromosome only in cases where it has been found cytogenetically.[76] PCR investigation of childhood ALL confirmed the low incidence of Ph+ in this age group (1.2%).[40] Failure to detect the mRNA in remission did not necessarily indicate that the clone had been eliminated, suggesting that mRNA may not be expressed in dormant cells which may ultimately lead to relapse.[40]

The commoner breakpoint in childhood and in adults is m-BCR which has been found in 68% of Ph+ cases detected by PCR.[74,75,77] Additional chromosomal change occurs equally in M- and m-bcr cases (own observation). Clinically, the site of the breakpoint appears to have little effect with no difference in the age distribution in adults, or in immunophenotype C-ALL or pre-B ALL. There appears, however, to be an association between high leucocyte counts and M-bcr. Conversion from Ph+ ALL to CML chronic phase has been described, to my knowledge, only in M-BCR cases.[78,79] Heterogeneity of the target cell for chromosomal change has been shown by cell colony and cell separation studies in both m-BCR and M-BCR Ph+ ALL. Approximately half the M-BCR cases and a minority of m-BCR cases[80–82] have been shown to arise in a pluripotent stem cell suggesting affinity with CML. The remaining cases involve only cells of the lymphoid lineage indicative of true ALL.[82,83]

Prognosis for Philadelphia positive ALL is poor. This is particularly marked in childhood series when 90–99% of children achieve remission and >60% of patients are cured. Remission is achieved in 78% to 80% of cases but median event-free survival is only 12–18 months.[67,71] In adults,

L M Secker-Walker

Ph+ cases fare worse than Ph− cases in terms of remission achievement and survival, but in this age group, when overall prognosis is poor, the effect is less marked than in childhood.[10,84,85] The concurrence of partial or total monosomy 7 with t(9;22) appears to signal a particularly poor prognosis.[86] Prognosis is unrelated to the location of the breakpoint M-BCR or m-BCR.[10,82,87] There is, however, a suggestion that event-free survival may be better in cases which arise in a pluripotent stem cell than in cases arising in a lymphoid committed progenitor regardless of breakpoint location.[83] Occasionally long-term survival (>5 years) has been recorded[71,88] but it is unlikely that these patients can be cured by chemotherapy alone. Some measure of success has been achieved with bone marrow transplantation.[67,89]

Translocations in mature-B ALL: t(8;14)(q24;q32); t(2;8)(p12;q24); t(8;22)(q24;q11)

Burkitt-type ALL, FAB type L3, represents an acute leukaemic presentation of Burkitt's lymphoma.[90,91] The three translocations found in Burkitt's lymphoma are also found in mature B-ALL in the ratios 85:8:12, but have never been found in B-precursor ALL.[92] Additional chromosome change is found at diagnosis in more than half the reported cases with a predominance of trisomy 1q and abnormalities of chromosome seven.[92–94]

This subgroup has been described in patients aged 4–65 years, predominantly in males, leucocyte count is low (median 10×10^9/l), blasts express surface immunoglobulin (SIg), but the proportion of L3 blasts may be low. Extramedullary disease is frequent. In adults, an incidence of 5% with t(8;14) or t(8;22) has been reported with median age and sex ratio not significantly different from those without 8q24 abnormalities.[95] In childhood, clinical features are similar to those in adults, but there is a markedly high male /female ratio, and patients are older than those without 8q24 abnormalities.[96] In

Table 2. *Genes involved in B lineage acute lymphoblastic leukaemia*

Chromosomal rearrangement	Genes	
t(1;19)(q23;p13)	PBX1	E2A
t(17;19)(q22;p13)	HLF	E2A
t(4;11)(q21;q23)	ALL1	
t(5;14)(q31;q32)	IL3	IGH
t(2;8)(p12;q24)	IGK	MYC
t(8;14)(q24;q32)	MYC	IGH
t(8;22)(q24;q11)	MYC	IGL
t(9;22)(q34;q11)	ABL	m-BCR/M-BCR
t(11;14)(q13;q32)	BCL1	IGH

Reference[27].

adults and in children, remission rate and median survival compare unfavourably with those lacking 8q24 abnormalities.[95,96]

The translocations have in common a breakpoint at 8q24, site of the oncogene *MYC*, and a second breakpoint at the site of an immunoglobulin chain gene the heavy chain *IGH* at 14q32, or the light chain genes kappa *IGK* at 2p12 or lambda *IGL* at 22q11. The recombination of *MYC* and the *IG* genes appears to represent misrecognition of the *MYC* sequences by a recombinase involved in *IG* gene rearrangement.[97] The result of the translocations is to dysregulate *MYC* expression, bringing about uncontrolled cell proliferation.[98]

Prognosis for this subgroup is extremely poor. Half the cases fail to achieve remission and those that do relapse early. Median survival reported for these cases is <1 year.[2]

Translocations in T-ALL

Translocations in T-ALL frequently involve the sites of the T-cell receptor (*TCR*) genes namely alpha and delta *TCRA* and *TCRD* which map to 14q11–q13 and the beta and gamma chains *TCRB* and *TCRG* at 7q32–36 and 7p15, respectively. The involvement of TCR loci in T-ALL is found in <50% of cases unlike the situation for mature B-ALL which involves the IG loci in the majority of cases.[18] Known translocations are shown in Table 3, indicating the genes at the breakpoints where known.[99–104] Two of these are discussed in more detail.

t(1;14) (p34;q11)

This translocation is found in 3% of T-ALL cases and transposes the *TAL1* gene from 1p34 into the *TCRA/D* chain complex on 14q11. The particular

Table 3. *Genes involved in T lineage acute lymphoblastic leukaemia*

Chromosomal rearrangement	Genes	
t(1;14)(p32;q11)	TAL 1	TCRD
t(7;7)(p15;q11)	TCRG	
t(7;9)(q35–36;q34)	TCRB	
t(7;11)(q35;p13)	TCRB	RBTN2
t(7;19)(q35–36;p13)	TCRB	
t(8;14)(q24;q11)	MYC	TCRA
t(10;14)(q24;q11)	HOX11	TCRD
t(11;14)(p13;q11)	RBTN2	TCRD
t(11;14)(p15;q11)	TTG1	TCRA/D
inv(14)(q11q32)	TCRA	
inv(14)(q11q32)	TCRA	IGH

Reference[27].

interest in this gene and evidence if its involvement in T-cell leukaemogenesis comes from the demonstration that 25% of T-ALL patients exhibit a 90 base pair deletion of one allelle of *TAL1* in the absence of cytogenetic evidence of its rearrangement.[105,106]

t(8;14) (q24;q11)

This translocation brings *TCRA* into juxtaposition with *MYC* and brings about the downregulation of this gene. This mechanism is analogous to that with t(8;14) (q24;q32) in B-cell malignancies in which *C-MYC* is downregulated by the *IGH* gene.[102,107] A survey of 15 childhood cases described as having paediatric leukaemia/lymphoma with this translocation, gave an estimated incidence of 1% of cases. The disease is characterized by male predominance (10/15), a median age of 5.5 years (range 1.8–17 years), high white blood count (median $95 \times 10^9/1$), central nervous system involvement and extramedullary leukaemia. Immunophenotype is commonly T-cell, but at least one patient with B lineage precursor ALL has been described. Prognosis is generally poor with a median event-free survival of 4 months.[102]

Deletion of 6q

Loss of sequences from the long arm of chromosome 6 result from proximal breakpoints between 6q13 and q21 and distal breakpoints at q21 and q23 with common loss of band q21.[108,109] Deletion of 6q is found as the only change in approximately 3% of cases but occurs more frequently with other changes giving an overall incidence of 8% to 13% of childhood cases[2, 13, 16] and 6% of adults (own data). Of particular interest is its association with both T-ALL and C-ALL immunophenotypes in all age groups.[14,17] The data from my laboratory suggest that 6q− is considerably more frequent in T− than in C-ALL (see Table 4). Patients with 6q abnormalities do not differ clinically from those without, neither has any prognostic significance been demonstrated for this abnormality.[109]

Table 4. *Incidence of 6q and 9p abnormalities and of 'normal' cases in C-ALL and T-ALL in adults and children analysed in the cytogenetics laboratory at The Royal Free Hospital*

	C-ALL	T-ALL
Total cases	194	55
	No. (%)	No. (%)
del (6q)	6 (4)	9 (16)
t/del 9p/i9q	9 (5)	5 (9)
Normal	30 (16)	14 (26)

The location of the oncogene *MYB* at 6q22–24, and an observation that cell lines bearing 6q− had elevated levels of c-*MYB* compared to those of non-6q− cell lines at the same stage of development, suggested a role for this oncogene in these cases.[108] However, no rearrangement of the gene itself or of adjoining sequences has been demonstrated.[110]

Deletions and translocations of 9p

Abnormalities of 9p have been described in approximately 13% of ALL cases and are found in both T− and C-ALL. Abnormalities of sequences from 9p21–p22 include loss of sequences by deletion or unbalanced translocation. Abnormalities of 9p were originally described in patients with massive lymphadenopathy, splenomegaly, CNS disease and a high peripheral leucocyte count.[111,112] Loss of 9p also occurs in patients without lymphomatous disease[113–116] but a recent report suggests 9p loss may be twice as common in T-ALL[17] (also see Table 4). The impact of 9p loss on prognosis is unclear.[114,116]

The genes for alpha and beta interferon *INFA* and *INFB* have been mapped to 9p21–9p22. The importance of these genes or a closely linked gene in the aetiology of ALL, and their involvement in cases lacking cytogenetic evidence of 9p involvement, is suggested by the demonstration of hemizygous and less commonly homozygous loss of *INFA* and *INFB* in patients with, and without, apparent 9p loss.[117,118] Two important established changes which result in 9p loss are i(9) (q10q10) and dic(9;12).

Isochromosome 9q

Isochromosome 9q, i(9)(q10) results in the short arms of one homologue of chromosome 9 accompanied by duplication of the long arms.[114] Cases reported range from 3–35 years, WBC from 1.4–250 × 10^9/l and have been seen in cases with blast cell immunophenotypes C−, Pre-B or T-ALL. It is probably more common among childhood than adult cases; there is no evidence that it is associated with a poor prognosis.[119]

dic(9; 12) (p11–13; p11–12)

This translocation occurs in B-precursor ALL with an incidence of <1% in childhood.[46,120–123] A review and update of some 15 published cases with dic(9;12) showed an age range of 3–24 years (median 7 years), WBC 0.8–132 median 8.2 × 10^9/l and an excess of males:females (12:3). These patients appear to have an excellent prognosis, with all 15 patients in continuous remission at 0–93 months with a median follow-up of 57+ months.[122,123]

Deletions and translocations of 12p

An abnormality of 12p has been found in 8% to 10% of childhood ALL[17,44,124,125] and in 5% of adults (own data). Immunophenotypes include

L M Secker-Walker

C-ALL, pre-B, and infrequently T-ALL. No case with hyperdiploidy >50 has been found, and the median leucocyte count (30 × 10⁹/1) is higher than cases lacking these abnormalities. An association of 12p abnormalities with central nervous system relapse has been reported.[14] Abnormalities include deletions, balanced and unbalanced translocations.[115] Of the recurring translocations, dic(7;12)(p11;p12), dic(9;12)(p11–13;p11–12), t(12;13)(p13;q14), t(12;17)(p13;q21) and dic(12;17)(p11;p11–12) few have been studied in detail. The t(12;17) (p13;q21) occurs in childhood early B lineage ALL with an incidence of <0.5%.[125]

Numerical change – ploidy groups (see Table 5)

Hypodiploidy

Hypodiploidy, clonal loss of one or more chromosomes accounts for between 5% and 8% of reported series[3,4,13,14,16,17,18,46,47,126,127] and 9% of adults.[128] There is little consistency in the clinical features of these cases. One survey indicates that it is commoner in C-ALL (10%) than in T-ALL (4%).[126] Prognosis for this group is variable; it has been associated with an excellent prognosis;[14,129] with a prognosis no worse than any other ploidy group except hyperdiploid >50,[127] and with a poor prognosis.[85] These conflicting outcomes confirm the heterogeneity of the hypodiploidy group which include patients with <30 chromosomes (near haploidy) and those with less than and greater than 40 chromosomes[130].

Near-haploidy 23–34 chromosomes

Near-haploidy is marked by the gain from haploidy (23 chromosomes) chiefly of chromosomes 10,14,18,21 and the presence of both sex chromosomes, XX or XY. The reported incidence ranges from 0.7% to 2.4%.[127,131] The oldest reported patient with near haploidy is 19 years. Female predominance has been described in some, but not all, surveys.[130] A median WBC 14 × 10⁹/l and B-precursor ALL further characterize the group.[131] This group has a particularly poor prognosis with median survival of 11 months. Two long-term survivors have been reported; one in first remission at 7 years, the other in second remission at 10 years. A near haploid clone may duplicate to hyperdiploidy.[130–132] The importance of distinguishing true hyperdiploidy from duplicated near-haploidy cannot be over-emphasized in view of the different prognoses for the two groups.

Pseudodiploidy

Pseudodiploidy describes a clone with a 'false' diploid complement of 46 chromosomes. The vast majority of pseudodiploid clones are formed by structural change of one or more chromosomes. In rare cases a pseudodiploid clone arises by gain of one chromosome and loss of another. Pseudodiploidy

Table 5. *Ploidy groups in acute lymphoblastic leukaemia*

Ploidy	Immuno-phenotype	Associated features	Incidence
Near-haploidy 23–30	C-ALL	WBC: 14 × 10⁹/l AGE: <19yrs	0.7%–2.4%
Hypodiploidy 30–45	C-ALL/ (T-ALL)	–	5%–9%
Pseudodiploidy 46R	–	–	C[1]: 40% A[2,3]: 9–11%
Low hyperdiploidy 47–50	–	–	C[1]: 11%–15% A[2]: 8%–11%
High hyperdiploidy >50	C-ALL	WBC: <10 × 10⁹/l Age: C[1]: 2–9 y A[2]: 16 y	C[1]: 16%–27% A[2]: 4%–5%
Triploidy/tetraploidy	T-ALL/ C-ALL	Age: C[1]: 8.6 y	C[1]: 1% A[2]: 7%

[1]= childhood; [2]= adult; [3]= excluding translocation subgroups.

accounts for 10% to 40% of recent childhood series.[3,4,13,16,17,18] In adults classified on a hierarchical system, it occurs in between 9% and 24% of cases[11,128] (see Table 6).

Low hyperdiploidy 47–50 chromosomes

The most frequent gains are of chromosomes 21, X, 8, and 10; structural change is common and includes abnormalities of 1q, 6q 12p and 19p. There is little consistency in the clinical and blast cell findings of this group. The incidence in childhood ranges from 11% to 15%[3,4,17,18,133] and in adults between 8% and 11%[11, 128] (Table 6). The heterogeneous nature of the group is highlighted by a variable prognosis. With short-term follow-up in patients entered to IWCL3, the low hyperdiploid group appeared to be relatively poor risk[2] but after minimum follow-up at 6 years low hyperdiploid cases fared almost as well as those in the high hyperdiploid group.[85] Van der Plas has also shown an outcome as good as that for high hyperdiploidy in children with other good risk features.[14] In contrast, Jackson et al described it as a poor risk group.[18] Prognosis for this group may be improved by contemporary treatment.[133] Trisomy 21 as the sole acquired karyotypic change may be associated with a favourable prognosis.[134] In adults, low hyperdiploidy is relatively good risk.[128]

Table 6. *Established change: incidence in childhood and adult cases of B-lineage ALL analysed in the cytogenetics laboratory at The Royal Free Hospital*

Chromosome category	Adults 140		Children 54	
	Number	%	Number	%
t(1;19)	4	(2.8)	4	(7.4)
der(19)	3	(2.1)	49	(7.4)
del(6q)	6	(4.3)	1	(1.9)
t(4;11)	6	(3.8)	0	(0)
t(9;22)	35	(25.0)	1	(1.9)
del9p/i9q	6	(3.8)	3	(5.5)
11q23	0	(0)	1	(1.9)
t/del(12p)	4	(2.8)	0	(0)
tdic(9;12)	2	(1.4)	1	(1.9)
TT65+	10	(7.2)	0	(0)
51–65	7	(5.0)	19	(35.2)
47–50	13	(9.3)	3	(5.5)
Ps	13	(9.3)	8	(14.8)
<46	7	(5.0)	1	(1.9)
Haploid	1	(0.5)	1	(1.9)
Normal	23	(16.4)	7	(13.0)

High hyperdiploidy 51–65 chromosomes

Chromosomal gain in high hyperdiploidy is nonrandom with an excess gain of chromosomes X, 4, 6, 10, 14, 17, 18 and 21. The incidence in childhood series (16% to 27%)[3,4,13,14,17] is at least 6 times greater than in adults (4%–5%)[11,128] Table 6. This group is associated with other known good risk factors namely age 2–9 years or in adults age <18 years; leucocyte counts <10 × 10^9/l; female sex; C-ALL immunophenotype; FAB type L1. In all surveys reported to date, patients with 51–60 chromosomes have had the best prognosis. Three recent childhood surveys have had an average 5-year event-free survival of 72%.[14, 18, 135] The benefit of hyperdiploidy >50 was emphasized in a recent study of childhood ALL with follow-up of 12–18 years. This showed karyotype and treatment alone to be of prognostic importance with overall survival in patients with >50 chromosomes to be significantly better than that of all other groups.[13] Survival in adults is not as good as in children but is still significantly better than that of other ploidy groups.[128]

Within this good risk subgroup, up to 30% of children succumb to the disease. A small but important group have been shown to suffer a first relapse as late as 5 years from diagnosis.[13] There is evidence that HeH patients enjoy long and possibly lasting second remissions.[29] Nevertheless the early identification of patients who may relapse is clearly of paramount importance.

There is some evidence that, within this subgroup, patients with trisomy 6[18] or with trisomies 4 and 10[22] have the best prognosis. These trisomies are themselves strongly associated with high hyperdiploidy but these reports would repay examination in other series of patients. Possibly more convincingly, two surveys have recently shown an adverse effect of structural change with comparative event-free survival of 82% for patients with numerical change only, and 62% for patients with structural as well as numerical change.[14, 135] It has been observed that children in this subgroup with structural change are older than those without.[17]

One characteristic which distinguishes patients with HeH is their response to the folate antagonist methotrexate (MTX) used in all treatment regimes. Improved survival has been demonstrated in patients whose lymphoblasts have the ability to accumulate high levels of methotrextate and methotrexate polyglutamate in vitro. This ability has been shown to be greatest in lymphoblasts from children with high hyperdiploidy.[136]

Elimination of the leukaemic clone appears to be most effective if the mitotic activity of the blasts is high. Moreover, patients who fail to achieve clinical remission (<5% blasts) after 28 days of treatment have a poorer prognosis than those showing early elimination of the leukaemic cells. Heterogeneity of these two aspects of the leukaemic clone has been examined in children with high hyperdiploidy. Heerema et al, combining metaphase cytogenetics with interphase cytogenetics, using chromosome-specific centromeric probes (FISH), have demonstrated heterogeneity both in the mitotic index of the clone and in the elimination of the clone after 28 days of treatment. This technique will detect approximately 1/1000 clonal cells. The prognostic importance of these findings awaits further investigation.[137]

Triploidy/tetraploidy

Cases with >65 chromosomes represent a minority of cases in ALL with an incidence in childhood of approximately 1%. In this subgroup in children, T-cell immunophenotype was more frequent than C-ALL and the median age was high (8.7 years).[138] Near triploidy/tetraploidy is as common in adults as high hyperdiploidy (7%)[3,128] (Table 6). The prognostic significance in children awaits clarification but, in adults, these patients appear to do almost as well as those with 51–60 chromosomes.

Summary

Cytogenetics of ALL continues to be an important and independent prognostic indicator in spite of continuous adjustments to treatment regimens. There is evidence that new treatment protocols have improved the survival of some chromosomal subgroups but this, and suggestions that differences between chromosomal subgroups may be ironed out by more intensive or innovative treatment regimens, will need to be examined after longer follow-up. An ever-increasing understanding of the genetic consequences of translocations and other chromosmal change is extending the role of metaphase and interphase cytogenetics both in patient management and in increasing our understanding of the biology of the disease. Thus, while the initiating events of leukaemogenesis continue to defy explanation, treatment tailored to, and targeted at the acquired genetic lesion could become a reality in the not too distant future.

References

(1) Secker-Walker LM, Lawler SD, Hardisty RM. Prognostic implications of chromosomal findings in acute lymphoblastic leukaemia at diagnosis. *Br Med J* 1978; 2: 1529–30.

(2) IWCL3. Third International Workshop on Chromosomes in Leukemia (1980): Clinical significance of chromosomal abnormalities in acute lymphoblastic leukemia. *Cancer Genet Cytogenet* 1981; 4: 111–37.

(3) Secker-Walker LM. Prognostic and biological importance of chromosome findings in acute lymphoblastic leukemia. 10th anniversary article. *Cancer Genet Cytogenet* 1990; 49: 1–13.

(4) Pui CH, Crist WM, Look AT. Biology and clinical significance of cytogenetic abnormalities in childhood acute lymphoblastic leukemia. *Blood* 1990; 76: 1449–63.

(5) Rowley JD. Human oncogene locations and chromosome aberrations. *Nature* 1983, 301: 290–1.

(6) Erikson J, Ar Rushdi A, Drwinga HL, Nowell PC, Croce CM. Transcriptional activation of the translocated c-myc oncogene in Burkitt lymphoma. *Proc Natl Acad Sci USA* 1983; 80: 820–4.

(7) Klein G. The role of gene dosage and genetic transpositions in carcinogenesis. *Nature* 1981; 294: 313–8.

(8) Chessells JM. Acute lymphoblastic leukemia. *Semin Hematol* 1982; 19: 155–71.

(9) Secker-Walker, LM, Chessells JM, Stewart EL, Swansbury GJ, Richards S, Lawler SD. Chromosomes and other prognostic factors in acute lymphoblastic leukaemia: a long-term follow-up. *Br J Haematol* 1989; 72: 336–42.

(10) Secker-Walker LM, Craig JM, Hawkins JM, Hoffbrand AV. Philadelphia positive acute lymphoblastic leukemia in adults: age distribution, BCR breakpoint and prognostic significance. *Leukemia* 1991; 5: 196–9.

(11) Walters R, Kantarjian HM, Keating MJ et al. The importance of cytogenetic studies in adult acute lymphocytic leukemia. *Am J Med* 1990; 89: 579–87.

(12) Williams DL, Raimondi S, Rivera G, George S, Berard CW, Murphy SB. Prescence of clonal chromosome abnormalities in virtually all cases of acute lymphoblastic leukemia. *N Engl J Med* 1985; 313: 640–1.

(13) Dastugue N, Robert A, Payen C et al. Prognostic significance of karyotype in a twelve-year follow-up in childhood acute lymphoblastic leukemia. *Cancer Genet Cytogenet* 1992; 64: 49–55.

(14) Van der Plas DC, Hahlen K, Hagemeijer A. Prognostic significance of karyotype at diagnosis in childhood acute lymphoblastic leukemia. *Leukemia* 1992; 6: 176–84.

(15) Fenaux P, Lai JL, Morel P et al. Cytogenetics and their prognostic value in childhood and adult acute lymphoblastic leukemia (ALL) excluding L3. *Hematol Oncol* 1989; 7(4): 307–17.

(16) Crist WM, Carroll AJ, Shuster JJ et al. Poor prognosis of children with pre-B acute lymphoblastic leukemia is associated with the t(1;19)(q23;p13): A Pediatric Oncology Group study. *Blood* 1990; 76: 117–22.

(17) GFCH. Groupe Français de cytogenetique hématologique: Collaborative study of karyotypes in childhood acute lymphoblastic leukemias. *Leukemia* 1993; 7: 10–9.

(18) Jackson JF, Boyett J, Pullen J et al. Favorable prognosis associated with hyperdiploidy in children with acute lymphocytic leukemia correlates with extra chromosome 6. *Cancer* 1990; 66: 1184–9.

(19) Raimondi SC, Behm FG, Roberson PK et al. Cytogenetics of childhood T-cell leukemia. *Blood* 1988; 72: 1560–6.

(20) Pui C-H, Behm FG, Singh B et al. Heterogeneity of presenting features and their relation to treatment outcome in 120 children with T-cell acute lymphoblastic leukemia. *Blood* 1990; 75: 174–9.

(21) Hook EB. Exclusion of chromosomal mosaicism: tables of 90%, 95% and 99% confidence limits and comments on use. *Am J Hum Genet* 1977; 29: 94–7.

(22) Harris MB, Shuster JJ, Carroll A et al. Trisomy of leukemic cell chromosomes 4 and 10 identifies children with B-progenitor cell acute lymphoblastic leukemia with a very low risk of treatment failure: a Pediatric Oncology Group study. *Blood* 1992; 79: 3316–24.

(23) Schiffer CA, Larson RA, Bloomfield CD. Cancer and leukemia group B (CALGB) studies in adult acute lymphocytic leukemia. *Leukemia* 1992; 6: 171–4.

(24) Wodzinski MA, Watmore AE, Lilleyman JS, Potter AM. Chromosomes in childhood acute lymphoblastic leukaemia: karyotypic patterns in disease subtypes. *J Clin Pathol* 1991; 44: 48–51.

(25) Williams DL, Harris A, Williams KJ, Brosius MJ, Lemonds W. A direct bone marrow chromosome technique for acute lymphoblastic leukemia. *Cancer Genet Cytogenet* 1984; 13: 239–57.

(26) Stewart EL, Secker-Walker LM. Detection of the chromosomally abnormal clone in acute lymphoblastic leukemia. *Cancer Genet Cytogenet* 1986; 23: 25–35.

(27) Hawkins JM, Secker-Walker LM. Evaluation of cytogenetic samples and pertinent technical variables in adult acute lymphocytic leukemia. *Cancer Genet Cytogenet* 1991; 52: 79–84.

(28) Mitelman F, Kaneko Y, Trent J. Report of the committee on chromosome changes in neoplasia, Human Gene Mapping 11 (1991). *Cytogenet Cell Genet* 1991; 58: 1053–79.

(29) Secker-Walker LM. The prognostic implications of chromosomal findings in acute lymphoblastic leukemia. *Cancer Genet Cytogenet* 1984; 11: 233–48.

(30) Shikano T, Kaneko Y, Takazawa M, Ueno N, Ohkawa M, Fujimoto T. Balanced and unbalanced 1;19 translocation-associated acute lymphoblastic leukemias. *Cancer* 1986; 58: 2239–43.

(31) Michael PM, Levin MD, Garson OM. Translocation 1; 19 – a new cytogenetic abnormality in acute lymphocytic leukemia. *Cancer Genet Cytogenet* 1984; 12: 333–41.

(32) Carroll AJ, Crist WM, Parmley RT, Roper M, Cooper MD, Finley WH. Pre-B cell leukemia associated with chromosome translocation 1; 19. *Blood* 1984; 63: 721–4.

(33) Williams DL, Look AT, Melvin SL et al. New chromosomal translocations correlate with specific immunophenotypes of childhood acute lymphoblastic leukemia. *Cell* 1984; 36: 101–9.

(34) Secker-Walker LM, Berger R, Fenaux P et al. Prognostic significance of the balanced t(1;19) and unbalanced der(19)t(1;19) translocations in acute lymphoblastic leukemia. *Leukemia* 1992; 6: 363–9.

(35) Raimondi SC, Behm FG, Roberson PK et al. Cytogenetics of pre-B-cell acute lymphoblastic leukemia with emphasis on prognostic implications of the t(1;19). *J Clin Oncol* 1990; 8: 1380–8.

(36) Raimondi S, Roberson P, Behm FG, Pui C-H, Crist WM, Rivera GK. Clinical significance of the t(1;19) (q23;p13) in childhood acute lymphoblastic leukemia. *Proc Am Assoc Cancer Res* 1990; 31: 26.

(37) Nourse J, Mellentin JD, Galili N et al. Chromosomal translocation t(1;19) results in synthesis of a homeobox fusion mRNA that codes for a potential chimeric transcription factor. *Cell* 1990; 60: 535–45.

(38) Hunger SP, Galili N, Carroll AJ, Crist WM, Link MP, Cleary ML. The t(1;19) (q23;p13) results in consistent fusion of E2A and PBX1 coding sequences in acute lymphoblastic leukemias. *Blood* 1991; 77: 687–93.

(39) Mellentin JD, Murre C, Donlon TA et al. The gene for enhancer binding proteins E12/E47 lies at the t(1;19) breakpoint in acute leukemias. *Science* 1989; 246: 379–82.

(40) Izraeli S, Janssen JWG, Haas OA et al. Detection and clinical relevance of genetic abnormalities in pediatric acute lymphoblastic leukemia: a comparison between cytogenetic and polymerase chain reaction analyses. *Leukemia* 1993; 7: 671–8.

(41) Lai JL, Fenaux P, Estienne MH et al. Translocation t(1;19) (q23;p13) in acute lymphoblastic leukemia. A report on six new cases and an unusual t(17;19) (q11;q13), with special reference to prognostic factors. *Cancer Genet Cytogenet* 1989; 37: 9–17.

(42) Hunger SP, Ohyashiki K, Toyama K, Cleary ML. Hlf, a novel hepatic bZIP protein, shows altered DNA-binding properties following fusion to E2A in t(17;19) acute lymphoblastic leukemia. *Genes & Development* 1992; 6: 1608–20.

(43) Yamada T, Craig JM, Hawkins JM, Janossy G, Secker-Walker LM. Molecular investigation of 19p13 in standard and variant translocations: the E12 probe recognizes the 19p13 breakpoint in cases with t(1;19) and acute leukemia other than pre-B immunophenotype. *Leukemia* 1991; 5: 36–40.

(44) Raimondi SC, Privitera E, Williams DL et al. New recurring chromosomal translocations in childhood acute lymphoblastic leukemia. *Blood* 1991; 77: 2016–22.

(45) Mirro J, Kitchingman G, Williams D et al. Clinical and laboratory characteristics of acute leukemia with the 4;11 translocation. *Blood* 1986; 67: 689–97.

(46) Secker-Walker LM, Stewart EL, Chan L, O'Callaghan U, Chessells JM. The (4;11) translocation in acute leukaemia of childhood: the importance of additional chromosomal aberrations. *Br J Haematol* 1985; 61: 101–11.

(47) Prigogina EL, Puchkova GP, Mayakova SA. Nonrandom chromosomal abnormalities in acute lymphoblastic leukemia of childhood. *Cancer Genet Cytogenet* 1988; 32: 183–203.

(48) Hagemeijer A, van Dongen JJ, Slater RM et al. Characterization of the blast cells in acute leukemia with translocation (4;11): report of eight additional cases and of one case with a variant translocation. *Leukemia* 1987; 1:24–31.

(49) Pui C-H, Frankel LS, Carroll AJ et al. Clinical characteristics and treatment outcome of childhood acute lymphoblastic leukemia with t(4;11)(q21;q23): a collaborative study of 40 cases. *Blood* 1991; 77:440–7.

(50) Gu Y, Nakamura T, Alder H et al. The t(4;11) chromosome translocation of human acute leukemias fuses the ALL-1 gene, related to *Drosophila trithorax*, to the AF-4 gene. *Cell* 1992; 71:701–8.

(51) Djabali M, Selleri L, Parry P, Bower M, Young BD, Evans GA. A trithorax-like gene is interrupted by chromosome 11q23 translocations in acute leukaemias. *Nature Genet* 1992; 2:113–8.

(52) Tkachuk DC, Kohler S, Cleary ML. Involvement of a homolog of *Drosophila trithorax* by 11q23 chromosomal translocations in acute leukemias. *Cell* 1992; 71:691–700.

(53) Brizard A, Tanzer J, Huret JL. Prognosis in children with the t(4;11)(q21;q23) acute leukemia. *Blood* 1991; 78:2471–3.

(54) Secker-Walker LM, Stewart EL, Todd A. Acute lymphoblastic leukaemia with t(4;11) follows neuroblastoma: a late effect of treatment? *Med Pediatr Oncol* 1985; 13:48–50.

(55) Auxenfants E, Morel P, Lai JL et al. Secondary acute lymphoblastic leukemia with t(4;11): report on two cases and review of the literature. *Ann Hematol* 1992; 65(3):143–6.

(56) Lennard A, Jackson GH, Carey PJ, Bown N, Middleton P, Proctor SJ. Secondary acute lymphoblastic leukaemia with 4:11 translocation following treatment for Hodgkin's disease: case report and review of the literature. *Leukemia* 1991; 5:624–7.

(57) Morgan GJ, Cotter F, Katz FE et al. Breakpoints at 11q23 in infant leukemias with the t(11;19)(q23;p13) are clustered. *Blood* 1992; 80:2172–5.

(58) Huret JL, Brizard A, Slater R et al. Cytogenetic heterogeneity in t(11;19) acute leukemia: clinical, hematological and cytogenetic analyses of 48 patients – updated published cases and 16 new observations. [Review]. *Leukemia* 1993; 7:152–60.

(59) Kardon NB, Slepowitz G, Kochen JA. Childhood acute lymphoblastic leukemia associated with an unusual 8;14 translocation. *Cancer Genet Cytogenet* 1982; 6: 339–43.

(60) Secker-Walker LM, Hawkins JM, Prentice HG, Mackie PH, Heerema NA, Provisor AJ. Two Down syndrome patients with an acquired translocation, t(8;14)(q11;q32), in early B-lineage acute lymphoblastic leukemia. *Cancer Genet Cytogenet* 1993; 70: 148–50.

(61) Nowell PC, Hungerford DA. A minute chromosome in human granulocytic leukemia. *Science* 1960; 132: 1497.

(62) Rowley JD. Letter: A new consistent chromosomal abnormality in chronic myelogenous leukaemia identified by quinacrine fluorescence and Giemsa staining. *Nature* 1973; 243: 290–3.

(63) Richman CM, Rowley JD, Golomb HM. Chronic granulocytic leukemia: epidemiology and etiology, pathogenesis, cytogenetics, in vitro studies and clinical features. In: Goldman JM, Preisler HD, eds. *Hematology leukemias*. London: Butterworths International Medical Reviews, 1984: 208–224.

(64) Hagemeijer A. Chromosome abnormalities in chronic myeloid leukemia. *Baillières Clin Haematol* 1987; 1: 963–81.

(65) Secker-Walker LM, Summersgill BM, Swansbury GJ, Lawler SD, Chessells JM, Hardisty RM. Philadelphia-positive blast crisis masquerading as acute lymphoblastic leukaemia in children. *Lancet* 1976; 2: 1405.

(66) Ribeiro RC, Abromowitch M, Raimondi SC, Murphy SB, Behm F, Williams DL. Clinical and biologic hallmarks of the Philadelphia chromosome in childhood acute lymphoblastic leukemia. *Blood* 1987; 70: 948–53.

(67) Crist W, Carroll A, Shuster J et al. Philadelphia chromosome positive childhood acute lymphoblastic leukemia: clinical and cytogenetic characteristics and treatment outcome. A Pediatric Oncology Group study. *Blood* 1990; 76: 489–94.

(68) Catovsky D. Ph1-positive acute leukaemia and chronic granulocytic leukaemia: one or two diseases? *Br J Haematol* 1979; 42: 493–8.

(69) Sessarego M, Defferrari R, Fugazza G, Comelli A, Salvidio E, Ajmar F. Involvement of the short arm of the derivative chromosome 9 in Philadelphia-positive acute lymphoblastic leukemia. *Cancer Genet Cytogenet* 1991; 52: 43–9.

(70) Rieder H, Fonatsch C, Freund M. Abnormalities of the short arm of chromosome 9. A nonrandom secondary aberration in Philadelphia chromosome-positive acute lymphoblastic leukemia (ALL). *Cancer Genet Cytogenet* 1991; 53: 139–42.

(71) Fletcher JA, Tu N, Tantravahi R, Sallan SE. Extremely poor prognosis of pediatric acute lymphoblastic leukemia with translocation (9;22): updated experience. *Leuk Lymphoma* 1992; 8: 75–79.

(72) Santana VM, Dodge RK, Crist WM et al. Presenting features and treatment outcome of adolescents with acute lymphoblastic leukemia. *Leukemia* 1990;4: 87–90.

(73) Kurzrock R, Talpaz M. The genetics of the Philadelphia chromosome. In: Burnett A, Newland A, Keating A, eds. *Haematological oncology*, Volume 1. Cambridge University Press, 1991:79–110.

(74) Berger R, Chen SJ, Chen Z. Philadelphia-positive acute leukaemia. Cytogenetic and molecular aspects. *Cancer Genet Cytogenet* 1990;44:143–52.

(75) Maurer J, Janssen JW, Thiel E et al. Detection of chimeric BCR-ABL genes in acute lymphoblastic leukaemia by the polymerase chain reaction. *Lancet* 1991;337:1055–8.

(76) Janssen JW, Fonatsch C, Ludwig WD, Rieder H, Maurer J, Bartram CR. Polymerase chain reaction analysis of BCR-ABL sequences in adult Philadelphia chromosome-negative acute lymphoblastic leukemia patients. *Leukemia* 1992;6:463–4.

(77) Westbrook CA, Stock W. Clinical and molecular aspects of Philadelphia chromosome positive acute lymphoblastic leukemia. In: Keating A, ed. *Haematological oncology*, Vol. 2. Cambridge, England: Cambridge University Press, 1992: 157–68.

(78) Secker-Walker LM, Cooke HM, Browett PJ et al. Variable Philadelphia breakpoints and potential lineage restriction of bcr rearrangement in acute lymphoblastic leukemia. *Blood* 1988;72:784–91.

(79) Kalousek DK, Dube ID, Eaves CJ, Eaves AC. Cytogenetic studies of haemopoietic colonies from patients with an initial diagnosis of acute lymphoblastic leukaemia. *Br J Haematol* 1988;70:5–11.

(80) Jackson GH, Middleton P, Prince R, Bown N, Kernahan J, Reid MM. Philadelphia positive acute leukaemia with minor breakpoint cluster rearrangement may be a stem cell disease. *Br J Haematol* 1992;81:77–80.

(81) Sadamura S, Umemura T, Hirata J et al. P190-type bcr/abl expressed in myeloid colonies in a patient with Phl-positive acute lymphoblastic leukemia. *Leukemia* 1992;6:791–5.

(82) Tien HF, Wang CH, Chuang SM et al. Characterization of Philadelphia-chromosome-positive acute leukemia by clinical, immunocytochemical, and gene analysis. *Leukemia* 1992; 6: 907–14.

(83) Secker-Walker LM, Craig JM. Prognostic implications of breakpoint and lineage heterogeneity in Philadelphia-positive acute lymphoblastic leukemia: a review. *Leukemia* 1993; 7: 147–51.

(84) Gotz G, Weh HJ, Walter TA et al. Clinical and prognostic significance of the Philadelphia chromosome in adult patients with acute lymphoblastic leukemia. *Ann Hemat* 1992; 64: 97–100.

(85) Bloomfield CD, Secker-Walker LM, Goldman AI et al. Six-year follow-up of the clinical significance of karyotype in acute lymphoblastic leukemia. From the Sixth International Workshop on Chromosomes in Leukemia 1987. *Cancer Genet Cytogenet* 1989; 40: 171–85.

(86) Russo C, Carroll A, Kohler S et al. Philadelphia chromosome and monosomy 7 in childhood acute lymphoblastic leukemia: a Pediatric Oncology Group study. *Blood* 1991; 77: 1050–6.

(87) Lin M-T, Tien H-F, Wang Y-C, Lin D-T, Lin K-H. bcr rearrangements in Philadelphia chromosome-positive acute lymphoblastic leukemia. A study of five Chinese patients in Taiwan. *Cancer Genet Cytogenet* 1990; 47: 29–39.

(88) Fisher TC, Patil SR, Edwards R, Gingrich RD, Burns CP. Cytogenetic analysis of adult acute lymphoblastic leukemia including a Ph+ case surviving more than 5 years. *Cancer Genet Cytogenet* 1986; 23: 245–51.

(89) Barrett AJ, Horowitz MM, Ash RC et al. Bone marrow transplantation for Philadelphia chromosome-positive acute lymphoblastic leukemia. *Blood* 1992; 79: 3067–70.

(90) Berger R, Bernheim A, Brouet JC, Daniel MT, Flandrin G. t(8;14) translocation in a Burkitt's type of lymphoblastic leukaemia (L3). *Br J Haematol* 1979; 43: 87–90.

(91) Mitelman F, Andersson Anvret M, Brandt L et al. Reciprocal 8;14 translocation in EBV-negative B-cell acute lymphocytic leukemia with Burkitt-type cells. *Int J Cancer* 1979; 24: 27–33.

(92) Berger R, Bernheim A. Cytogenetic studies on Burkitt's lymphoma-leukemia. *Cancer Genet Cytogenet* 1982; 7: 231–44.

(93) Knuutila S, Elonen E, Heinonen K et al. Chromosome abnormalities in 16 Finnish patients with Burkitt's lymphoma or L3 acute lymphocytic leukemia. *Cancer Genet Cytogenet* 1984; 13: 139–51.

(94) Secker-Walker LM, Stewart E, Norton J et al. Multiple chromosome abnormalities in a drug resistant TdT positive B-cell leukemia. *Leukemia Res* 1987; 11: 155–61.

(95) Davey FR, Lawrence D, MacCallum J et al. Morphologic characteristics of acute lymphoblastic leukemia (ALL) with abnormalities of chromosome 8, band q24. *Am J Hematol* 1992; 40: 183–91.

(96) Rosanda C, Cantu Rajnoldi A, Invernizzi R et al. B-cell acute lymphoblastic leukemia (B-ALL): a report of 17 pediatric cases. *Haematologica* 1992; 77: 151–5.

(97) Haluska FG, Finver S, Tsujimoto Y, Croce CM. The t(8;14) chromosomal translocation occurring in B-cell malignancies results from mistakes in V–D–J joining. *Nature* 1986; 324: 158.

(98) Croce CM, Nowell PC. Molecular basis of human B cell neoplasia. *Blood* 1985; 65: 1–7.

(99) Xia Y, Brown L, Tsan JT et al. The translocation (1;14) (p34;q11) in human T-cell leukemia: chromosome breakage 25 kilobase pairs downstream of the TAL1 protooncogene. *Genes Chromosom Cancer* 1992; 4: 211–6.

(100) Raimondi SC, Pui CH, Behm FG, Williams DL. 7q32–q36 translocations in childhood T cell leukemia: cytogenetic evidence for involvement of the T cell receptor beta-chain gene. *Blood* 1987; 69: 131–4.

(101) Kaneko Y, Maseki N, Homma C et al. Chromosome translocations involving band 7q35 or 7p15 in childhood T-cell leukemia/lymphoma. *Blood* 1988; 72: 534–8.

(102) Lange BJ, Raimondi SC, Heerema N et al. Pediatric leukemia/lymphoma with t(8;14) (q24;q11). *Leukemia* 1992; 6: 613–8.

(103) Dube ID, Kamel-Reid S, Yuan CC et al. A novel human homeobox gene lies at the chromosome 10 breakpoint in lymphoid neoplasias with chromosomal translocation t(10;14). *Blood* 1991; 78(11): 2996–3003.

(104) Foroni L, Boehm T, Lampert F, Kaneko Y, Raimondi S, Rabbitts TH. Multiple methylation-free islands flank a small breakpoint cluster region on 11p13 in the t(11;14)(p13;q11) translocation. *Genes Chromosom Cancer* 1990;1:301.

(105) Brown L, Cheng J-T, Chen Q et al. Site-specific recombination of the tal-1 gene is a common occurrence in human T cell leukemia. *EMBO J* 1990;9: 3343–51.

(106) Carroll AJ, Crist WM, Link MP et al. The t(1;14) (p34;q11) is nonrandom and restricted to T-cell acute lymphoblastic leukemia: A pediatric oncology group study. *Blood* 1990;76:1220–4.

(107) Finger LR, Harvey RC, Moore RC, Showe LC, Croce CM. A common mechanism of chromosomal translocation in T- and B-cell neoplasia. *Science* 1986;234:982–85.

(108) Barletta C, Pelicci PG, Kenyon LC, Smith SD, Dalla Favera R. Relationship between the c-myb locus and the 6q-chromosomal aberration in leukemias and lymphomas. *Science* 1987;235:1064–7.

(109) Hayashi Y, Raimondi SC, Look AT et al. Abnormalities of the long arm of chromosome 6 in childhood acute lymphoblastic leukemia. *Blood* 1990;76: 1626–30.

(110) Park JG, Reddy EP. Large-scale molecular mapping of human c-myb locus: c-myb proto-oncogene is not involved in 6q-abnormalities of lymphoid tumors. *Oncogene* 1992;7:1603–9.

(111) Kowalczyk JR, Grossi M, Sandberg AA. Cytogenetic findings in childhood acute lymphoblastic leukemia. *Cancer Genet Cytogenet* 1985;15:47–64.

(112) Chilcote RR, Brown E, Rowley JD. Lymphoblastic leukemia with lymphomatous features associated with abnormalities of the short arm of chromosome 9. *N Engl J Med* 1985;313:286–91.

(113) Carroll AJ, Castleberry RP, Crist WM. Lack of association between abnormalities of the chromosome 9 short arm and either 'lymphomatous' features or T cell phenotype in childhood acute lymphocytic leukemia. *Blood* 1987;69: 735–8.

(114) Pollak C, Hagemeijer A. Abnormalities of the short arm of chromosome 9 with partial loss of material in hematological disorders. *Leukemia* 1987;1:541–8.

(115) UKCCG. United Kingdom Cancer Cytogenetics Group. Translocations involving 9p and/or 12p in acute lymphoblastic leukemia. *Genes Chromosom Cancer* 1992;5:255–9.

(116) Murphy SB, Raimondi SC, Rivera GK et al. Nonrandom abnormalities of chromosome 9p in childhood acute lymphoblastic leukemia: association with high-risk clinical features. *Blood* 1989;74:409–15.

(117) Diaz MO, Rubin CM, Harden A et al. Deletions of interferon genes in acute lymphoblastic leukemia. *N Engl J Med* 1990; 322: 77–82.

(118) Middleton PG, Prince RA, Williamson IK et al. Alpha interferon gene deletions in adults, children and infants with acute lymphoblastic leukemia. *Leukemia* 1991; 5: 680–2.

(119) Shippey CA, Lawlor E, Secker-Walker LM. Isochromosome 9q in acute lymphoblastic leukemia: a new non-random finding. *Leukemia* 1989; 3: 195–9.

(120) Carroll AJ, Raimondi SC, Williams DL et al. tdic(9;12): a nonrandom chromosome abnormality in childhood B-cell precursor acute lymphoblastic leukemia: a Pediatric Oncology Group Study. *Blood* 1987; 70: 1962–5.

(121) Secker-Walker LM, Shippey CA, Hoffbrand AV, Williams AT, Shey SA. Two breakpoints on 9p in translocation-dicentric chromosomes in B-lineage acute lymphoblastic leukemia. *Cytogenet Cell Genet* 1989; 51: 1076.

(122) Mahmoud H, Carroll AJ, Behm F et al. The non-random dic(9;12) translocation in acute lymphoblastic leukemia is associated with B-progenitor phenotype and an excellent prognosis. *Leukemia* 1992; 6: 703–7.

(123) Huret JL, Heerema NA, Brizard A et al. Two additional cases of tdic(9;12) in acute lymphocytic leukemia (ALL): prognosis in ALL with dic(9;12). *Leukemia* 1990; 4: 423–5.

(124) Raimondi SC, Williams DL, Callihan T, Peiper S, Rivera GK, Murphy SB. Nonrandom involvement of the 12p12 breakpoint in chromosome abnormalities of childhood acute lymphoblastic leukemia. *Blood* 1986; 68: 69–75.

(125) Krance RA, Raimondi SC, Dubowy R et al. t(12;17)(p13;q21) in early pre-B acute lymphoid leukemia. *Leukemia* 1992; 6: 251–5.

(126) Uckun FM, Gajl Peczalska KJ, Provisor AJ, Heerema NA. Immunophenotype-karyotype associations in human acute lymphoblastic leukemia. *Blood* 1989; 73: 271–80.

(127) Pui CH, Williams DL, Raimondi SC et al. Hypodiploidy is associated with a poor prognosis in childhood acute lymphoblastic leukemia. *Blood* 1987; 70: 247–53.

(128) Secker-Walker LM, Hawkins JM, Janossy G, Hoffbrand AV. Independent prognostic significance of karyotype in adults with acute lymphoblastic leukemia and an increase in poor risk chromosome features with advancing age at diagnosis. *Blood* 1990; 76: 319a.

(129) Secker-Walker LM, Swansbury GJ, Hardisty RM et al. Cytogenetics of acute lymphoblastic leukaemia in children as a factor in the prediction of long-term survival. *Br J Haematol* 1982; 52:389–99.

(130) Callen DF, Raphael K, Michael PM, Garson OM. Acute lymphoblastic leukemia with a hypodiploid karyotype with less than 40 chromosomes: the basis for division into two subgroups. *Leukemia* 1989; 3:749–52.

(131) Gibbons B, MacCallum P, Watts E et al. Near haploid acute lymphoblastic leukemia: seven new cases and a review of the literature. *Leukemia* 1991; 5:738–43.

(132) Onodera N, McCabe NR, Nachman JB et al. Hyperdiploidy arising from near-haploidy in childhood acute lymphoblastic leukemia. *Genes Chromosom Cancer* 1992; 4:331–6.

(133) Raimondi SC, Roberson PK, Pui CH, Behm FG, Rivera GK. Hyperdiploid (47–50) acute lymphoblastic leukemia in children. *Blood* 1992; 79:3245–52.

(134) Raimondi SC, Pui CH, Head D et al. Trisomy 21 as the sole acquired chromosomal abnormality in children with acute lymphoblastic leukemia. *Leukemia* 1992; 6(3):171–5.

(135) Pui CH, Raimondi SC, Dodge RK et al. Prognostic importance of structural chromosomal abnormalities in children with hyperdiploid (greater than 50 chromosomes) acute lymphoblastic leukemia. *Blood* 1989; 73:1963–67.

(136) Whitehead VM, Vuchich MJ, Lauer SJ et al. Accumulation of high levels of methotrexate polyglutamates in lymphoblasts from children with hyperdiploid (greater than 50 chromosomes) B-lineage acute lymphoblastic leukemia: a Pediatric Oncology Group study. *Blood* 1992; 80:1316–23.

(137) Heerema NA, Argyropoulos G, Weetman R, Tricot G, Secker-Walker LM. Interphase in situ hybridization reveals minimum residual disease in early remission and return of the diagnostic clone in karyotypically normal relapse of the acute lymphoblastic leukemia. *Leukemia* 1993; 7:537–43.

(138) Pui C-H, Carroll AJ, Head D et al. Near-triploid and near-tetraploid acute lymphoblastic leukemia of childhood. *Blood* 1990; 76:590.

Fungal infections

T R ROGERS

Introduction

Infection has long been recognized to be a major complication of the treatment of haematological malignancies, with a high attributable mortality.[1] The nature of the underlying disease, as well as the intensity of immunosuppression induced by treatment, determine in large part the types, incidence and severity of opportunistic infection encountered. Over the past decade there has been a noticeable change in the pattern of infectious complications, perhaps brought about by the availability of potent antibacterial agents, such as newer cephalosporins and quinolones, which have dramatically reduced the likelihood of fatal bacterial sepsis. The net effect of this is that more intensive immunosuppression is feasible, but as a consequence, patients are subjected to more prolonged periods of profound immunodeficiency. This development has coincided with the emergence of fungi as opportunistic pathogens.[2] There is little doubt that this is a cause and effect relationship, although a heightened awareness of the risk of fungal infection on the part of haematologists, microbiologists and infectious disease physicians may also be relevant.

Incidence and risk factors

The underlying disease has a bearing on the incidence of opportunistic fungal infections, for instance, they are more common in leukaemia than in lymphoma or solid tumours with a reported incidence of 7.9%, 3.9% and 4.1%, respectively.[3] Bodey estimated that, at MD Anderson Hospital, fungi accounted for 20 to 30% of fatal infections in leukaemic patients, compared to 10 to 15% in lymphoma patients and 5% in solid tumour cases.[4]

The T-cell immunodeficiency associated with lymphoma or steroid use predisposes to candidosis and cryptococcosis. Infections with *Aspergillus* are

All correspondence to: Dr T R Rogers, Department of Infectious Diseases and Bacteriology, Royal Postgraduate Medical School, Hammersmith Hospital, Ducane Road, London W12 ONN, UK.

Cambridge Medical Reviews: Haematological Oncology Volume 3

also described in patients who are chronically immunosuppressed including those being treated for chronic graft versus host disease (GVHD) after bone marrow transplantation (BMT). The principal risk factors are summarized in Table 1.

Profound neutropenia ($<0.1 \times 10^9$/l) is the dominant risk factor for fungal infection in leukaemic patients, especially when this state persists for 3 weeks or longer during the course of remission induction treatment[5] (RIT) or BMT.[6]

Analyses of factors related to invasive mycoses with, eg *Candida*[7] and *Aspergillus*[8] point to the contributory role of broad spectrum antibiotics, which facilitate colonization of the skin and mucosal surfaces of the gastrointestinal and respiratory tracts including the sinuses. Damage to mucosal integrity by viruses such as cytomegalovirus or herpes simplex virus allows local invasion with the risk of bloodstream dissemination. Indwelling vascular or urinary catheters may also provide portals of entry for fungal pathogens.[9] Parenteral nutrition is particularly associated with yeast fungaemia, or rarely infection with *Malassezia furfur*.[10] Diabetes mellitus increases susceptibility to yeast infection and also mucormycosis. Unusually, marijuana and heroin abuse have been incriminated as the source of *Aspergillus* that resulted in rhinocerebral infection.[11]

Fungal pathogens: ecology and epidemiology

Although several different species of *Candida* have been found to cause infections in leukaemia and lymphoma patients,[12] by far the most frequently documented and characterized of these is *C. albicans*. Next in frequency is *C. tropicalis*. Both species are normal constituents of the resident bowel flora. Overgrowth progressing to local infection or thrush is therefore usually an infection of endogenous origin. There is evidence that local invasion in the bowel follows a process of translocation of yeasts across the mucosal barrier which is brought about by prior removal of the resident bacterial flora. Occa-

Table 1. *Risk factors for systemic fungal infections*

Prolonged, profound neutropenia
T-cell immunodeficiency
Diabetes mellitus
Corticosteroids
Broad-spectrum antibiotics
Indwelling vascular lines
Parenteral nutrition
Cytomegalovirus/herpes simplex virus infection
Hospital building/maintenance work
Marijuana/heroin abuse

sional clustering of cases of candidosis on high risk units suggests that certain *Candida* strains have the potential to cause outbreaks as a consequence of cross-infection. In the past few years there has been a noticeable increase in frequency of infections due to non-albicans *Candida* species.[13] Most important are *C. krusei* and *C. glabrata* which, by virtue of their inherent drug resistance, have probably been selected out as a result of increased azole use.[14] A recent report of an outbreak of *C. krusei* infection on a BMT unit where fluconazole was extensively used, highlights the capacity of this species to cause nosocomial infections under suitable conditions.[15] Of other yeasts reported in the setting of leukaemia therapy, *Trichosporon* spp. are best recognized,[16] although this is a relatively uncommon pathogen. It typically causes infections that are mistakenly diagnosed as candidosis due to the similar pattern of clinical presentation. It is unresponsive to amphotericin B therapy.

Aspergillus fumigatus and *A. flavus* are the species most often responsible for aspergillosis[17] although others are occasionally encountered.[18] These organisms are widely distributed in the environment and fungal spore counts can vary considerably according to seasonal factors, the activity of staff on the ward who may shed spores from their clothes, and local building work.[19] Several major outbreaks of aspergillosis have been associated with demolition of walls, maintenance work, and faulty air conditioning on BMT units.[20–22]

Mucor,[23] *Fusarium*[24] and *Cryptococcus*[25] are also environmental organisms which are usually acquired by inhalation, as are some of the rarer fungal pathogens (Table 2). *Histoplasma*, *Blastomyces* and *Coccidioides* are encountered as opportunistic pathogens typically in patients who have lived or travelled to endemic areas which include the mid West and west coast of the United States, Central and South America, the Middle East and Africa.[26]

Antifungal drugs
Amphotericin B (AMB), a polyene antibiotic, inhibits fungal growth by binding to ergosterol, with consequent disruption of the cell membrane permeability barrier. It has fungicidal action in vitro but this is difficult to demonstrate in vivo. It has a broad spectrum of antifungal activity[27], which includes most *Candida* spp., *Aspergillus* spp. and *Cryptococcus neoformans*, and is widely viewed as the 'gold standard' of therapy against which all new agents must be compared. Primary or inherent resistance to AMB is rare, with the exception of *Candida lusitaniae* and *Pseudoallescheria boydii*, but resistance developing during treatment occasionally does occur.[28]

There is minimal absorption of the drug following oral administration and it has to be given parenterally for treatment of systemic infection in a single daily dose of up to 1 mg/kg. Drug concentrations are highest in the lungs, kidneys and hepatosplenic tissues, while penetration of the central nervous system (CNS) is less good. The total quantity of AMB given in a course of treatment should generally not exceed 2–3 g because of cumulative toxicity,

Table 2. *Opportunistic fungi and associated infections in leukaemia and lymphoma patients*

Fungi	Associated clinical features
Frequent:	
Candida spp.	Candidaemia, septic skin lesions, pneumonia, hepatic, brain abscesses
Aspergillus spp.	Pneumonia, with cavitation, haemorrhagic skin lesions, brain, renal abscesses, endocarditis
Infrequent:	
Cryptococcus neoformans	Meningitis of insidious onset, fungaemia, skin, brain abscesses
Mucor	Palatal eschar, with sinus, brain, eye invasion
Fusarium	Pulmonary and skin lesions mimicking aspergillosis
Rare:	
Trichosporon	Fungaemia, skin lesions mimicking candidosis.
Pseudoallescheria	Pulmonary, brain, skin lesions mimicking aspergillosis
Paecilomyces	Endophthalmitis
Alternaria *Curvularia*	Nasal septum lesions
Histoplasma *Blastomyces* *Coccidioides*	Pulmonary infiltrates, skin, bone lesions
Malessezia furfur	Fungaemia, mycotic thrombi, endocarditis

probably explained by the long half-life. The duration of treatment in established infection is generally 6 to 8 weeks. On first administration, a test dose of 1 mg should be given over 30 to 60 minutes and, if tolerated, the full dose can then be given in the same infusion. Current evidence suggests that this is as safe as the previous approach of using a dose escalation regimen over several days.[29] Acute side-effects include fever, rigors, less commonly cardiac arrythmias and rarely anaphylaxis. Febrile reactions accompanying infusions can be suppressed by co-administration of iv hydrocortisone. The most frequently encountered toxicity due to AMB is renal impairment, which may be complicated by hypokalaemia and hypomagnesaemia specifically related to renal tubular damage. Amiloride at a dose of 10–20 mg/day may help to prevent the tubular loss of potassium. When there are concerns about renal toxicity, because of rising serum creatinine levels, the daily dose should be halved or the dosing interval increased to alternate days. If there is insufficient clinical evidence to support its further use, the drug should be stopped.

Although renal function may improve, permanent nephrotoxicity can result.

There is no indication for measuring serum AMB levels during therapy because they do not correlate with renal toxicity. Where toxicity precludes the use of AMB therapy, despite a need to continue treatment, liposomal AMB (AmBisome) is justified, despite its expense. Daily doses of up to 3 mg/kg have been well tolerated[30] with apparently equivalent efficacy and minimal nephrotoxicity compared with conventional AMB. The reason why it is less nephrotoxic is unclear, as is its precise mode of action. Peak serum concentrations are up to 10-fold those of conventional AMB, but its half-life is considerably shorter. Tissue concentrations are also different to those found with conventional AMB; higher concentrations are obtained in the liver and spleen compared to the lungs, kidneys and CNS. Liposomal AMB may also be the preferred choice in patients with a history of earlier AMB toxicity who require a further course of treatment.

Fluconazole is a new synthetic bis triazole whose development represents an important breakthrough in antifungal therapy. It is fungistatic by virtue of inhibition of a critical step in ergosterol synthesis, the target being fungal cytochrome p450. It is most active against *Candida albicans*, *C. tropicalis*, and *Cryptococcus neoformans*, but *Candida krusei* and *C. glabrata* are resistant.[31] There is also little useful activity against *Aspergillus* spp. In AIDS patients exposed to the drug over prolonged periods resistant strains of *C. albicans* have emerged indicating that secondary resistance does occur. This is most likely when there is a heavy fungal load, such as occurs in AIDS but, to date, this has not been recognized as a problem in neutropenic patients. Whether fluconazole is active against the less frequently occurring fungal species (Table 2) needs to be determined.

The availability of an oral as well as intravenous route of administration, with excellent bioavailability, make this a much easier drug to use than AMB. Furthermore, serious toxic side-effects, even when using higher than normal doses of the drug are very rare. It is widely distributed throughout the body with good penetration of the CNS, and is excreted largely as active drug through the kidneys. There is minimal hepatic metabolism. The normal therapeutic dose is in the range of 200 to 400 mg daily which has been shown to be effective in a variety of local and systemic yeast infections. The dose should be reduced in the presence of renal failure, and after dialysis a repeat dose should be given. There is no indication for measuring serum levels.

Itraconazole is a synthetic dioxolane triazole with a similar mode of action to fluconazole. It has a broad spectrum of activity against *Candida* species including most strains of *C. glabrata* and *C. krusei* and it is also active against *Aspergillus* spp. and *Cryptococcus neoformans*. Acquired resistance seems to be rare. Despite this attractive profile, the widespread use of itraconazole has been limited by lack of a parenteral formulation (due to its poor water solubility) and variable, often poor bioavailability with the oral capsule formulation,[32] such that subtherapeutic serum and tissue concentrations frequently occur, particularly after BMT. Absorption of the drug is also reduced as a consequence of hypochlorhydria following H-2 receptor antagonist use. For treatment an initial loading dose of 600 mg should be given followed by dosing in the range 200 to 400 mg/day. Serum levels should be monitored weekly: peak concentrations 2–4 hours post dose should exceed 0.25 mg/l.

The problem of poor bioavailability should be overcome with a new cyclodextrin formulation; the preliminary results of pharmacokinetic studies are very encouraging.[33] Itraconazole is well distributed in the tissues, including the brain, despite low concentrations in cerebrospinal fluid. There is virtually no renal excretion of the drug. It is metabolized in the liver and the drug and its metabolites are excreted into the bowel. Side-effects are usually minor although caution is required if hepatic function is impaired. Hypertension has been reported with doses in excess of 400 mg/day. Further information on side-effects related to use of the cyclodextrin formulation is awaited.

Flucytosine (5-fluorocytosine, FC) is a synthetic fluorinated pyrimidine which acts by inhibiting both RNA and DNA synthesis in the fungal cell. It is fungistatic. The spectrum of activity is limited to *Cryptococcus neoformans* and *Candida* spp., and a proportion of both species are inherently resistant to the drug. Furthermore, drug resistance can also develop during the course of therapy especially if FC is given alone. For this reason it should normally only be used in combination with AMB. Oral and intravenous formulations are both available, and serum levels obtained with either route of administration are comparable. The distribution of the drug is good and relatively high concentrations are achieved in the CNS. Virtually all of the drug is excreted unchanged through the kidneys. Therefore, if renal function is impaired, there is a danger of accumulation in the blood and consequent toxicity, particularly on the bone marrow. This is usually manifested as neutropenia and thrombocytopenia and is thought to be due principally to metabolites such as 5-fluorouracil. Other side-effects of FC are nausea, vomiting and diarrhoea, and occasional hepatotoxicity.

Treatment by the oral route of administration is usual using a daily dose of up to 150 mg/kg in four divided doses. However, in the event of renal impairment, the maximum dose should be 100 mg/kg/day with close monitoring of serum levels: these should be kept within the range 70–80 mg/l peak and 30–40 mg/l trough.[34] Algorhythms are available for guidance about dosing according to creatinine clearance, but these should not replace serum monitoring.

Combination therapy

In general, a suspected or proven fungal infection is treated by a single agent, either AMB, fluconazole or itraconazole. Some clinical studies have shown that, in cryptococcosis and *Candida* endophthalmitis, combination therapy with AMB and FC is more effective than use of AMB alone. Again, serum levels of FC need to be carefully monitored because of AMB induced nephrotoxicity. There are conflicting in vitro data on the effects of combining an azole with AMB but, in view of their mode of action, there is at least the theoretical possibility of antagonism, and therefore their combined use is not recommended. Although FC and an azole are likely to be at least additive when used together, there is no proven clinical indication for this combination.

Drug interactions

Prescribers should be aware of possible adverse effects of giving any of the above antifungals with other drugs commonly used in patients with haematological malignancy. The principal interactions are listed in Table 3.

New antifungals

Several new formulations of AMB either prepared in liposomes[35] (ABCD, 'Amphocil', Zeneca) or lipid complexes[36] (ABLC, Liposome Company) are in the early stages of clinical evaluation. One way of formulating a much

Table 3. *Interactions between antifungal and other drugs used in neutropenic patients*

Antifungal	Interaction with	Effect
Amphotericin B	Diuretics Aminoglycosides Antineoplastic drugs Corticosteroids	Nephrotoxicity
	Digoxin	Enhanced effect of digoxin due to hypokalaemia
Fluconazole	Warfarin	Enhanced anticoagulation
	Oral hypoglycaemics Phenytoin	Delayed excretion of these drugs
Flucytosine	Amphotericin B	Nephrotoxicity Bone marrow suppression
Itraconazole	H-2 receptor antagonists Antacids	↓ Itraconazole absorption
	Rifampicin Phenytoin	↓ Itraconazole serum levels
	Terfenadine Cyclosporin A Digoxin	↑ serum levels of these drugs

needed intravenous preparation of itraconazole might be to incorporate the drug into liposomes; as yet no such preparation has been developed. UK109, 496 (Pfizer) is a new triazole with the promise of good activity against *Aspergillus* spp. as well as other medically important species. An open clinical study of its efficacy and safety in aspergillosis is planned, and the results are awaited with interest.

Preventive strategies

Careful clinical assessment before the initiation of immunosuppressive therapy is important to detect established infection early on. Particular attention must be given to the mouth, teeth, skin and perineum, with X-rays of the chest and nasal sinuses, and a full microbiological screen to identify colonization by potential pathogens.

Chemoprophylaxis

Heavy fungal colonization of the oro-gastro-intestinal tract poses a threat of systemic infection, and the traditional approach has been to suppress resident yeasts for the duration of neutropenia. Orally administered antifungals have been incorporated into non-absorbable regimens,[37] and have included nystatin suspension, AMB lozenges and suspension, miconazole gel and clotrimazole troches. They are often poorly tolerated and furthermore, there is very little evidence that any of them, either given alone or in combination, are able to prevent local or systematic fungal infections. Therefore their use is not recommended. However, chlorhexidine mouth gargles may help to prevent oral candidosis.[38]

Ketoconazole was important as the first orally administered antifungal that was also systemically absorbed. Several prophylaxis studies demonstrated a reduction in oropharyngeal, oesophageal and vaginal candidosis, but significantly there was no reduction in systemic mycoses.[39] Most of the patients were receiving leukaemia chemotherapy. Special problems arose in BMT as a result of significantly impaired absorption of the drug which was exacerbated by co-administration of H-2 receptor antagonists or antacids.[40] Two particular problems that were encountered have restricted its use. First, an interaction with cyclosporin A leading to nephrotoxicity[41] and hypertension in BMT patients and secondly, hepatotoxicity.[42] An increased rate of colonization by *Candida glabrata* was also seen in some units. In view of this doubtful efficacy and risk of complications, ketoconazole cannot be recommended.

One of the new triazoles, fluconazole or itraconazole, is a better choice. Considerable experience has been gained with fluconazole given in doses ranging from 50 to 400 mg daily. In cancer patients, 50 mg daily significantly reduced oropharyngeal candidosis when compared to placebo[43] and has also been shown to be more effective than oral polyenes.[44] More recently, Winston

232

et al[45] assessed a 400 mg daily dose in neutropenic RIT patients. In addition to a reduction in local candidosis, there were fewer systemic yeast infections compared to the group receiving oral polyenes; however, this difference was not statistically significant nor was there any reduction in mortality between the two groups. Goodman et al[46] compared fluconazole 400 mg daily to placebo in BMT patients, and found that, in addition to a reduction in episodes of systemic candidosis (15.8% vs 28%), there was a reduction in attributable mortality. Concerns have emerged from these and other related studies because of an increased incidence of colonization by resistant *Candida krusei*, complicated in some instances by bloodstream infections with this organism. Also there was no reduction in the occurrence of invasive aspergillosis.

In the case of itraconazole, comparatively few studies have been performed in neutropenic patients, but from the information that is available from these and studies in AIDS patients, the drug does appear to be effective for prevention of localized candida infections. More data are needed to determine efficacy in protecting against systemic infections. Studies are in progress using the oral cyclodextrin preparation at a daily dose of 400 mg.

The important potential advantage of itraconazole is its superior activity against *Aspergillus* compared with other azoles. In one study that is often cited[47] itraconazole, 200 mg 12-hourly, was significantly better than ketoonazole, 200 mg 12-hourly, at preventing aspergillosis. A criticism of this study is that itraconazole was compared to a historical group of ketoconazole recipients who could have had greater exposure to nosocomial acquisition of *Aspergillus*. Nevertheless, the further observation of a reduced mortality (9% vs 57%) due to aspergillosis in the itraconazole patients was impressive. Another important finding in this study was that, when peak serum itraconazole levels were maintained above 0.25 mg/l, the risk of aspergillosis was lowest. There can be wide variations in itraconazole levels even in the same patient.

Amphotericin B has also been evaluated for prophylaxis using either intermittent intravenous dosing (3 times weekly)[48] or as a nebulized preparation.[49,50] Unfortunately, even though there have been trends to suggest protection against *Aspergillus*, most of the studies done to date have used historical controls, and so no confident recommendation can be made. Nevertheless, for patients exposed to the risk of nosocomial acquisition of *Aspergillus*, for example during adjacent building work, and where a HEPA filtered room is not available, the use of prophylactic AMB would be justified. Preliminary evidence from recent studies using prophylactic liposomal AMB suggests that it is effective.[51] However, the cost of the drug is considerable and its prophylactic use should be restricted to selected high risk patients.

Choice of antifungal for prophylaxis

For patients who are receiving chemotherapy only, the most likely complicating fungal infection is candidosis, and therefore fluconazole is to be recommended. A dose of 100 mg daily is commonly used and may be more effective in preventing systemic candidosis than a dose of 50 mg. Whether even higher doses, as used in some American studies, are even better remains to be established. The same applies to autologous or HLA-matched sibling BMT, although there have been fewer studies in BMT patients to justify this choice. Whenever the duration of neutropenia exceeds 3 weeks, a switch to itraconazole 200 mg/day should be considered because of the greater risk of aspergillosis. Itraconazole is preferable for patients receiving mismatched or unrelated transplants, because of the greater risk of aspergillosis, but an alternative would be nebulized or iv AMB.

Duration of prophylaxis Where possible, patients should start antifungal prophylaxis at least 4 days before the expected onset of neutropenia and 48 hours before antibacterial prophylaxis is commenced because use of an antibacterial alone suppresses bacterial growth and may allow overgrowth of yeast in the bowel. If a patient on oral fluconazole develops bad mucositis, a switch to iv fluconazole is warranted. Prophylaxis should be continued until circulating neutrophils exceed $1\times10^9/l$, with the likelihood of full marrow recovery. In BMT patients with GVHD, antifungal prophylaxis should be continued until steroid immunosuppression has been stopped. Prophylaxis should be stopped if it is necessary to start empirical antifungal therapy in a febrile patient because of the possibility of drug antagonism. Prophylaxis should be restarted once the therapeutic drug has been stopped.

A detailed recommendation for antifungal prophylaxis has recently been published by the BSAC Working Party[52] and a modified version of this is shown in Table 4.

Table 4. *Recommendations for chemoprophylaxis of fungal infections during neutropenia*

Patient group	Regimen
Remission induction therapy	Fluconazole, oral, 100 mg daily
(Neutropenia >7 days	Start 4 days before anticipated
Consolidation therapy	onset of neutropenia
Autologous BMT	Stop when neutrophils $>1 \times 10^9/l$
HLA matched sibling BMT	Stop if AMB given for therapy
Neutropenia >21 days	Use/change to itraconazole oral, 200 mg daily
HLA mismatched BMT	or
Local building works	Nebulized AMB and/or intermittent iv AMB
GVHD; receiving steroids	

Colony stimulating factors (CSF)

The use of colony stimulating factors such as G-CSF has been shown to accelerate bone marrow recovery after RIT and BMT[53, 54] with a coincident reduction in febrile episodes and bacterial infections. No clear evidence is available to show that the incidence of fungal infections is also significantly reduced, although this might be expected. CSFs are also being investigated as an adjunct to AMB in the treatment of established fungal infection in neutropenic patients; the results are awaited with interest.

Protective environment

Patients with profound neutropenia should be cared for in a single room with reverse barrier nursing precautions. This has the additional advantage of preventing nosocomial acquisition of *Candida* even though there have been few reports of outbreaks of candidosis on leukaemia units. The inclusion of HEPA filtration, and the maintenance of positive pressure in the room, can protect high risk patients from *Aspergillus*. These are expensive facilities to build and maintain but the cost can be justified on the basis of the findings of several studies.[55] In any newly designed transplant ward of, say, eight beds, at least two should each have both positive and negative pressure facilities for protective isolation as well as barrier nursing as, and when, required.

Clinical presentations and management of fungal infections

The febrile neutropenic patient

The most common initial presentation of fungal infection is fever persisting in spite of broad spectrum antibiotics, and the absence of localized physical signs. The patient should be examined carefully, on a daily basis, for development of chest signs and skin lesions indicative of fungal sepsis. Full microbiological investigations should include cultures of blood, sputum and urine, and any suspected lesions on the skin should be biopsied and cultured. In the early stages of pulmonary infection the chest X-ray may be normal or show non-specific changes; here, a CT-scan may reveal the presence of cavitating lesions indicative of *Aspergillus* infection.

Fever continuing undiagnosed for 96 hours necessitates empirical antifungal therapy.[56,57] There is good evidence that early treatment reduces mortality from invasive fungal infections.[58,59] Amphotericin B has to be the drug of choice (Table 5) as there are inadequate data on the use of azoles in this situation and, furthermore, the patient is likely to have been receiving azoles for chemoprophylaxis.

Patients who respond to empirical AMB often have a coincident recovery of neutrophils which allows treatment to be stopped once the patient becomes afebrile. However, in persistently febrile patients with continuing profound

Table 5. *Strategies for antifungal therapy in the febrile neutropenic patient*

1. Patient febrile for 96 hours and unresponsive to antibiotics:
   - Start empirical amphotericin B (1 mg/kg/day)
   - Continue therapy until: (a) bone marrow recovery occurs
                                          or
                             (b) patient has been afebrile for at least 7 days and no infection has been documented
2. A fungal infection has been documented:
   - Candidosis: treat with amphotericin B (0.5–1 mg/kg/day) or fluconazole* 200–400 mg/day. Remove intravenous line if implicated
   - Aspergillosis: treat with amphotericin B (1 mg/kg/day), or liposomal AMB (3 mg/kg/day) in presence of renal impairment, or itraconazole (200–400 mg/day)
   - Other mycosis: treat according to known susceptibility for antifungal agents. Refer isolate to reference laboratory for sensitivity tests

* Only patients not receiving fluconazole prophylaxis.

neutropenia AMB should be continued. If significant renal toxicity occurs, liposomal AMB may have to be considered. When the cause of the infection is microbiologically documented, the approach to treatment depends on the causative organism. Bodey[4] reviewed 188 cases of candidosis. Candidaemia was present in 99 but in only 44 out of the 133 patients who had an invasive infection. No patients with persistent neutropenia survived their infection. This study underlines the importance of neutrophil recovery in the outcome of invasive candida infection and supports the recommendation of continuing antifungal treatment until marrow recovery occurs. The organs that may be involved in invasive candidosis include lungs, kidneys, heart and central nervous system including the eye.

The development of pulmonary infiltrates in a persistently febrile neutropenic patient is strongly suggestive of pulmonary aspergillosis. Although definitive diagnosis can only be made on tissue biopsy, this is not always feasible for clinical reasons but should be attempted whenever possible. The isolation of an *Aspergillus* sp. in sputum or a lavage specimen is strong supportive evidence. The results of preliminary studies with fungal antigen detection tests[60,61] and polymerase chain reaction[62] are promising but, as yet, these tests are not readily available to most leukaemia units. Antibody tests are of no value in diagnosis.[63]

In 20% of patients with pulmonary aspergillosis, the infection disseminates to extrapulmonary sites including skin, kidneys, heart and central nervous system.[64] Infection at those sites is also very difficult to diagnose without biopsy; however, CT-scan may provide strong supportive evidence when localized signs are present, eg fitting or hemiparesis as an indication of CNS infection.[65]

A microbiologically documented infection necessitates prolonged treatment of at least 6 weeks duration, although a decision on when to stop the antifungal will depend on the individual case. Recently, successful surgical resection of pulmonary aspergillomas has been reported[66] and may become part of the established management of aspergillosis.

Mucormycosis may present initially with involvement of the palate, facial oedema, blurring of vision,[67] and, in advanced infection, neurological signs consistent with extension of the infection to the frontal lobes of the brain. Diagnosis is made on biopsy of an oral lesion if present. Surgical debridement of necrotic infected tissue should be carried out, and antifungal therapy is usually given although conventional AMB and azoles are ineffective in this infection which carries a high mortality. Liposomal AMB may be worth using but no data are available. Fusarium infection[68] can mimic aspergillosis; typically, skin lesions are present and biopsy of these establishes the diagnosis. AMB is the therapeutic drug of choice. *Pseudoallescheria boydii* may present in a similar fashion.[69] However, it is resistant to AMB, and this is one of the few occasions where miconazole therapy is indicated.

Hepatosplenic candidosis This is an uncommon presentation of candida infection, often at a time when neutrophil recovery is established after leukaemia therapy. CT-scan of the liver typically shows multiple lesions. Treatment is often not very effective but there are recent reports of success with high doses of fluconazole[70] or liposomal AMB.[71]

Fungal infection in chronically immunocompromised patients

Invasive aspergillosis occurs in patients who are chronically immunocompromised, particularly those with chronic GVHD after BMT who are receiving steroid immunosuppression. Typically, it presents as either a pulmonary or disseminated infection but involvement of the CNS is also well described. Conventional AMB or itraconazole are both suitable agents to use. *Candida* occasionally presents in a similar manner.

Cryptococcosis is also an infection of the chronically immunocompromised,[72] particularly lymphoma patients. Although it is a systemic infection with fungaemia, it usually presents with signs of meningitis. Diagnosis can usually be readily confirmed by examination of cerebrospinal fluid. Microscopy typically reveals a lymphocytosis and cryptococci. Cryptococcal antigen detection and culture should be performed. The cryptococcal antigen test should also be carried out on blood. Occasionally skin lesions are present. These should be biopsied.

Before the AIDS epidemic, the treatment of choice for cryptococcal infection was a combination of AMB + FC.[73] However, recent experience suggests that fluconazole is as effective and less toxic than combination therapy.[74] Once patients have recovered from their acute infection, they should continue on long-term fluconazole (200 mg daily) until immunological recovery has occurred.

References

(1) Young LS. Management of infections in leukemia and lymphoma. In: Rubin RH, Young LS, eds. *Clinical approach to infection in the compromised host*. New York: Plenum Medical 1988: 467–501.

(2) Bodey GP. The emergence of fungi as major hospital pathogens. *J Hosp Infect* 1988; 11 (suppl A): 411–26.

(3) Pizzo PA, Robichaud RN, Wesley R, Commers JR. Fever in the pediatric and young adult patient with cancer. *Medicine* 1982; 61: 153–65.

(4) Bodey GP. Infection in cancer patients: a continuing association. *Am J Med* 1986; 81: 11–26.

(5) Gerson SL. Prolonged granulocytopenia: the major risk factor for invasive pulmonary aspergillosis in patients with acute leukemia. *Ann Intern Med* 1984; 100: 345–51.

(6) Pirsch JD, Maki DG. Infectious complications in adults with bone marrow transplants and T-cell depletion of donor marrow. *Ann Intern Med* 1986; 104:619–31.

(7) Karabinis A, Hill C, Leclercq B, Tancrède C, Baume D, Andremont A. Risk factors for candidemia in cancer patients: a case-control study. *J Clin Microbiol* 1988; 26: 4219–32

(8) Sherertz RJ, Belani A, Kramer BS et al. Impact of air filtration on nosocomial aspergillus infections: unique risk of bone marrow transplant recipients. *Am J Med* 1987; 83: 709–18.

(9) Allo MD, Miller J, Townsend T, Tan C. Primary cutaneous aspergillosis associated with Hickman intravenous catheters. *N Engl J Med* 1987; 317: 1105–8.

(10) Garcia CR, Johnston BL, Corvi G, Walker LJ, George WL. Intravenous catheter-associated Malassezia furfur fungemia. *Am J Med* 1987; 83: 790–2

(11) Leen CLS, Brettle RP. Fungal infections in drug users. *J Antimicrob Chemother* 1991; 28 (suppl A): 83–96.

(12) Meunier F. Fungal infections in the compromised host. In: Rubin RH, Young LS, eds. *Clinical approach to infection in the compromised host*. New York: Plenum Medical 1988: 193–220.

(13) Merz WG, Karp JE, Schron D, Saral R. Increased incidence of fungaemia caused by *Candida krusei*. *J Clin Microbiol* 1986; 24: 581–4.

(14) Wingard JR, Merz WG, Rinaldi MG, Miller CB, Karp JE, Saral R. Association of *Torulopsis glabrata* infections with fluconazole prophylaxis in neutropenic bone marrow transplant patients. *Antimicrob Agents Chemother* 1993; 37: 1847–9.

(15) Wingard JR, Merz WG, Rinaldi MG, Johnson TR, Karp JE, Saral R. Increase in *Candida krusei* infection among patients with bone marrow transplantation and neutropenia treated prophylactically with fluconazole. *N Engl J Med* 1991; 325: 1274–7.

(16) Hoy J, Hau K-C, Rolston K, Hopfer RL, Luna M, Bodey GP. *Trichosporon beigelli*. *Rev Infect Dis* 1986; 8: 959–67.

(17) Rinaldi MG. Invasive aspergillosis. *Rev Infect Dis* 1983; 5: 1061–77.

(18) Moore CK, Hellreich MA, Coblentz CL, Roggli VL. *Aspergillus terreus* as a cause of invasive pulmonary aspergillosis. *Chest* 1988; 94: 889–91.

(19) Rhame FS. Prevention of nosocomial aspergillosis. *J Hosp Infect* 1991; 18 (suppl A): 466–72.

(20) Sarubbi FA, Kopf HB, Wilson B, Mc Ginnis MR, Rutala WA. Increased recovery of *Aspergillus flavus* from respiratory specimens during hospital construction. *Am Rev Resp Dis* 1982; 125: 33–8.

(21) Ruutu P, Valtonen V, Tutanen L et al. An outbreak of invasive aspergillosis in a haematologic unit. *Scand J Infect Dis* 1987; 19: 347–51.

(22) Rogers TR, Barnes RA. Prevention of airborne fungal infection in immunocompromised patients. *J Hosp Infect* 1988; 11 (suppl A): 15–20.

(23) Skahan KJ, Wong B, Armstrong D. Clinical manifestations and management of mucormycosis in the compromised patient. In: Warnock DW, Richardson MD, eds. *Fungal infections in the compromised patient*. 2nd edn. Chichester: John Wiley and Sons 1991: 153–90.

(24) Meyer D, Rosen P, Armstrong D. Phycomycosis complicating leukemia and lymphoma. *Ann Intern Med* 1972; 77: 872–9.

(25) Richardson MD, Warnock DW. *Fungal infection: diagnosis and management.* 1st ed. Oxford: Blackwell Scientific Publications 1993: 115.

(26) Sarosi GA, Davies SF. Clinical manifestations and management of histoplasmosis in the compromised patient. In: Warnock DW, Richardson MD. *Fungal infection in the compromised patient.* Chichester: John Wiley and Sons 1982: 187–98.

(27) Gallis H, Drew, R, Pickard W. Amphotericin B: 30 years of clinical experience. *Rev Infect Dis* 1990; 12: 308–20.

(28) Powderly WG, Kobayashi GS, Herzig GP, Medoff F. Amphotericin B resistant yeast infection in severely immunocompromised patients. *Am J Med* 1988; 84: 826–32.

(29) British Society for Antimicrobial Chemotherapy Working Group. Therapy of deep fungal infection in haematological malignancy 1994. Submitted for publication.

(30) Meunier F, Prentice HG, Ringdén O. Liposomal amphotericin B (AmBisome): safety data from a phase II/III clinical trial. *J Antimicrob Chemother* 1991; 28 (suppl B): 83–91.

(31) Warnock DW, Burke J, Cope NJ, Johnson EM, vonFraunhofer NA, Williams EW. Fluconazole resistance in *Candida glabrata*. *Lancet* 1988; ii: 1310.

(32) Bradford CR, Prentice AG, Warnock DW, Copplestone, JA. Comparison of multiple dose pharmacokinetics of two formulations of itraconazole during remission induction for acute myeloblastic leukaemia. *J Antimicrob Chemother* 1991; 28: 555–60.

(33) Prentice AG, Warnock DW, Johnson SAN, Oliver DA. Multiple dose pharmacokinetics of a new cyclodextrin solution formulation of itraconazole in patients undergoing remission induction chemotherapy for acute myeloid leukaemia. (Abstract 744). In: *Program and abstracts of the 32nd interscience conference on antimicrobial agents and chemotherapy*. Anaheim: American Society for Microbiology 1992; 234.

(34) British Society for Antimicrobial Chemotherapy Working Party. Laboratory monitoring of antifungal chemotherapy. *Lancet* 1991; 337: 1577–80.

(35) Fromtling RA. Amphotericin B cholesterol sulfate complex. *Drugs of Future* 1993; 18: 303–6.

(36) Kan V, Bennett J, Amantea M et al. Comparative safety, tolerance and pharmacokinetics of amphotericin B lipid complex and amphotercin B deoxycholate in healthy male volunteers. *J Infect Dis* 1991; 164: 418–21.

(37) Rogers TR. Prevention of infection in neutropenic bone marrow transplant patients. In: Schönfeld H, Hahn FE, eds. *Antibiotics and chemotherapy*. Basel: Karger, 1985; 90–113.

(38) Ferretti GA, Ash RC, Brown AT, Parr MD, Romond, EH, Lillich, TT. Control of oral mucositis and candidiasis in marrow transplantation: a prospective double-blind trial of chlorhexidine digluconate oral rinse. *Bone Marrow Transpl* 1988; 3: 483–93.

(39) Hann IM, Prentice HG, Corringham R et al. Ketoconazole versus nystatin plus amphotericin B for fungal prophylaxis in severely immunocompromised patients. *Lancet* 1982; 1: 826–9.

(40) Hann IM, Prentice HG, Keaney M et al. The pharmacokinetics of ketoconazole in severely immunocompromised patients. *J Antimicrob Chemother* 1982; 10: 489–496.

(41) Morganstern GR, Powles R, Robinson B, Mc Elwain TJ. Cyclosporin interaction with ketoconazole and melphalan. *Lancet* 1982; ii: 1342.

(42) Lewis JH, Zimmerman HJ, Benson GD, Ishak, KG. Hepatic injury associated with ketoconazole therapy: analysis of 33 cases. *Gastroenterology* 1984; 86: 503–13.

(43) Samonis G, Rolston K, Karl C, Miller P, Bodey GP. Prophylaxis of oropharyngeal candidiasis with fluconazole. *Rev Infect Dis* 1990; 12 (suppl 3): S369–73.

(44) Brammer KW. A comparison of fluconazole and oral polyenes in the prevention of fungal infection during neutropenia. In: *Proceedings of trends in the management of systemic fungal infections*. Nijmegen 1991. Abstract no 13.

(45) Winston DJ, Chandrasekar PH, Lazarus HM et al. Fluconazole prophylaxis of fungal infections in patients with acute leukemia: results of a randomized placebo controlled, double blind, multicenter trial. *Ann Intern Med* 1993; 118: 495–503.

(46) Goodman JL, Winston DJ, Greenfield RA et al. A controlled trial of fluconazole to prevent fungal infections in patients undergoing bone marrow transplantation. *N Engl J Med* 1992; 326: 845–851.

(47) Tricot G, Joosten E, Boogaerts MA, Vande Pitte J, Cauwenbergh G. Ketoconazole vs. itraconazole for antifungal prophylaxis in patients with severe granulocytopenia: preliminary results of two nonrandomised studies. *Rev Infect Dis* 1987; 9 (suppl 1): 594–9.

(48) Bodey GP, Anaissie EJ. Fluconazole vs intravenous amphotericin B for antifungal prophylaxis in leukemic patients. In *Proceedings of the seventh international congress of chemotherapy*. Berlin 1991. Munich Futuramed Abstract 1964.

(49) Conneally E, Cafferkey MT, Daly PA, Keane CT, McCann SR. Nebulized

amphotericin B prophylaxis against invasive aspergillosis in granulocytopenic patients. *Bone Marrow Transpl* 1990; 5: 403–6.

(50) Jeffrey GM, Beard ME, Ikram RB, et al. Intranasal amphotericin B reduces the frequency of invasive aspergillosis in neutropenic patients. *Am J Med* 1991; 90: 685–92.

(51) Tollemar J, Ringdén O, Andersson S et al. Prophylactic use of amphotericin B (AmBisome) against fungal infections: a randomized trial in bone marrow transplant recipients. *Transpl Proc* 1993; 25: 1495–7.

(52) British Society for Antimicrobial Chemotherapy Working Party Report. Chemoprophylaxis for candidosis and aspergillosis in neutropenia and transplantation: a review and recommendations. *J Antimicrob Chemother* 1993; 32: 5–21.

(53) Groopman JE, Molina J-M, Scadden DT. Hematopoietic growth factors: biology and clinical applications. *N Engl J Med* 1989; 321: 1449–59.

(54) Sheridan WP, Morstyn G, Wolf M et al. Granulocyte colony stimulating factor and neutrophil recovery after high-dose chemotherapy and autologous bone marrow transplantation. *Lancet* 1989; 334: 891–5.

(55) Barnes RA, Rogers TR. Control of an outbreak of nosocomial aspergillosis by laminar air flow isolation. *J Hosp Infect* 1989; 14: 89–94.

(56) EORTC International Antimicrobial Therapy Cooperative Group. Empiric antifungal therapy in febrile granulocytopenic patients. *Am J Med* 1989; 86: 668–72.

(57) Barnes RA, Rogers TR. Response rates to a staged antibiotic regimen in febrile neutropenic patients. *J Antimicrob Chemother* 1988; 22: 759–63.

(58) Pizzo PA, Robichaud KJ, Gill FA, Witebsky FG. Empiric antibiotic and antifungal therapy for cancer patients with prolonged fever and granulocytopenia. *Am J Med* 1982; 72: 101–11.

(59) Burch PA, Karp JE, Merz WG, Kuhlman JE, Fishman EK. Favorable outcome of invasive aspergillosis in patients with acute leukemia. *J Clin Oncol* 1987; 5: 1985–93.

(60) Rogers TR, Haynes KA, Barnes RA. Value of antigen detection in predicting invasive pulmonary aspergillosis. *Lancet* 1990; 336: 1210–3.

(61) Haynes KA, Latge JP, Rogers TR. Detection of *Aspergillus* antigens associated with invasive infection. *J Clin Microbiol* 1990; 28; 2040–4.

(62) Tang CM, Holden DW, Aufauvre-Brown A, Cohen J. The detection of *Aspergillus* spp. by the polymerase reaction and its evaluation in bronchoalveolar lavage fluid. *Am Rev Resp Dis* 1993; 148: 1313–7.

(63) Young RC, Bennett JE. Invasive aspergillosis: absence of detectable antibody response. *Am Rev Resp Dis* 1971: 104: 710–6.

(64) Young RC, Bennett JE, Vogel CL, Carbone PP, De Vita VT. Aspergillosis: the spectrum of the disease in 98 patients. *Medicine* 1970; 49; 147–73.

(65) Walsh TJ, Hier DB, Caplan LR. Aspergillosis of the central nervous system: clinicopathological analysis of 17 patients. *Ann Neurol* 1985; 18: 574–82.

(66) Prentice HG. Personal communication.

(67) Hyatt DS, Young YM, Haynes KA, Taylor JM, Mc Carthy DM, Rogers TR. Rhinocerebral mucormycosis following bone marrow transplantation. *J Infect* 1992; 24: 67–71.

(68) Cofrancesco E, Boschetti C, Viviani MA. Efficacy of liposomal amphotericin B (AmBisome) in the eradication of fusarium infection in a leukaemic patient. *Haematologica* 1992: 77: 280–3.

(69) Guyotat D, Piens MA, Bouvier R, Fiere D. A case of disseminated *Scedosporium apiospermum* infection after bone marrow transplantation. *Mykosen* 1987; 30: 151–4.

(70) Flannery MT, Simmons DB, Saba H, Altus P, Wallach PM, Adelman HM. Fluconazole in the treatment of hepatosplenic candidiasis. *Arch Intern Med* 1992; 152: 406–8.

(71) Hudson J, Scott GL, Warnock DW. Treatment of hepatic candidosis with liposomal amphotericin B in patient with acute leukaemia. *Lancet* 1991; 338: 1534–5.

(72) Hay RJ. Clinical manifestations and management of cryptococcosis in the compromised patient. In: Warnock DW, Richardson MD, eds. *Fungal infections in the compromised host*. 2nd edn. Chichester: John Wiley and Sons, 1991: 85–115.

(73) Bennett JE, Dismukes WE, Duma RJ et al. A comparison of amphotericin alone and combined with flucytosine in the treatment of cryptococcal meningitis. *N Engl J Med* 1979; 301: 126–81.

(74) Lapidus WI, Saag M. Cryptococcal meningitis. In: Powderly WG, van't Wout JW, eds. *Fluconazole*. Lancashire: Marius Press, 1992: 133–51.

Index

Page numbers in *italic* refer to figures and/or tables